D1567374

# AN ENUMERATION OF CHINESE MATERIA MEDICA

## 中 藥 詞 彙

# An Enumeration of Chinese Materia Medica

## Second Edition

### Shiu-ying Hu

With editorial assistance from

Y.C. Kong and Paul P.H. But

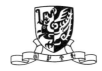

## The Chinese University Press

ISBN 962–201–803–3

First edition 1980
*Second edition* 1999

**THE CHINESE UNIVERSITY PRESS**
The Chinese University of Hong Kong
SHA TIN, N.T., HONG KONG
Fax: +852 2603 6692
      +852 2603 7355
E-mail: cup@cuhk.edu.hk
Web-site: http://www.cuhk.edu.hk/cupress/w1.htm

Printed in Hong Kong

敬獻吾師

莫 古 禮 博 士

Dedicated to

Dr. Floyd A. McClure

In appreciation of his guidance and encouragement in
medicinal plant research, beginning in 1935 at
Lingnan University, Canton
China

# CONTENTS

# FOREWORD

MAN has sought agents from nature to relieve his ills and discomforts probably from his earliest years of experimentation with what his environment provided. As he turned instinctively to his ambient vegetation for food, putting everything possible into his mouth to assuage hunger, he naturally soon discovered plants with striking psychic and physical effects. He then began to recognize medicinal, narcotic and poisonous plants. At first subconsciously and slowly, later consciously and more expeditiously, he bent many of these plants with their remarkable properties to his use. And very early in the development of human cultures they became everywhere intimately associated with magic and religion and provided a mainstay for the growth of shamanism.

When cultures evolved far enough to throw off most of the throes of shamanism, much if not most of the knowledge of medicine—accumulated and passed on orally over the millenia—persisted in folklore. It was passed down, still orally, from generation to generation, until finally much of it could be reduced to written records and thus preserved for posterity.

It is natural to presume that those regions where man's cultural history is oldest should have inherited perhaps the richest store of such knowledge. If this be true, then China must take its place as one of the parts of the world with a rich store of ethnopharmacological tradition. It is common knowledge, I believe, that China does indeed have one of the world's most extensive, most elaborate and most complex bodies of folk medicine or ethnopharmacology. The home of an ancient system of writing, the region where paper was invented, a country long famous for conservation of tradition and inhabited by a people known for their dedication to learning, China by all arguments had to possess a rich and carefully preserved heritage of the healing arts.

The recent upsurge of interest in China itself in the technical investigation of many of its ancient folk remedies is heartening. Ethnopharmacology has experienced a new and encouraging rebirth in scientific circles around the world. Medicine will not soon forget, for example, the meteoric rise of ephedrine, isolated from a plant employed for millenia by simple country folk in the interior of China. Yet the scientific world finds it difficult to cope with the extensive Chinese folk pharmacopoeia, mainly because of the language barrier. Since the investigation into new medicinal agents has perforce to be an international effort, this hindrance is, from the point of view of progress in the health of mankind, lamentable.

It is primarily because of the extraordinary contribution towards elimination or lessening of this barrier that botany, pharmacology, chemistry and medicine will welcome Dr. Shiu Ying Hu's present work: An *Enumeration of Chinese Materia*

*Medica.* It is much more than its title implies. I am not aware of any similar treatise. Offering the Chinese names of medicines in Chinese and transliterated and the English equivalent, the list appends the "pharmaceutical name" as well. The scientific name of the plants involved is also available. Thus, it is an easy task to find quickly the source of Chinese medicines.

The amount of labor devoted to the preparation of this enumeration was obviously very great. And it could not have been done by anyone. Dr. Hu is an accomplished botanist, at home both in her science and in her native language. Furthermore, she is not only a taxonomic botanist who has given years to the study of the Chinese flora but an economic botanist who has to her credit many publications on food and medicinal plants of China. For the growing interest in ethnopharmacological circles in Chinese medicine, it is fortunate that a scientist of her capabilities has undertaken the task. She deserves a warm expression of thanks.

I am certain that Hu's *An Enumeration of Chinese Materia Medica* will quickly earn a lasting place on the reference shelves of botany, pharmacology, chemistry and medicine.

RICHARD EVANS SCHULTES
Paul C. Mangelsdorf Professor
of Natural Sciences and
Director, Botanical Museum,
Harvard University

# PREFACE

ON many occasions in the past I would have first consulted *An Enumeration of Chinese Materia Medica,* if it had only been available! I recall Chinese friends asking me for the English identification of Oriental plants believed to be of high economic or medicinal value; or responding to a local Poison Control Center requesting the identification of the Chinese herbal names printed on the medication belonging to a person admitted for emergency treatment; or the many occasions when trivial Oriental names were referred to in conversations or the literature that I was unable to transpose into a genus or species name. This book goes beyond providing answers to such difficult questions about the identity of Oriental medicinal plants. It enables a person knowledgeable only in the English language to write and pronounce the Chinese names for a known species and, if desired, to establish the identity of other Oriental plants similar to the species of interest. It is also a unique, informative experience simply to browse through this treasure-book of information.

E. JOHN STABA
Professor and Director
Graduate Studies in Pharmacognosy
Department of Pharmacognosy
College of Pharmacy
University of Minnesota

# ACKNOWLEDGMENTS

DEEP appreciation is due to Dr. Lily M. Perry of the Arnold Arboretum, Harvard University, for reading the entire manuscript and for many helpful suggestions; to Dr. H. M. Chang, Director of the Institute of Science and Technology, The Chinese University of Hong Kong, for encouragement and for the arrangement with the University Press for the publication of the work; to both Dr. Y. C. Kong, Department of Biochemistry, and Dr. Paul P.H. But, Chinese Medicinal Material Research Centre, Institute of Science and Techno-logy, The Chinese University of Hong Kong, for editorial assistance; to Dr. Richard E. Schultes, Professor of Economic Botany and Director of the Botanical Museum, Harvard University, for the foreword; to Dr. E. John Staba, Professor and Director of Graduate Studies in Pharmacognosy, for the preface; to Dr. C. Y. Chen and Prof. S. C. Cheung for their enthusiastic support; to Mr. William Ho and Mr. L. H. Shen of The Chinese University of Hong Kong for the preparation of the Chinese index; and to Dr. Peter F. Stevens, Assistant Professor of Biology and Assistant Curator of the Arnold Arboretum, Harvard University, for helpful suggestions.

# INTRODUCTION

THE embryonic form of this book has been a personal companion and a ready source of assistance to the author in the identification of Chinese medicinal plants. Naturally the consulters will find the same usefulness in its more complete state and handier form. It contains a time-saving device for the identification of the Chinese materia medica. It has two principal parts and four appendices. Part I consists of an alphabetic list of more than 2,000 Chinese medicines with the botanical names, and their equivalents in English and in pharmaceutical usage. Part II is a systematic arrangement of the plants, animals, minerals, and miscellaneous preparations, with each item carrying one to several numbers referring to the names in Part I. The book is intended to help people in science and medicine, to facilitate their work of writing by supplying them with the scientific and vernacular names of the subject matter of their research. Guided by this goal, brevity of form, simplicity in structure, and convenience for consultation have been the criteria for the selection of items for entry, and the information supplied. The book is in fact a forerunner of a more comprehensive illustrated work on the botany of the Chinese materia medica.

The work began as a list of Chinese medicines for quick reference to meet personal needs. The increasing interest in Chinese medicine outside China has created an ever-growing demand on the author's time for the identification of Chinese medicinal plants. Requests from physicians, pharmacologists, phytochemists, botanists in various disciplines of economic botany, and from business firms come continually. Normally, one to several names are involved. In 1977, a psychiatrist interested in Chinese remedies for mental patients asked for the identification of fifty odd ingredients involved in twenty different kinds of pills, powder, or liquid preparations currently used in China. It took the author a whole week to complete the identification and to translate the explanations concerning these drugs. In the summer of 1978, a more time consuming request had to be answered. A famous Chinese physician in Hong Kong who is preparing a book on his experience in the use of 700 common Chinese medicines asked for assistance in checking the botanical identification and in supplying the English equivalents of the names. It took a month to perform a professional courtesy of this magnitude. Consequently, from the results of this research, and from the aggregated information obtained in the translation of the ancient and recent multiple recipes prepared in connection with the articles on the contributions to our knowledge of the Chinese motherwort, of ginseng, and of eucommia, a list for a quick identification of Chinese materia medica emerged.

The list was first constructed over a xeroxed copy of the *List of Chinese Medicines* published by the order of the

Inspector General of Customs of China in 1889. The Chinese names of the medicines and their transliterations were used as a basis for corrections of the scientific identifications and for additions of new material. Consequently so many revisions and additions were made that it became difficult to decipher (Fig. 1). It was typed and made legible. In September 1978, the author was invited to speak on the ecology and phytogeography of ginseng in an International Ginseng Symposium which took place in Seoul, Korea. A xeroxed copy of the clean list was presented to Dr. H. M. Chang, Director of the Institute of Science and Technology, The Chinese University of Hong Kong, for advice and for consideration of publication. Dr. E. John Staba, Director of Graduate Studies in Pharmacognosy, University of Minnesota, saw the manuscript in that preliminary state. The encouragement of these two scientists-administrators incited the author to plunge into the laborious task of checking and rechecking, and of preparing Part II and the appendices.

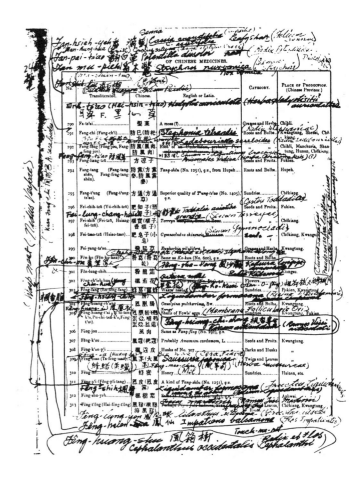

FIGURE 1. A page of the xeroxed copy of the *List of Chinese Medicines* published in 1889, showing the degree of revision and addition needed for bringing up-to-date the identifications of the Chinese materia medica.

## Selection

It is neither expedient, advisable, nor possible for a dictionary to include all the words known to a language for which it is prepared. A lexicographer has to use his judgement to select entries for inclusion that would fit with the purpose of the work. The knowledge of Chinese materia medica is in a state of flux. New discoveries and new information are added continually. The number of articles for which medicinal value has been claimed is very large. The most recent work on the subject published in Shanghai in 1977, *Chung-yao ta tz'ŭ-tien* 中葯大辭典 [An Encyclopedia of Chinese Medicines], contains 5,767 items. Many of these articles represent obscure plants mentioned in local manuals, or animals raised or hunted primarily for food. Items of this nature are inappropriate for the purpose at hand. They do not come up to the criteria of utility and usability. The names that are likely to be consulted fit with the principle of utility. These are selected. The names that are not likely to be needed for consultation are omitted. Their entry would make the book too cumbersome to be a handy reference for quick identification of the Chinese materia medica.

*The List of Chinese Medicines* published in 1889 by the Chinese Maritime Customs Service is considered a very useful reference. It contains 19 individual lists of drugs examined in port cities between November 1884 and October 1885. The localities of the ports extended north-southward from Newchwang ( 牛莊, Long. 121°30′ E, Lat. 38°30′ N) to Pakhoi ( 北海, 109°05′ E, 21°20′ N) and Kiungchow ( 瓊州, 110°25′ E, 20°02′ N), and east-westward from Ichang ( 宜昌, 111°15′ E, 30°15′ N) in the interior, to Takow ( 打狗＝高雄 Kao-hsiung, 120°11′ E, 20° N) and Tamsui ( 淡水, 121°22′ E, 25°10′ N) in Taiwan (Fig. 2). As a conclusion, there is a *General Alphabetical List of Chinese Medicines* which contains all the articles reported in the 19 local lists. The articles in this general list are significant in four respects. First, they represent the drugs of commercial value used at a time when Chinese medicine was hardly influenced by Western science. Secondly, they were produced in a wide range of territories within the country. In addition to being instrumental to the well-being of the people, they had a considerable influence on the economy of the land. Thirdly, they are the names which are likely to be seen in classical records and current prescriptions. Fourthly, there was a great deal of movement of materia medica within China and to its neighboring countries at that early date. For example, take Szechuan lovage ( 川芎, Ch'uan-hsiung, *Ligusticum wallichii*). In the 12 months when observations were made, 480 piculs of the dry root worth 290 taels of silver were carried overland to Newchwang, and 8,385 piculs worth 49,638 taels were transported over the Yangtze River by boat to Shanghai for distribution to consumers in eastern China and Japan. During the same period, 12 piculs of dried

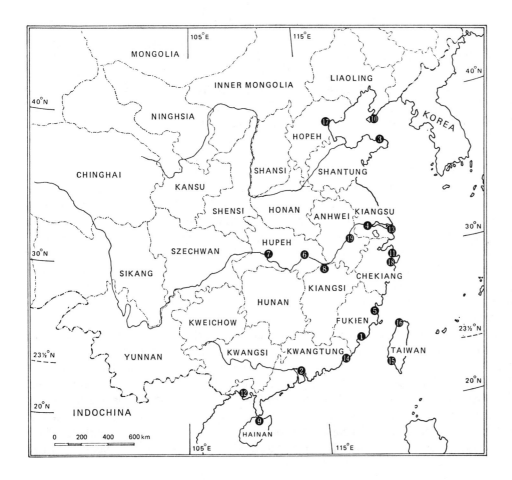

FIGURE 2. A portion of the map of China showing the 19 port cities from which information of 1,575 articles of Chinese medicines was collected between November 1884 and October 1885. All these articles that can be identified are incorporated in the present work.

1. Amoy
2. Canton
3. Chefoo
4. Chinkiang
5. Foochow
6. Hankow
7. Ichang
8. Kiukiang
9. Kiungchow
10. Newchwang
11. Ningpo
12. Pakhoi
13. Shanghai
14. Swatow
15. Takow
16. Tamsui
17. Tientsin
18. Wenchow
19. Wuhu

honeysuckle flowers (銀花, Yin-hua, *Lonicera japonica*) worth 87 taels, produced in Kiangsu and Hupeh provinces, were shipped to Amoy via Shanghai for distribution in Manila and Singapore. Material was also moved in reverse directions. For example, 34 piculs of Betel-Nut (檳榔, Ping-lang, *Areca catechu*) worth 136 taels were shipped from southeastern Asia, via Canton and Hankow, to Ichang for distribution in the interior of China. Likewise, 1.5 piculs of Seahorse (海馬, Hai-ma) worth 348 taels were delivered from Hainan Island and Singapore to Shanghai for distribution in China. All the items that can be identified in this general list are incorporated in the book. The products of animal and mineral origin are also included. The author, being a professional plant taxonomist, has neither the facilities nor the time to check for the correct application of scientific names of these zoological articles. For this reason, the scientific names of animals are omitted.

Regarding the more recent publications, the more outstanding ones are consulted. Pioneer Chinese scientists began to investigate the material used in traditional Chinese medicine in the 1930s. Their efforts were obscured by the introduction of Western medicine, and their progress was hampered by the Sino-Japanese War. After the 1950s, explosive activities in field investigation, laboratory experiments, and clinical applications of the Chinese materia medica took place within China. Rapid changes were made. New information concerning the source material of medicine, scientific identification, and chemical contents was acquired continually. The results of the investigations made before the 1960s were summarized in two classical works. These are the *Chung-yao chih* 中藥誌 [New Chinese Materia Medica], in four volumes, 1959-61, and *Yao-ts'ai hsüeh* 藥材學 [Chinese Pharmacognosy], in one large volume by Hsü *et al.* in 1961. In 1976 and 1977, two comprehensive works were published which include more recent findings as well as ancient documents. These are *Zhong cao yao xue* 中草藥學 (Chung ts'ao-yao hsüeh) [Chinese Pharmacology], volume II, 1976, and *Chung-yao ta tz'ŭ-tien* 中藥大辭典 [An Encyclopedia of Chinese Medicines], volumes I and II, 1977 and III, 1978. Important items in these four monumental works have been selected for inclusion. Meanwhile, numerous manuals and handbooks have been published for regional or provincial use. The contents of three more widely used ones published between 1969 and 1971 are also incorporated. These are *Chang-yung Chung-ts'ao-yao shou-ts'ê* 常用中草藥手冊 [A Handbook of Common Medicines], 1969; *Chang-yung Chung-ts'ao-yao t'u-p'u* 常用中草藥圖譜 [Colored Illustrations of Common Medicines], 1970; and *Pei-fang chang-yung Chung-ts'ao-yao shou-ts'ê* 北方常用中草藥手冊 [A Handbook of Northern Common Medicines], 1971. Special articles published in the *Acta Phytotaxonomica Sinica* dealing with the nomenclature and the classification of

Chinese medicinal plants have been reviewed, and many names have been selected for inclusion.

## Structure

The book contains approximately two thousand articles, many of which have more than one name. When an article has two or more names, the more familiar one is entered as a major name and the others as alternative names. Some articles also have minor names. Alternative names are placed in parentheses while minor names are not. An example will make this structure clear. In *Sapindus mukorosii*, Mu-huan-tzŭ 木槵子 is treated as the major name, (Mu-yüan-tzŭ 木圓子 and Wu-huan-tzŭ 無槵子 ) are its alternative names, and Mu-huan-jou 木槵肉 and Mu-huan-kên 木槵根 are its minor names. A reference number is attached to a major name for cross-reference with the systematic arrangement of the species in Part II.

There are five columns per page in Part I. On the left, two columns are devoted to the Chinese names which are transliterated in Roman alphabets by the Wade system as it appears in Mathews' *Chinese-English Dictionary* (revised American edition, Harvard University Press). This system is chosen primarily for its wide application in large Chinese libraries in the United States. The Chinese collection in the Library of Congress, the Library of Harvard-Yenching Institute at Harvard University, the Gest Oriental Library at Princeton University, and the East Asian Collection of Hoover Institution at Stanford University are good examples. Moreover, the system was used by authors of most early English publications on Chinese materia medica, such as that of Bretschneider's *Botanicum Sinicum,* Stuart's *Chinese Materia Medica, Vegetable Kingdom,* and Read's *Chinese Medicinal Plants from the Pên Ts'ao Kang Mu.* In addition, there is a more practical reason for the author to adopt the Wade system, i.e., the economy of time. The *List of Chinese Medicines* published by the Chinese Maritime Customs in 1889 contains 1,575 items. The names and synonyms of this list are romanized by the Wade system. All the items that can be identified in modern terms are cited in the present work, and the spelling of the names and synonyms is taken as it appeared in the original form. A tremendous amount of time was saved in the preparation of the manuscript of this book, for the checking of the transliteration was limited to the articles added to the 1889 list.

A consulter who can read and pronounce the Chinese name of a drug can locate its position in Part I and thus find its identification rather easily, or with some practice. For the people who are not very familiar with the Wade system of romanization, a guide to the syllables with examples drawn largely from Part I is provided in Appendix I-A.

The botanical epithets, printed in bold-face type, follow

the Chinese names. A complete botanical name consists of two Latin words or latinized forms which represent the genus and the species respectively. In taxonomic literature, for the sake of clarity, the author or authors who first described the species are placed after the scientific epithet. For the purpose at hand, such a practice is not absolutely necessary, and for the economy of space, the authors' names are omitted in Part I.

For reasons explained already, an open space is left after the names of an animal, a mineral, or a miscellaneous product. In the same column, there are many incidences where one article may have two or more specific names. This is a natural consequence of compiling information for a big country such as China. Apparently, in many cases people with similar cultural background have gathered closely related species and used them as remedies for similar ailments and called them by the same name. *Aconitum delavayi, A. hemsleyanum, A. sunpanense,* etc. for Ts'ao-wu-t'ou 草烏頭, *Bupleurum falcatum, B. chinense,* and *B. scorzoneraefolium* for Ch'ai-hu 柴胡, and *Typha angustata* and *T. latifolia* for Hsiang-p'u 香蒲, are some good examples. In some cases, it appears that people in different areas have gathered unrelated species and called them the same name independently. For example, Hai-fêng-t'êng 海風藤 is used for *Ficus maritinii* of Moraceae, *Piper kadsura* of Piperaceae, *Akebia quinata* of Lardizabalaceae, and for *Usnea diffracta,* a lichen. Names of this type are very confusing. Many of the confused names can be clarified by adding modifiers to the basic name. For example, in Niu-hsi 牛膝, Huai-niu-hsi 懷牛膝 refers to *Achyranthes bidentata,* T'u-niu-hsi 土牛膝 to *A. aspera,* and Ch'uan-niu-hsi 川牛膝 to *Cyathula capitata.* However, some confusion still awaits future investigation.

The column for English equivalents contains two elements. The citations printed in capitals and small capitals are the vernacular names adapted from Bailey's *Manual of Cultivated Plants,* Fernald's *Gray's Manual of Botany,* eighth edition, Hill's *Economic Botany,* Hu's *Enumeration of the Vascular Plants of Hong Kong,* Kingsbury's *Poisonous Plants of the United States and Canada,* Peck's *Manual of the Higher Plants of Oregon,* Neal's *In Gardens of Hawaii,* Rehder's *Manual of Cultivated Trees and Shrubs,* and Steward's *Manual of Vascular Plants of the Lower Yangtze Valley, China.* The phrases in normal print are descriptive terms. The vernacular names carrying the asterisk (*) represent epithets used for the first time. Many of these names are adapted directly from the generic names. This is a common practice in horticulture where *Chrysanthemum, Eucommia, Forsythia,* and *Magnolia* have all become common names. Other new vernacular names in this column represent the romanized short Chinese names. In the English language there are already many common names of fruits which have this origin. Kumquat (金橘), Loquat (魯橘), Lichee (荔枝), Longan (龍眼), and Wampee (黃

皮）are some examples. In medicine, ginseng, the French spelling of the Chinese drug 人参 (Jên-shen by the Wade system of romanization) is now used internationally. It seems that for short names such as Kuei-hua 桂花, La-mei 蠟梅, Mei 梅, Pai-shu 白朮, San-ch'i 三七, and Tsang-shu 蒼朮 there are no better terms than those adapted from the romanized Chinese names. In adapting the romanized syllables of a drug name for an English common name, the pronunciation symbols and hyphens are dropped. For example, Fêng-t'êng 風藤 becomes Fengteng for *Piper kadsura* and Pai-ch'ien 白前 becomes Paichien for *Cynanchum stautonii*. In very few cases where the alternative names are easier to pronounce than the major name for non-Chinese speaking people, the common name is derived from the former. For example, in *Gynura segetum*, the name Tusanchi derived from the alternative name is chosen in preference of the word Sanchitsao from the major name. Other new common names are constructed or adapted by the author in accordance to the general practices observed in the manuals mentioned above. Some of them are derived from the translation of the scientific name or part of it, such as Citrus-scented Angelica for *Angelica citriodora,* Shield Kadsura for *Kadsura peltifera*, and Dragon's Head for *Dracocephalum ruyschiana*. Some others are translations of the Chinese names, such as Ginger Sanchi 薑三七 for *Stahlianthus involucratus,* Golden Dendrobium 金石斛 for *Dendrobium linawianum,* and Iron Holly 鐵冬青 for *Ilex rotunda.* Still others are coined from the author's knowledge of the nature of the species. For example, Red Magnolia is given to *Magnolia liliflora* for its unique deep red flowers, and Chinese Chive is adapted for *Allium chinese* because of its dwaf habit, its slightly enlarged bulbs, and its fistulose leaves. In these three respects, the species is close to the common chive. Tamala is used for *Cinnamomum tamala.* When Francis Hamilton described the species, he took up the local name *tamala* for the specific epithet. It is fitting therefore, to use Tamala as the vernacular name of the species.

The column on the right is devoted to names used by pharmacists. A major portion of these names are taken from the *New Chinese Materia Medica* and the *Chinese Pharmacognosy.* The names of articles that are not included in these books are provided by the author. They are adapted from the scientific names of the objects and the parts used in accordance to the rules of botanical Latin. The procedure of preparing these names is complex, because Latin is a highly inflected language with genders, numbers and cases that must all agree. Space does not allow the explanation of details here. It suffices to point out that in each name, the part used is a substantive in the singular number and nominative case, and the scientific name (or part of it) that follows must agree with the noun in number, but it is in the genitive case. The reader is advised to refer to Stearn's *Botanical Latin* (1973) for further information.

Part II is a systematic summary of the entries of Part I. It covers 1,716 species of plants, about 120 items of animals, 79 minerals, and 41 miscellaneous preparations. Each entry is linked up with the citations of Part I by one or more numbers placed in the parentheses after it.

A relatively small number of plant species are non-vascular, the thallophytes and bryophytes. These are arranged in groups higher than the family rank. Each group carries a few letters for the purpose of cross-reference. These abbreviations are: (Alg) = algae, (A-myc) = ascomycetes, (B-myc) = basidiomycetes, (G-myc) = gasteromycetes, (Lich) = lichens, and (Bryo) = bryophytes.

The species of vascular plants are arranged by their families. Fifty-eight of these are ferns and fern-allies (pteridophytes). They are placed in families as they appear in *Iconographia Cormophytorum Sinicorum* (*1*: 107-284. 1972). Each family carries a number (F1–F50) for the purpose of cross-reference. The spermatophytes are arranged in families by the Engler system. The family numbers are adopted from the Enumeratio Familiarum Siphonogamarum which appear in Dalla Torre and Harms' *Genera Siphonogamarum ad Systema Englerianum Conscripta* (pp. v–vii. 1900). These reference numbers are extensively used for filing specimens in large herbaria throughout the world.

The species within a family are arranged alphabetically. The family that has the largest number of species used for medicine in China is Leguminosae. One hundred and five species have been recorded. The next large family is Compositae which has 99 species of medicinal plants. The other large families are Liliaceae with 66 species, Ranunculaceae with 57 species, Rosaceae and Umbelliferae each with 46 species, Euphorbiaceae with 37 species, Rutaceae with 35 species, Gramineae with 30 species, Araliaceae with 28 species, and Orchidaceae with 27 species.

Consulters who can read Chinese may find that some of the botanical names used in this work differ from the ones printed in the outstanding references mentioned above. All these names have been carefully checked with the original publications, and found to be more accurate according to existing rules of botanical nomenclature, and current taxonomic practice.

**Appendices**

Four appendices are provided in this book to help the consulters to locate the names quickly. Appendix I contains two sections. Section A (Appendix I-A) is a guide to the Wade system of romanization. It is prepared to assist the people who can read Chinese, but who are not familiar with the northern pronunciation and the Wade system. It gives a bird's-eye view of all the syllables with examples of Chinese characters. Section B (Appendix I-B) is prepared for people who have the names of Chinese herbs or crude drugs with the Pinyin system of romanization, and who want the scientific identification of the material and/or the English equivalents of the names. The table of conversion of the Pinyin to the Wade system is sufficient to help these people to solve their problems.

Appendix II is prepared for people who know the botanical names and want to look up the Chinese and English equivalents or the pharmaceutical terms. It contains two alphabetic lists: A. List of the families or higher groups of plants, and B. List of the genera of plants. Each family or generic name is followed by a family reference number or an abbreviation as stated above. From one of these lists, a consulter can find the plant name in Part II, and by the reference number it carries, he can look up the Chinese, English, or the pharmaceutical terms in Part I.

Appendix III is prepared for people who have difficulties in classical Chinese characters. Many of the names in the outstanding references mentioned above are printed in simplified Chinese characters. It took the author months to become familiar with this type of printing. The young people in China would have equal difficulty with the printing in classical references. For them and those of future generations who are not familiar with classical printing, a list for the conversion of simplified Chinese characters into the older types is provided in Appendix III.

Appendix IV is an index of Chinese names. They are arranged in the order of the number of strokes of each character. Their respective reference numbers in Part I are given immediately after the Chinese.

A notion for preparing two more appendices (one on an index to the English names, and the other on an index to the pharmaceutical terms) was contemplated but discarded on the criteria of utility and usability. This book has the function of a check list. It is not, and it should not be regarded as a source book. People who know the common English names or the pharmaceutical terms of plants and animals etc. are likely to look for information in a source book, not a check list. For the sake of usability, it is rational not to increase the volume and cost of printing by adding more indices which will have little likelihood of consultation.

**Literature cited**

In this Introduction, the sources of literature cited are incomplete. For the readers who would like to have more information, a complete list is provided. The anonymous items are entered by their dates of publication.

ANONYMOUS. *List of Chinese Medicines.* x, 493. China Imperial Maritime Customs. III. Miscellaneous Series No. 17. Shanghai. 1889.

————. *Chung-yao chih* 中葯誌 [A New Chinese Materia Medica]. I. Root and Rhizomes. 1-564, *figs.* 359, *pl.* 41, *photos* 179. 1959. II. Seeds and Fruits. 1-530, *figs.* 298, *pl.* 23, *photos* 202. 1959. III. Whole Herbs, Leaves Flowers, Barks, Lianas, Resins, Algae and Fungi, Miscellaneous plant products. 1-677, *figs.* 422, *pl.* 26, *photos* 222. 1961. IV. Animals, Insects and Minerals. 1-326, *figs.* 52, *pl.* 14, *photos* 117. 1961. Peking: People's Health Press, 1959-1961.

————. *Chang-yung Chung ts'ao-yao shou-ts'ê* 常用中草藥手冊 [A Handbook of Common Medicines]. [23], 1-1040, *figs.* [422]. Peking: People's Health Press, 1969.

————. *Chang-yung Chung ts'ao-yao t'u-p'u* 常用中草藥圖譜 [Colored Illustrations of Common Medicines]. [20], 1-396, *pl.* 1-228, 1-64. Peking: People's Health Press, 1970.

————. *Pei-fang chang-yung Chung ts'ao-yao shou-ts'ê* 北方常用中草藥手冊 [A Handbook of Northern Common Medicines]. [19], 1-1055. Peking: People's Health Press, 1971.

————. *Chung-kuo kao-têng chih-wu t'u-chien* 中國高等植物圖鑒 [Iconographia Cormophytorum Sinicorum]. 1: iv-v. 107-284. Peking: Science Press, 1972.

————. *Zhong cao yao xue* 中草藥學 (Chung ts'ao-yao hsüeh) [Chinese Pharmacology]. II. 1-897, *figs.* 726. Nanking College of Pharmacy. Kiangsu People's Press, 1976.

————. *Chung-yao ta tz'ŭ-tien* 中藥大辭典 [An Encyclopedia of Chinese Medicines]. I. vi, 15, 1-1489. II. 13, 1491-2754. Shanghai People's Press, 1977. III. 1-764. Shanghai Science Technology Press, 1978.

BAILEY, L. H. *Manual of Cultivated Plants.* 1-1116. New York: Macmillan, 1949.

BRETSCHNEIDER, E. V. Botanicum Sinicum. Notes on Chinese botany from native and Western sources. I. *Journ. N. China Branch Roy. Asiat. Soc.* n. ser. **16**: 18-230. 1882. II. *ibid.* **25**: i-ii, 1-468. 1893. III. *ibid.* **29**: 1-623. 1896.

DALLA TORRE, C. G. and H. HARMS. *Genera Siphonogamarum ad Systema Englerianum Conscripta.* 1-720. 1900. 721-921. 1907. Lisiae, 1900-1907.

FERNALD, M. L. *Gray's Manual of Botany.* 8th ed. i-lxiv, 1-1613. New York: American Book, 1950.

HILL, A. F. *Economic Botany.* i-xii, 1-560. New York: McGraw-Hill, 1952.

HSÜ, K. C. *et al. Yao-ts'ai hsüeh* 藥材學 [Chinese Pharmacognosy]. 1-1416. Peking: People's Health Press, 1960.

HU, S. Y. *Enumeration of the Vascular Plants of Hongkong.* i-ii, 1-100, index. Biol. Dept. Chinese University of Hong Kong, 1972.

————. A contribution to our knowledge of Leonurus L., *I-mu-ts'ao,* the Chinese motherwort. *Journ. Chin. Univ. Hong Kong* 2(**2**): 335-387. 1974.

————. A contribution to our knowledge of ginseng. *Am. Journ. Chin. Med.* **5**(**1**): 1-23. 1977.

————. A contribution to our knowledge of Tu-chung—*Eucommia ulmoides. Am. Journ. Chin. Med.* **7**(**1**): 5-37.

1979.

____. Herbal teas and populace health care in tropical China. Am. Journ. Chin. Med. **25(1)**: 103-104. 1997

JAEGER, E. C. *A Source-book of Biological Names and Terms.* 2nd ed. i-xxxv, 1-287. 1954.

KINGSBURY, J. M. *Poisonous Plants of the United States and Canada.* i-xiii, 1-626. New Jersey: Prentice-Hall, 1964.

MATHEWS, R. H. *A Chinese-English Dictionary.* i-xxi, 1-1226. Shanghai: China Inland Mission and Presbyterian Mission Press, 1931. Am. ed. Harvard Univ. Press, 1943.

NEAL, M. C. *In Gardens of Hawaii.* Rev. ed. i-xix, 1-924. Honolulu: Bishop Museum, 1968.

PECK, M. E. *A Manual of the Higher Plants of Oregon.* 2nd ed., 1-926. Binfords and Mort. Oregon State Univ., 1961.

READ, B. E. *Chinese Medicinal Plants from the Pên Ts'ao Kang Mu.* i-xvi, 1-389. Peking, 1936.

REHDER, A. *Manual of Cultivated Trees and Shrubs.* 2nd ed., i-xxx, 1-996. New York: Macmillan, 1940.

SMITH, A. W. *A Gardener's Book of Plant Names,* i-xix, 1-428. New York: Harper & Row, 1963.

STEARN, W. T. *Botanical Latin.* 2nd ed. 1-xiv, 1-566. Newton Abbot, England: David & Charles, 1973.

STEWARD, A. N. *Manual of Vascular Plants of the Lower Yangtze Valley, China.* 1-621. Corvallis: Oregon Univ., 1958.

STUART, G. A. *Chinese Materia Medica. Vegetable Kingdom.* [1-2], 1-558, i-vi. Shanghai, 1910.

# INTRODUCTION TO SECOND EDITION

THE term, Chinese materia medica, was used for ben-cao (本草) by G. A. Stuart in 1910 when he reported about his work on *Ben-cao Gong-mu* (本草綱目) [Compendium of Materia Medica] of Li Shi-zhen. Presently, in American academic and trading communities, the general term used for ben-cao is Chinese herbal medicines.

The first edition of *An Enumeration of Chinese Materia Medica* is out of print. Time has proved that its usefulness exceeded the original target set for it, "to help people in science and medicine, to facilitate their work of writing by supplying them with the scientific and vernacular names of the subject matter of their research." Actually, in fields outside science and medicine, there are sinologists who keep the book on their desks. They have found it being the only lexicon in which they can find many names of flowers and plant products mentioned in Chinese literature and culture. It seems that good news spread fast. On the other side of the globe, in Boston, Chinese practitioners wanted to purchase the book. They need it for the English names in their communication with the American patients.

As the academic world outside China becomes interested in Chinese herbal medicines, the usefulness of this book extends to the collection, identification and curatorial work of market material available in their local drug stores. The proprietors and clerks of the drug stores dealing with Chinese herbal medicines outside China operate in Chinese language. When a researcher purchases any herbal Chinese Medicine, he/she can ask the pharmacist to write the name on each package. By using Appendix IV and Part I, he/she can get the scientific identification, the English and the pharmaceutical names of the specimens. With the scientific names he/she can use Appendix II-B and Part II in the book to file the specimens in a systematic order by the Englerian System, the system used in the Flora Reipublicae Popularis Sinicae and the Flora of China.

The items included in the second edition has been my deep concern. It took me much time and thought to fight with the temptation of adding more items to the book than what is done, after reviewing over 40 recent publications from China. Between 1970 and 1997 there was a great proliferation of simple illustrated books on Chinese herbal medicines. In the first two years of 1970s, handbooks and/or manuals for the identification of local medicinal plants were published for every province or special political area in China. These tool books were small (13 x 9 cm), handy, and each containing 300–500 source species with line drawings. In the 1980s, several resourceful large (25 x 18 cm or 28 x 21 cm) materia medica, encyclopedia and coloured photographic icones of nationwide magnitude, each covering 5,000 to 6,000 source species were published. Between 1990 and 1997, many medium-sized books, skillfully prepared and illustrated with colored photographs for the identification of source species and for distinguishing genuine and false market products were published. These tool books are prepared by experienced practitioners of traditional Chinese medicine, professors of pharmacognosy in pharmaceutical universities and health officers of the central government. These tool books cover between 400 and 500 items. Evidently, one unique character of tool books for the general public is handiness. I finally decide that the size of a lexicon of this nature is determined by its usefulness to the people it serves. Following the principle of utility and usability set for selecting items included in the original edition, I decided to keep the book as close to the first edition as possible.

Three conditions are set for making alterations: (1) nomenclatural changes caused by botanical revisions of the genera concerned; (2) addition of source species to items enriched due to area extension explored in China; and (3) correction and clarification of the text of any original item. Following these guiding principles, in the second edition, 26 items have changed scientific names, 40 new sources species are added and one correction with explanation is made to the original text.

Example of the nomenclatural change is found in Wu-chu-yü 吳茱萸. In the original edition, its scientific name is *Evodia rutaecarpa* (Juss.) Bentham. It is changed to *Tetradium rutaecarpum* (Juss.) Hartley. Between 1950 and 1970s phytochemists working on the active compositions of Wu-chu-

yü isolated and named evoden, evodin, evodol hydroxy-evodiamine, evocarpine, isoevodiamine, and evodinone. In botanical nomenclature, the change of the scientific epithet of a species does not affect its vernacular name. Similar condition happened with Wu-chia-p'i 五加皮 where the generic name was changed from Acanthopanax to Eleutherococcus. In both cases, the former generic names, Acanthopanax and Evodia, are used as the English common names of the source species. This will help future workers to recognize the root of chemicals associated with Wu-chu-yü.

Example for the second condition is found in Huang-ch'i 黄芪. In the original edition, the source species are *Astragalus membranaceus* (Fischer) Bunge and *A. mongolicus* Bunge, both from northern China. Now, this item is enriched by adding *A. tongolensis* Ilbr. from Sichuan, and adjacent areas in Gansu, Qinghai and Tibet (543a), *A. floridus* Benth. (543b) from Sichuan and adjacent areas in Tibet and Qinghai and *Hedysarum polybotrus* Hand.-Mazz. from Gansu (543c).

Shên-ch'ü ( 神麴, shen-qu in *An Encyclopedia of Chinese Medicines*, entry 3573) needs clarification. The original treatment contains two elements. Shên-ch'ü from northern China and Chien-ch'ü 建麴 from Fujian in southeastern China. In traditional Chinese medicine, shên-ch'ü is a yeast cake prepared from six source species (Hu, 1997, p. 117), three of which are fresh wild plants and the other three are products of cultivated plants. The ingredients are: 3 kg each of ground rice bean (*Delanda umbellata* [Thunb.] S. Y. Hu) and apricot seed (*Prunus armeniaca* L., soaked and seed coat removed); 6 kg each of chopped fresh Chinese wormwood (*Artemisia apiacea* Hance), smartweed (*Polygonum hydropiper* L.) and cocklebur (*Xanthium sibiricum* Patrin ex Widder); and 50 kg of wheat flour (*Triticum aestivum* L.). The process of production consists of mixing the above ingredients with water to make a soft dough. Use a piece of the dough, knead it smooth and press it into a cake, approximately 1 cm thick. In a warm, poorly ventilated room, the cakes are piled up and covered with wheat (millet or rice) straw to undergo fermentation by yeast cells attached to the fresh plants and/or by air-borne spores of micro-organisms. When the cakes appear yellow, they are separated, cut into serving sizes, dried and stored for distribution.

Shiu Ying Hu
Herbarium, Department of Biology
The Chinese University of Hong Kong
Hong Kong

# PART I

# An Alphabetic List of Chinese Medicines

With the Botanical Names and Their Equivalents in
English and in Pharmaceutical Usage

# AN ALPHABETICAL LIST OF CHINESE MEDICINES

| Transliteration | Chinese | Botanical Name | English | Pharmaceutical | A |
|---|---|---|---|---|---|
| 0001 A-chiao | 阿膠 | — | Ass-hide glue | Gelatinum Asini | |
| 0002 A-huang | 阿黃,阿磺 | — | Sulphur preparation | — | |
| 0003 A-la-pai-chiao | 阿拉伯膠 | **Acacia senegal** | GUM ARABIC | Gummi Arabicum | |
| 0004 A-pien (A-fu-yung) | 阿片(阿芙蓉) | **Papaver somniferum** | Opium | Morphine, Opium | |
| 0005 A-wei | 阿魏 | **Ferula assafoetida** | ASAFETIDA | Asafetida | |
| −a  Hsin-chiang-a-wei | 新疆阿魏 | **F. conocaula** **F. sinkiangensis** | CHINESE ASAFETIDA | | |
| 0006 Ai (Wu-yüeh-ai) | 艾(五月艾) | **Artemisia vulgaris** **A. argyi** | COMMON MUGWORT | Herba Artemisiae | |
| 0007 Ai-fên | 艾粉 | **Blumea balsamifera** | Powdered extract of *Blumea* | — | |
| 0008 Ai-jung (Ai-mien) | 艾絨(艾綿) | **Artemisia vulgaris** **A. argyi** | Mugwort (tender) | — | |
| 0009 Ai-na-hsiang | 艾納香 | **Blumea balsamifera** | Extract of *Blumea* | — | |
| 0010 Ai-t'iao | 艾條 | **Artemisia vulgaris** **A. argyi** | Mugwort (shoot) | Caulis Artemisiae | |
| 0011 Ai-yeh | 艾葉 | Same as the above | Mugwort (leaf) | Folium Artemisiae | |
| 0012 Ai-yu | 艾油 | **Blumea balsamifera** | Oil of *Blumea* | Oleum Blumeae | |
| 0013 Ai-yu-tzǔ | 愛玉子 | **Ficus pumila** | JELLY-SEED | Semen Fici Pumilae | |
| 0014 An-hsi-hsiang | 安息香 | **Styrax benzoin** | SUMATRA BENZOIN | Benzoinum | |
| | | **S. hypoglaucus** **S. macrothyrsus** **S. subniveus** | CHINESE BENZOIN | Benzoinum | |
| | | **S. tonkinensis** | SIAM BENZOIN | Benzoinum | |

| Transliteration | Chinese | Botanical Name | English Name | Pharmaceutical |
|---|---|---|---|---|
| 0015 An-yeh | 桉葉 | **Eucalyptus globulus** | EUCALYPTUS | Folium Eucalypti |
| 0016 Cha-jou | 楂肉,查肉 | **Crataegus pinnatifida** (see Shan-cha-jou) | Dried Hawthorn (fruit) | Fructus Crataegi |
| 0017 Cha-ping (Cha-jou, Shan-cha-ping) | 楂餅(楂肉,山楂餅) | **Crataegus pinnatifida** | Hawthorn (cake) | Pericarpium Crataegi |
| 0018 Ch'a (Ming) | 茶(茗) | **Camellia sinensis** | TEA | Folium Camelliae |
| 0019 Ch'a-tzŭ-ping | 茶子餅 | **C. oleifera** | Tea-oil (cake) | Fructus Camelliae Oleifera |
| 0020 Ch'a-yeh | 茶葉 | **C. sinensis** | Tea (leaves) | Folium Camelliae |
| 0021 Ch'ai-hu (Ch'ai-hu-t'ou, Ch'ai-t'ou) | 柴胡(柴胡頭,柴頭) | **Bupleurum falcatum** **B. scorzoneraefolium** | HARE'S EAR (root) | Radix Bupleuri |
| −ª Pai-ch'ai-hu | 北柴胡 | **B. chinense** | CHINESE HARE'S EAR | Radix Bupleuri |
| 0022 Ch'ai-p'i-chang (Pao-p'i-chang) | 豺皮樟(豹皮樟) | **Actinodaphne chinensis** | LEOPARD CAMPHOR | Radix Actinodaphnes |
| 0023 Ch'an-ch'u-kan | 蟾蜍乾 | — | Dried toad | Bufo Siccus |
| 0024 Ch'an-hua | 蟬花 | **Cordyceps scotianus** | Sclerotia of infested Cicada | Cordyceps Cicadae |
| −ª Hsiao-ch'an-hua | 小蟬花 | **C. sobolifera** | | |
| 0025 Ch'an-kao | 潺槁 | **Litsea glutinosa** | POND SPICE | Radix, Cortex et Folium Litseae Glutinosae |
| 0026 Ch'an-shui (Ch'an-t'ui, Ch'an-t'o, Ch'an-i) | 蟬蛻(蟬退,蟬脫,蟬衣) | — | Exuviae of Cicada | Peristracum Cicadae |
| 0027 Ch'an-su | 蟾酥 | — | Cake of toad skin secretion | Secretio Bufonis |

| Transliteration | Chinese | Botanical Name | English | Pharmaceutical |
|---|---|---|---|---|
| 0028 Chang-ch'ai | 樟柴 | **Cinnamomum camphora** | CAMPHOR TREE (twigs) | Caulis Cinnamomi |
| 0029 Chang-liu-t'ou (Pi-hsiao-chiang) | 樟柳頭(閉鞘薑) | **Costus speciosus** | CRAPE GINGER | Rhizoma Costi |
| 0030 Chang-mu | 樟木 | **Cinnamomum camphora** | Wood of Camphor Tree | Lignum Cinnamomi |
| 0031 Chang-mu-p'i | 樟木皮 | **Cinnamomum camphora** | Bark of Camphor Tree | Cortex Cinnamomi |
| 0032 Chang-mu-tzŭ | 樟木子 | **Cinnamomum camphora** | Fruit and seed of Camphor Tree | Fructus et Semen Cinnamomi |
| 0033 Chang-nao | 樟腦 | **Cinnamomum camphora** | Camphor | Camphora |
| 0034 Chang-nao-yu | 樟腦油 | **Cinnamomum camphora** | Camphor oil | Oleum Camphorae |
| 0035 Chang-p'ien (Chang-nao-p'ien) | 樟片(樟腦片) | **Cinnamomum camphora** | Refined Camphor | Camphora Depurata |
| 0036 Ch'ang-ch'un-hua | 長春花 | **Catharanthus roseus** | MADAGASCAR PERIWINKLE | Herba Catharanthi |
| 0037 Ch'ang-ch'un-t'êng | 常春藤 | **Hedera helix** **H. nepalensis** var. **sinensis** | COMMON IVY EVERGREEN IVY | Caulis Hederae |
| 0038 Ch'ang-p'u | 菖蒲 | **Acorus calamus** | SWEETFLAG, CALAMUS | Rhizoma Calami |
| 0039 Ch'ang-shan (Ch'ang-shan-yeh) | 常山(常山葉) | **Dichroa febrifuga** or **Orixa japonica** | *CHINESE QUININE | Radix Dichroae |
| 0040 Ch'ao-wu (=Ho-shou-wu) | 潮烏(=何首烏) | **Polygonum multiflorum** | NIMBLE-WILL, CHINESE CORNBIND | Rhizoma Polygoni Multiflori |
| 0041 Chê-hsieh | 澤瀉 | **Alisma plantago-aquatica** | WATER-PLANTAIN | Rhizoma Alismatis |
| 0042 Chê-ku-ts'ai | 鷓鴣菜 | **Caloglossa leprieurii** | *CALOGLOSSA | Herba Caloglossae |
| 0043 Chê-lan (P'ê-lan) | 澤蘭(佩蘭) | **Eupatorium japonicum** | *EUPATORIUM | Herba Eupatorii |
| 0044 Chê-pei (Chê-pei-mu) | 浙貝(浙貝母) | **Fritillaria thunbergii** | CHEKIANG FRITILLARY | Bulbus Fritillariae Thunbergii |
| 0045 Chê-shih (Tai-chê-shih) | 赭石(代赭石) | — | Hematite | Hematitum |

5

| Transliteration | Chinese | Botanical Name | English | Pharmaceutical |
|---|---|---|---|---|
| 0046 Ch'ê-ch'ien-ts'ao (Ch'ien-kuan-ts'ao) | 車前草(錢貫草) | **Plantago major, or P. asiatica** | COMMON PLANTAIN | Herba Plantaginis |
| 0047 Ch'ê-ch'ien-tzǔ | 車前子(車前) | **Plantago major, or P. asiatica** | Seed of Plantain | Semen Plantaginis |
| 0048 Chên-chu | 珍珠(眞珠) | — | Pearls | Margarita |
| 0049 Chên-chu-mu (Chên-chu-p'ei) | 眞珠母(珍珠貝) | — | Mother of pearl | Concha Margaritifera Usta |
| 0050 Chên-chu-ts'ao | 珍珠草 | **Phyllanthus urinaria** | PHYLLANTHUS | Herba Phyllanthi |
| 0051 Chên-jên (Chên-tzǔ) | 榛仁(榛子) | **Corylus heterophylla** | HAZEL-NUTS | Fructus Coryli |
| 0052 Ch'ên-hsiang (Mi-hsiang) | 沉香(密香) | **Aquilaria agallocha** | ALOESWOOD, AGARU (Sans.) | Lignum Aquilariae |
| 0053 Ch'ên-p'i (Kuo-pi') | 陳皮(果皮) | **Citrus reticulata** | Mandarin Orange (peel) | Pericarpium Citri Reticulatae |
| 0054 Ch'ên-p'i-kao (Chih-ch'ên-p'i) | 陳皮膏(製陳皮) | **Citrus reticulata** | Tangerine (peel paste) | Extractus Pericarpii Citri Reticulatae |
| 0055 Ch'ên-sha | 辰砂 | — | High grade cinnabar | Cinnabaris |
| 0056 Ch'ên-tsung-t'an | 陳棕炭 | **Trachycarpus fortunei** | CHINESE PALM (petiole fiber charred) | Vagina Trachycarpi Carbonisata |
| 0057 Ch'êng-ch'ieh | 澄茄 | **Piper cubeba** | CUBEB | Fructus Cubebae |
| 0058 Ch'êng-liu (Kuan-yin-liu) | 檉柳(觀音柳) | **Tamarix chinensis** | TAMARISK | Ramulus Tamaricis cum Folio |
| 0059 Ch'êng-t'ung | 槙桐 | **Clerodendrum kaempferi** | PAGODA FLOWER | Radix et Folium Clerodendri Kaempferi |
| 0060 Chi-ch'ang-fêng | 鷄腸楓 | **Morinda officinalis** | *MORINDA (root) | Radix Morindae |

| Transliteration | Chinese | Botanical Name | English | Pharmaceutical |
|---|---|---|---|---|
| 0061 Chi-chao-san-chi | 鷄爪三七 | **Kalanchoe laciniata** | KALANCHOE | Herba Kalanchoes |
| 0062 Chi-chi | 及己 | **Chloranthus serratus** | *SERRATE-LEAVED CHLORANTHUS | Herba Chloranthi Serrati |
| 0063 Chi-chih | 齏汁 | — | Mixture of ginger and garlic juice | *Chi-chih |
| 0065 Chi-hsing-tzŭ (Chi-hsing, Fêng-hsien-tzŭ) | 急性子(急性, 鳳仙子) | **Impatiens balsamina** | GARDEN BALSAM, TOUCH-ME-NOT | Semen Impatientis |
| 0066 Chi-hsüeh-t'êng | 鷄血藤 | **Millettia reticulata** **M. dielsiana** **Spatholobus suberectus** | MILLETTIA SPATHOLOBUS | Radix Millettiae Reticulatae et Dielsianae Radix Spatholobi |
| 0067 Chi-hua (Chih-mo-hua) | 檵花(紙沫花) | **Loropetalum chinense** | STRAP FLOWER | Radix Loropetali |
| 0068 Chi-jou (Chi-ch'ang-fêng) | 戟肉(鷄腸楓) | **Morinda officinalis** | MORINDA (root) | Radix Morindae |
| 0069 Chi-ku-hsiang | 鷄骨香 | **Croton crassifolius** | THICK-LEAVED CROTON (root) | Radix Crotonis Crassifolii |
| 0070 Chi-ku-ts'ao | 鷄骨草 | **Abrus cantoniensis** | CHINESE PRAYER-BEADS | Frutex Abri |
| 0071 Chi-kuan-hua (Chia-kuan) | 鷄冠花(加冠) | **Celosia cristata** | COCKSCOMB | Flos et Semen Celesiae |
| 0072 Chi-li (Pai-chi-li, tz'ŭ-chi-li) | 蒺藜(白蒺藜, 刺蒺藜) | **Tribulus terrestris** | CALTROP | Fructus Tribuli |
| 0073 Chi-lien | 鷄連 | See Huang-lien | — | — |

| | Transliteration | Chinese | Botanical Name | English | Pharmaceutical |
|---|---|---|---|---|---|
| 0074 | Chi-nei-chin (Chi-chun-p'i, Nei-chin) | 鷄內金(鷄肫皮,內金) | — | Lining of chicken gizzard | Corium Stomachichum Galli |
| 0075 | Chi-nu (Liu-chi-nu) | 寄奴(劉寄奴) | **Artemisia anomala** | *LARGE-LEAVED ARTESIMIA | Herba Artemisiae Anomalae |
| 0076 | Chi-shêng (Pai-chi-shêng, Hu-chi-shêng) | 寄生(北寄生,槲寄生) | **Viscum coloratum** (see Sang-chi-shêng) | RED-FRUIT MISTLETOE | Ramus Visci Colorati |
| 0077 | Chi-shih-t'êng | 鷄屎藤(鷄矢藤) | **Paederia scandens** | CHICKEN-DUNG CREEPER | Radix et Ramus Paederiae |
| 0078 | Chi-ts'ai (Hsiang-Chi-ts'ai) | 薺菜(香薺菜) | **Capsella bursa-pastoris** | SHEPHERD'S PURSE | Herba Capsellae |
| 0079 | Chi-yen-ts'ao | 鷄眼草 | **Kummerowia striata** | Chicken-dung Creeper | Herba Kummerowiae |
| 0080 | Ch'i-ai (Fu-jung-chü) | 蘄艾(芙蓉菊) | **Crossostephium chinense** | *CROSSOSTEPHIUM | Herba Crossostephii |
| 0081 | Ch'i-chih-chüeh | 七指蕨 | **Helminthostachys zeylanica** | *HELMINTHOSTACHYS | Herba Helminthosta-chydis |
| 0082 | Ch'i-huang-ts'ao | 溪黃草 | **Plectranthus striatus** | *Plectranthus | Herba Plectranthi |
| 0083 | Ch'i-kan (Kan-ch'i) | 漆乾(干漆) | **Rhus verniciflua** | VARNISH TREE (dried varnish) | Lacca Sinica Exsiccata |
| 0084 | Ch'i-li-hsiang (Chiu-li-hsiang) | 七里香(九里香) | **Murraya paniculata** | *MURRAYA | Frutex Murrayae |
| 0085 | Ch'i-shê (Shê-kan, Pê-pu-shê) | 蘄蛇(祈蛇,蛇乾,百步蛇) | — | Dried venomous snake from Hupeh | Agkistrodon |

| Transliteration | Chinese | Botanical Name | English | Pharmaceutical |
|---|---|---|---|---|
| 0086 Ch'i-shih (Yang-ch'i-shih) | 起石(陽起石) | — | Actinolite | Actinolitum |
| 0087 Ch'i-ta-ku (Ch'i-ku-ch'a) | 漆大姑(漆姑茶) | **Glochidion eriocarpum** | RED-FRUITED GLOCHIDION | Ramus Glochidionis Eriocarpi |
| 0088 Ch'i-ts'ai (Yu-hsing-ts'ao) | 蕺菜(魚腥草) | **Houttuynia cordata** | FISH-SMELL HERB | Herba Houttuyniae |
| 0089 Ch'i-ts'ao (T'u-ts'an) | 蠐螬(土蠶) | — | Grubs of June Beetle | Holotrichia |
| 0090 Ch'i-tzǔ | 杞子 | See Kou-ch'i-tzǔ | — | — |
| 0091 Ch'i-yeh-i-chih-hua | 七葉一枝花 | **Paris polyphylla** | *PARIS | Rhizoma Paridis |
| 0092 Ch'i-yeh-lien (Ch'i-chia-p'i) | 七葉蓮(七加皮) | **Schefflera arboricola** | *TAIWAN SCHEFFLERA | Radix Schefflerae Arboricola |
| 0093 Chia-chu-t'ao | 夾竹桃 | **Nerium oleander (N. indicum)** | OLEANDER | Folium et Cortex Nerii Indici |
| 0094 Chia-chü (Pi-pa-tzǔ) | 假蒟(蓽茇子) | **Piper sarmentosum** | WILD PEPPER | Caulis et Fructus Piperis |
| 0095 Chia-fei | 咖啡 | **Coffea arabica** | COFFEE BEAN | Semen Coffeae |
| 0096 Chia-p'i (Tz'ǔ-wu-chia-p'i) | 加皮(刺五加皮) | **Eleutherococcus senticosus** (see Wu-chia-p'i) | ELEUTHERO | Radix Eleutherococci |
| 0097 Chia-p'ien | 甲片 | See Ch'uan-shan-chia-p'ien | — | — |
| 0098 Chiai-tzǔ | 芥子 | **Brassica juncea** | MUSTARD (seed) | Semen Brassicae Junceae |
| 0099 Chiai-tzǔ (Pai-chiai-tzǔ) | 芥子(白芥子) | **Brassica hirta** | MUSTARD (seed) | Semen Sinapis |

| | Transliteration | Chinese | Botanical Name | English | Pharmaceutical |
|---|---|---|---|---|---|
| 0100 | Chiang (Shêng-chiang, Kan-chiang) | 薑(生薑, 乾薑) | **Zingiber officinale** | GINGER (fresh or dry) | Rhizoma Zingiberis |
| 0101 | Chiang-ch'ung (Chiang-ts'an) | 彊蟲(彊蠶) | — | Dried sick Silkworm | Bombyx cum Batryte |
| 0102 | Chiang-hsiang (Chiang-chên-hsiang) | 降香(降真香) | **Dalbergia sissoo**<br>**D. odorifera**<br>**D. parviflora** | *SCENTED ROSEWOOD | Lignum Dalbergiae odoriferae |
| 0103 | Chiang-huang (Huang-chiang) | 薑黃(黃薑) | **Curcuma longa**<br>**(C. domestica)** | TURMERIC | Rhizoma Curcumae |
| 0103A | Chiang-li (Lung-hsü-tsai) | 江蘺(龍鬚菜) | **Gracilaria verrucosa** | *DRAGON WISKERS | Herba Gracilariae |
| 0104 | Chiang-p'i | 薑皮 | **Zingiber officinale** | Ginger (skin) | Cortex Zingiberis |
| 0105 | Chiang-san-ch'i | 薑三七 | **Stahlianthus**<br>**involucratus**<br>**Caulokaempferia**<br>**yunnanensis**<br>**(Camptandra**<br>**yunnanensis)** | *GINGER SANCHI | Rhizoma Stahlianthi vel Caulokaempferiae |
| 0106 | Chiang-ts'an | 彊蠶 | See Chiang-ch'ung | — | — |
| 0107 | Chiang-tzǔ | 江子 | **Croton tiglium** | CROTON (seed) | Semen Crotonis |
| 0108 | Chiang-yu | 薑油 | **Zingiber officinale** | Ginger oil | Oleum Gingiberis |
| 0109 | Ch'iang-huo | 羌活 | **Notopterygium incisium** | *CHIANGHUO | Radix Notopterygii |
| —a | Ch'uan-ch'iang | 川羌 | **N. franchetii** | SICHUAN CHIANGHUO | — |
| —b | Ts'an-ch'iang | 蠶羌 | **N. forbei** | *CH'INGHAI CHIANGHUO | — |
| 0110 | Ch'iang-lang (Shih-k'o-lang) | 蜣螂(屎蚵蜋) | — | Dung Beetle | Catharsius |
| 0111 | Ch'iang-wei-hua | 薔薇花 | **Rosa multiflora** | SEVEN-SISTERS ROSE | Flos Rosae Multiflorae |
| 0112 | Chiao-pai-tzǔ | 茭白子 | **Zizania canduciflora** | WILD RICE | Fructus Zizaniae |
| 0113 | Chiao-t'ou (Pa-chiao-kên) | 蕉頭(芭蕉根) | **Musa basjoo** | BANANA (stump) | Caudex Musae |

| Transliteration | Chinese | Botanical Name | English | Pharmaceutical | Ch'iao |
|---|---|---|---|---|---|

| Transliteration | Chinese | Botanical Name | English | Pharmaceutical |
|---|---|---|---|---|
| 0114 Chiao-tz'ŭ-p'ien | 角薊片 | See Tsao-chiao-tz'ŭ | — | — |
| 0115 Ch'iao-kan (Hsieh-pai) | 蕎乾(薤白) | **Allium chinense** | *CHINESE CHIVE (bulbs) | Bulbus Allii Chinensis |
| 0116 Ch'iao-mai (San-chiao-mai) | 蕎麥(三角麥) | **Fagopyrum esculentum** | BUCKWHEAT | Fructus Fagopyri |
| 0117 Ch'iao-mai-ch'i (Chi-hsüeh-ch'i, Wu-kung-ch'i) | 蕎麥七(鷄血七, 蜈蚣七) | **Polygonum amplexicaule** | *AMPLEXICAUL KNOTWEED | Caudex Polygoni Amplexicaulis |
| 0118 Chieh-hung (Chü-hung) | 桔紅(橘紅) | **Citrus erythrocarpa** | RED TANGERINE | Exocarpium Citri Erythrocarpae |
| 0119 Chieh-kêng | 桔梗 | **Platycodon grandiflorum** | BALLOON FLOWER | Radix Platycodonis |
| 0102 Chieh-ku-mu | 接骨木 | **Sambucus williamsii (S. racemosa)** | ASIATIC ELDER | Frutex Sambuci |
| 0121 Chieh-lo (Chieh-pai) | 桔絡(桔白) | **Citrus reticulata** | MANDARIN ORANGE (Vascular bundle) | Fasciculus Vascularis Pericarpii Citri |
| 0122 Chieh-p'i | 桔皮 | **Citrus reticulata** | MANDARIN ORANGE (peel) | Pericarpium Aurantii |
| 0123 Chieh-yeh | 桔葉 | **Citrus reticulata** | MANDARIN ORANGE (twig) | Ramus Citri |
| 0124 Ch'ieh | 茄 | **Solanum melongena** | EGG PLANT | — |
| Ch'ieh-chih | 茄枝 | ,,      ,, | EGG PLANT (branch) | Ramus Solani Melongenae |
| Ch'ieh-kên | 茄根 | ,,      ,, | EGG PLANT (root) | Ramus Solani Melongenae |
| Ch'ieh-p'i | 茄皮 | ,,      ,, | EGG PLANT (peel) | Pericarpium Solani Melongenae |
| 0125 Chien-chih | 建梔(建枝) | **Gardenia jasminoides** | GARDENIA (fruit from Fukien) | Fructus Gardeniae |

| | Transliteration | Chinese | Botanical Name | English | Pharmaceutical |
|---|---|---|---|---|---|
| 0126 | Chien-ch'ü | 建粬 | **Monascus purpureus** (see Shên-ch'ü) | *RED YEAST (from Fukien) | Massa Monasci purpurei |
| 0127 | Chien-ch'un-lo | 剪春羅 | **Lychnis coronata** | MULLEIN PINK | Herba Lychnis |
| 0128 | Chien-chün | 建君 | See Shih-chün-tzŭ | — | — |
| 0129 | Chien-hsieh | 建瀉 | **Alisma plantago-aquatica** | WATER PLANTAIN (from Fukien) | Rhizoma Alismatis |
| 0130 | Chien-hsüeh-fêng-hou | 見血封喉 | **Antiaris toxicaria** | *ANTIARIS | Latex et Semen Antiaris |
| 0131 | Chien-hua (K'uan-tung-hua) | 揀花(款冬花) | **Tussilago farfara** | *TUSSILAGO, COLT'S FOOT | Flos Farfarae |
| 0132 | Chien-shan-yao (Chien-shan) | 建山藥(見山) | **Dioscorea opposita** | YAM (from Fukien) | Radix Dioscoreae |
| 0133 | Chien-shui | 鹻水 | — | Lye or Potash | — |
| 0134 | Chien-ti-ku (Kou-ch'i-p'ien, Ti-ku-p'i) | 揀地骨(枸杞片, 地骨皮) | **Lycium chinense** | MATRIMONY VINE (bark of root, best quality) | Cortex Lycii Radicis |
| 0135 | Chien-wei-fêng | 尖尾楓 | **Callicarpa longissima** | *LONG-LEAVED CALLICARPA | Folium Callicarpae Longissimae |
| 0136 | Ch'ien-chang-chih (Mu-hu-tieh) | 千張紙(木蝴蝶) | **Oroxylum indicum** | TREE-OF-DAMOCLES | Semen Oroxyli |
| 0137 | Ch'ien-chin-pa (Chin-niu-wei) | 千斤拔(金牛尾) | **Moghania philippinensis** | *SMALL-LEAVED MOGHANIA | Radix Moghaniae |
| 0138 | Ch'ien-chin-t'êng | 千斤藤 | **Stephania japonica S. hernandifolia** | *STEPHANIA | Radix et Ramus Stephaniae |
| 0139 | Ch'ien-chin-tzŭ (Hsü-sui-tzŭ) | 千金子(續隨子) | **Euphorbia lathyris** | *LATHYROL SPURGE | Semen Euphorbia Lathyris |

12

| Transliteration | Chinese | Botanical Name | English | Pharmaceutical |
|---|---|---|---|---|
| 0140 Ch'ien-hu | 前胡 | **Peucedanum praeruptorum** | *PEUCEDANUM, MASTERWORT | Radix Peucedani |
| 0141 Ch'ien-jih-hung | 千日紅 | **Gomphrena globosa** | GLOBE-AMARANTH | Flos Gomphrenae |
| 0142 Ch'ien-kên | 茜根 | See Ch'ien-ts'ao | — | — |
| 0143 Ch'ien-li-kuang | 千里光 | **Senecio scandens** | RAGWORT | Herba Senecionis |
| 0144 Ch'ien-nien-chien | 千年見 | **Homalomena occulta** | *HOMALOMENA | Rhizoma Homalomenae |
| 0145 Ch'ien-niu-tzŭ | 牽牛子 | **Ipomoea nil (Pharbitis nil)** | MORNING GLORY | Semen Pharbitidis |
| 0146 Ch'ien-shih (Tz'ŭ-shih) | 茨實（茨實） | **Euryale ferox** | *EURYALE | Semen Euryalis |
| 0147 Ch'ien-ta-ch'iu | 千打錘 | **Lindera chunii** | CHUN'S ALLSPICE | Radix Linderae Chunii |
| 0148 Ch'ien-ts'ao (Ch'ien-kên, Hsüeh-chien-ch'ou, Ch'ien-ts'ao-kên) | 茜草（茜根，血見愁，茜草根） | **Rubia cordifolia** | MADDER | Radix Rubiae |
| 0149 Ch'ien-ts'êng-chih | 千層紙 | — | Pink-speckled mica | Muscovitum |
| 0150 Ch'ien-ts'êng-lou (Kuan-yeh-lien-ch'iao) | 千層樓（貫葉連翹） | **Hypericum perforatum** | *Perfoliate St. Johnswort | Herba Hyperici Perforati |
| 0151 Chih-ch'ên-p'i | 製陳皮 | — | Preserved peel of Citrus | — |
| 0152 Chih-chü (Chih-chü-tzŭ, Wan-tzŭ-kuo) | 枳具（枳椇，枳椇子，萬字果） | **Hovenia dulcis** | *HOVENIA | Semen Hoveniae |
| 0153 Chih-ho | 枝核 | See Li-chih-ho | — | — |

| | Transliteration | Chinese | Botanical Name | English | Pharmaceutical |
|---|---|---|---|---|---|
| 0154 | Chih-k'o | 枳殼(枳壳，枝殼) | **Citrus aurantium, C. wilsonii,** or **Poncirus trifoliata** | Peel of various Citrus fruit | Fructus Citri Immaturus Exsiccatus |
| 0155 | Chih-mu (Chu-mu) | 知母(猪母) | **Anemarrhena asphodeloides** | *ANEMARRHENA | Rhizoma Anemarrhenae |
| 0156 | Chih-shih | 枳實 | **Poncirus trifoliata** | TRIFOLIATE ORANGE | Fructus Ponciri |
| 0157 | Chih-tzŭ | 梔子(枝子) | **Gardenia jasminoides** | GARDENIA | Fructus Gardeniae |
| | Chih-tzŭ-kên (Chih-tzŭ-t'ou) | 梔子根(枝子頭) | „          „ | GARDENIA (root) | Radix Gardeniae |
| 0158 | Ch'ih-hsiao-tou (Hsiao-hung-tou) | 赤小豆(小紅豆) | **Delanda umbellata[1]** | Rice Bean SMALL RED-BEAN | Semen Delandae Umbellatae |
| 0159 | Ch'ih-shao (Ching-shao) | 赤芍(京芍) | **Paeonia lactiflora** or **P. obovata, P. veitchii** | PEONY (root) | Radix Paeoniae Lactiflorae |
| 0160 | Ch'ih-shih-chih (Shih-chih) | 赤石脂(石脂) | — | Halloysite | Halloysitum Rubrum |
| 0161 | Chin-ch'ai (Chin-ch'ai-hu) | 金釵(金釵斛) | **Dendrobium nobile** | *DENDROBIUM | Herba Dendrobii Nobilis |
| 0162 | Chin-ch'an-hua | 金蟬花 | — | Cicada with fungus growth | Cordyceps Cidadae |
| 0163 | Chin-chi-chao (Hsiang-pai-chih, Chi-chao-shên) | 金鷄爪(香白芷，鷄爪參) | **Angelica citriodora** | *CITRUS-SCENTED ANGELICA | Radix Angelicae Citriodorae |
| 0164 | Chin-chi-êrh | 錦鷄兒 | **Caragana sinica** | *CHINESE CARAGANA | Radix Caraganae Sinicae |

[1] Delanda umbellata (Thunb.) S. Y. Hu, nom nov. Dolichos umbellatus Thunb. in Trans. Linn. Soc. 2:339.1794.

| Transliteration | Chinese | Botanical Name | English | Pharmaceutical |
|---|---|---|---|---|
| 0165 Chin-chieh-kan (Chin-chü-kan) | 金桔乾(金橘乾) | **Fortunella margarita** | KUMQUAT (dried) | Fructus Fortunellae |
| 0166 Chin-ch'ien-sung-p'i | 金錢松皮 | **Pseudolarix amabilis** | GOLDEN LARCH | Cortex Pseudolaricis |
| 0167 Chin-ch'ien-ts'ao | 金錢草 | **Desmodium styracifolium** | *COIN-LEAVED DESMODIUM | Herba Desmodii Styracifolii |
| 0168 Chin-chih | 金汁 | — | Old liquid manure | — |
| 0169 Chin-chi-na-p'i | 金鷄納皮 | **Cinchona officinalis** or **C. calisaya** | CINCHONA BARK | Cortex Cinchonae |
| 0170 Chin-ching-shih (Shui-chin-yün-mu) | 金精石(水金云母) | — | Vermiculite | Vermiculitum |
| 0171 Chin-chu-ts'ai | 珍珠菜 | **Lysimachia clethroides** | *SUMMER-SWEET LYSIMACHIA | Radix Lysimachiae Clethroidis |
| 0172 Chin-chü-kan | 金橘乾 | **Fortunella margarita** | KUMQUAT (dried) | Fructus Fortunellae |
| 0173 Chin-êrh-huan | 金耳環 | **Asarum gracilipes A. insigne A. longepedunculatum** | GOLDEN EAR-RING | Herba Asari |
| 0174 Chin-fa-ts'ao (Chin-ssŭ-ts'ao) | 金髮草(金絲草) | **Pogonatherum paniceum** | GOLDEN-HAIR GRASS | Herba Pogonatheri |
| 0175 Chin- fu-hua | 金茯花 | See Hsüan-fu-hua | — | — |
| 0176 Chin-hsien-tiao-wu-kuei | 金綫吊烏龜 | **Stephania cepharantha** | *STEPHANIA | Radix Stephaniae Cephanathae |
| 0177 Chin-hsien-ts'ao | 金綫草 | **Antenoron neofiliforme** | JUMPSEED | Herba Antenoronis |

15

| Transliteration | Chinese | Botanical Name | English | Pharmaceutical |
|---|---|---|---|---|
| 0178 Chin-hua-ts'ao (K'ung-ch'ueh-wei) | 金花草(孔雀尾) | **Stenoloma chusana** | LACE FERN | Herba Stenolomatis |
| 0179 Chin-kang-t'êng | 金剛藤 | **Smilax china** | CHINESE GREENBRIER | Rhizoma Smilacis |
| 0180 Chin-kuo-lan (Chin-ku-lan, Chin-ku-yüan) | 金果欖(金果蘭,金古欖,金古杭) | **Tinospora capillipes** | *TINOSPORA | Radix Tinosporae |
| 0181 Chin-lien-hua | 金蓮花 | **Trollius chinensis** | *TROLLIUS | Flos Trollii |
| 0182 Chin-mao-kou-chi | 金毛狗脊 | **Cibotium barometz** | LAMB OF TARTARY | Rhizoma Cibotii |
| 0183 Chin-niu (Niu-ts'ao, Chin-niu-ts'ao) | 金牛(牛草,金牛草) | **Polygala telephioides** | *LESSER MILKWORT | Herba Polygalae Telephioidis |
| 0184 Chin-niu-k'ou (Shui-ch'ieh) | 金鈕扣(水茄) | **Solanum torvum** | WILD TOMATO | Radix Solani Torvi |
| 0185 Chin-po | 金薄 | — | Gold-leaf | — |
| 0186 Chin-pu-huan (Ta-chin) | 金不換(大金) | **Stephania sinica** | CHINESE STEPHANIA | Radix Stephaniae Sinicae |
| 0187 Chin-shih-hu (Chin-hu) | 金石斛(金斛) | **Dendrobium linawianum** | *GOLDEN DENDROBIUM | Herba Dendrobii Linawiani |
| 0188 Chin-suo-shih | 金鎖匙 | **Cocculus sarmentosus** | SNAIL SEED | Radix Cocculi Sarmentosi |
| 0189 Chin-ti-lo (Ti-lo) | 錦地蘿(錦地羅,地蘿) | **Drosera burmannii** | SUNDEW | Herba Droserae Burmannii |
| 0190 Chin-yin-hua (Mi-yin-hua, Shan-yin-hua, Yin-hua, Shuang-hua) | 金銀花(密銀花,山銀花,銀花,雙花) | **Lonicera japonica** | HONEYSUCKLE | Flos Lonicerae |

| Transliteration | Chinese | Botanical Name | English | Pharmaceutical |
|---|---|---|---|---|
| 0191 Chin-yin-hua-t'êng (Chin-yin-t'êng, Chin-yin-hua-yeh, Chin-yin-ts'ao) | 金銀花藤(金銀藤,金銀花葉,金銀草) | **Lonicera japonica** | HONEYSUCKLE | Ramus vel Folium Lonicerae |
| 0192 Chin-ying-jou (Chin-ying-tzǔ) | 金櫻肉(金櫻子) | **Rosa laevigata** | CHEROKEE ROSE (fruit) | Fructus Rosae Laevigatae |
| 0193 Chin-ying-kao | 金櫻羔(金櫻膏) | **Rosa laevigata** | Extract of Cherokee Rose | Praeparatus Rosae Laevigatae |
| 0194 Chin-ying-kên (Ying-kên, Chin-ying-t'ou) | 金櫻根(櫻根,金櫻頭) | **Rosa laevigata** | Root of Cherokee Rose | Radix Rosae Laevigatae |
| 0195 Chin-ying-tzǔ | 金櫻子 | **Rosa laevigata** | Fruit of Cherokee Rose | Fructus Rosae Laevigatae |
| 0196 Ch'in-chiao (Ch'in-chiao-p'i) | 秦艽(秦艽皮) | **Gentiana macrophylla** or **G. dahurica** | *LARGE-LEAVED GENTIAN | Herba Gentiana Macrophyllae |
| 0197 Ch'in-p'i | 秦皮 | **Fraxinus bungeana** or **F. rhynchophylla** | NORTHERN ASH (bark) | Cortex Fraxini |
| 0198 Ching-chiao | 京膠 | See O-chiao | — | — |
| 0199 Ching-chieh (Ching-chieh-sui, Ching-chieh-hua) | 荊芥(荊芥穗,荊芥花) | **Schizonepeta tenuifolia** See 0614A | *CHINGCHIEH | Herba Schizonepetae or Flos Schizonepetae |
| 0200 Ching-p'i (Tzǔ-ching-p'i) | 荊皮(紫荊皮) | **Kadsura peltigera** | *SHIELD-KADSURA (bark) | Cortex Kadsurae Peltigerae |
| 0201 Ching-san-lêng | 荊三稜 | **Scirpus yagara** | BULRUSH | Rhizoma Scirpi |
| 0202 Ching-shao | 京芍 | See Ch'ih-shao | — | — |

17

| | Transliteration | Chinese | Botanical Name | English | Pharmaceutical |
|---|---|---|---|---|---|
| 0203 | Ching-ta-chi (Lung-ya-ts'ao) | 京大戟(龍牙草) | **Euphorbia pekinensis** | PEKING SPURGE | Herba Euphorbiae Pekinensis |
| 0204 | Ching-t'ien-san-chi | 景天三七 | **Sedum aizoon** | ALPINE STONECROP | Herba Sedi Aizoon |
| 0205 | Ching-tzǔ (Man-ching-tzǔ) | 荊子(京子, 蔓荊子) | **Vitex trifolia** | *SEASHORE VITEX | Fructus Viticis |
| 0206 | Ch'ing-chiao | 清膠 | — | Gelatin | Gelatinum |
| 0207 | Ch'ing-chin-shih | 青金石 | — | Brown mica | Lapis Lazuli |
| 0208 | Ch'ing-chin-t'êng | 青筋藤 | **Ventilago leiocarpa** | *VENTILAGO | Radix Ventilaginis |
| 0209 | Ch'ing-chü | 青蒟 | **Piper betle** | BETEL PEPPER | Caulis Piperis Betlis |
| 0210 | Ch'ing-fan | 青礬 | — | Ferric ammonium sulphate | — |
| 0211 | Ch'ing-fên | 輕粉 | — | Calomel | Calomelas, or Hydrargyrum Chloratum |
| 0212 | Ch'ing-fêng-t'êng (Ch'ing-fêng-yeh) | 青風藤(青風葉) | **Sinomenium acutum** | *SINOMENIUM | Ramus Sinomenii |
| 0213 | Ch'ing-hao | 青蒿 | **Artemisia apiacea** | WORMWOOD | Herba Artemisiae Apiaceae |
| 0214 | Ch'ing-ho (Ho-yeh) | 青荷(荷葉) | **Nelumbo nucifera** | SACRED LOTUS | Folium Nelumbinis |
| 0215 | Ch'ing-hsiang-tzǔ (Ch'ing-hsiang, Ch'ing-hsien) | 青箱子(青箱, 青仙) | **Celosia argentea** | *CELOSIA | Semen Celosiae |
| 0216 | Ch'ing-hua | 青花 | — | Indigo mold | — |
| 0216A | Ch'ing-kuo | 青果 | See 0613 | | |
| 0217 | Ch'ing-lan | 青蘭 | **Dracocephalum ruyschiana** | DRAGON'S HEAD | Herba Dracocephali |

| | Transliteration | Chinese | Botanical Name | English | Pharmaceutical | Ch'ing |
|---|---|---|---|---|---|---|
| 0218 | Ch'ing-mêng-shih (Mêng-shih, Ming-shih) | 青礞石(礞石,明石) | See Mêng-shih | — | Lapis Chloritii | |
| 0219 | Ch'ing-mu-hsiang | 青木香 | **Aristolochia debilis** | BIRTHWORTH (root) | Radix Aristolochiae | |
| 0220 | Ch'ing-niang-tzŭ (Wan-ch'ing) | 青娘子(芫青) | — | Dried Beanbeetle | Cantharis | |
| 0221 | Ch'ing-p'i (Hsiao-ch'ing-p'i, Ching-p'i-tzŭ) | 青皮(小青皮,青皮子) | **Citrus sinensis** | Immature orange | Fructus Citri Sinensis Immaturis | |
| 0222 | Ch'ing-tai | 青黛 | See the following | Refuse of Indigo | Indigo Pulverata Levis | |
| −a | Liao-lan | 蓼藍 | **Polygonum tinctorium** | | | |
| −b | Ma-lan | 馬藍 | **Baphicacanthus cusia** | | | |
| −c | Mu-lan | 木藍 | **Indigofera tinctoria** | | | |
| −d | Sung-lan | 松藍 | Isatis tinctoria, I. indigotica | | | |
| 0223 | Ch'ing-t'êng | 青藤 | **Sinomenium acutum** | *SINOMENIUM | Ramus Sinomenii | |
| 0224 | Ch'ing-yeh-tan | 青葉膽 | **Swertia milensis** | *MILE SWERTIA | Herba Swertiae Mileensis | |
| 0225 | Ch'ing-yen (Jung-yen) | 青鹽(戎鹽) | — | Halite | Halitum (Sal Fossile) | |
| 0226 | Chiu-chieh-ch'a | 九節茶 | **Sarcandra glabra** | *SARCANDRA | Herba Sarcandrae | |
| 0227 | Chiu-chieh-ch'ang-p'u | 九節菖蒲 | **Anemone altaica** | ALTAI ANEMONE | Rhizoma Anemonis Altaicae | |
| 0228 | Chiu-hsiang-ch'ung | 九香虫(久香虫) | — | Dry Stinkbug | Aspongonpur or Coridius | |
| 0229 | Chiu-li-hsiang | 九里香 | **Murraya paniculata** | *MURRAYA | Ramus Murrayae | |

19

| | Transliteration | Chinese | Botanical Name | English | Pharmaceutical |
|---|---|---|---|---|---|
| 0230 | Chiu-li-ming (Ch'ien-li-kuang) | 九里明(千里光) | **Senecio scandens** | RAGWORT | Herba Senecionis |
| 0231 | Chiu-lung-kên | 九龍根 | **Bauhinia championii** | CHAMPION'S BAUHINIA | Radix Bauhiniae Championii |
| 0232 | Chiu-pi-ying (T'ieh-tung-ch'ing) | 救必應(鐵冬青) | **Ilex rotunda** | *IRON HOLLY | Cortex Ilicis Rotundae |
| 0233 | Chiu-ping-liang | 救兵粮 | **Pyracantha fortuneana** | FIRETHORN | Fructus Pyracanthae |
| 0234 | Chiu-ts'ai-tzŭ (Chiu-tzŭ) | 韭荣子(韭子) | **Allium tuberosum** | CHINESE LEEK | Fructus et Semen Allii Tuberosi |
| 0235 | Chiu-ts'êng-t'a (Hsiang-ts'ao, Lo-lê) | 九層塔(香草,羅勒) | **Ocimum basilicum** | SWEET BASIL | Herba Ocimi Basilici |
| 0236 | Ch'iu-shih | 秋石 | — | Urine deposit preparation | Depositum Urinae Praeparatum |
| 0237 | Ch'iu-yin (Ti-lung) | 蚯蚓(地龍) | — | Dry earthworm | Lumbricus |
| 0238 | Ch'iung-chih | 琼脂 | **Gelidium amansii** | Agar | Agar |
| 0239 | Ch'ou-mo-li | 臭茉莉 | **Clerodendrum fragrans** | FRAGRANT GLORYBOWER | Radix Clerodendri Fragrantis |
| 0240 | Ch'ou-niu (Êrh-ch'ou) | 丑牛(二丑) | **Ipomoea hederacea I. nil** | MORNING GLORY | Semen Ipomoeae |
| 0241 | Chu-êrh-shên (Niu-tzŭ-ch'i) | 珠兒參(扭子七) | **Panax major** | PEARL GINSENG | Rhizoma Panacis Majoris |
| 0242 | Chu-hsia | 菱夏 | **Pinellia ternata** or **P. pedatisecta** | PINELLIA (cooked tubers) | Cormus Pinelliae |
| 0243 | Chu-huang | 竹黃 | **Shiraia bambusicola** | Fungus infested bamboo | Sclerotia Shiraiae |

| Transliteration | Chinese | Botanical Name | English | Pharmaceutical |
|---|---|---|---|---|
| 0244 Chu-huang (T'ien-chu-huang) | 竺黄(竺箕，天竹黄) | **Bambusa textilis, Phyllostachys nigra, P. reticulata** | Tabasheer (siliceous secretion) | Concretio Silicea Bambusae |
| 0245 Chu-ju (Lu-chu-ju) | 竹茹(竹茹，綠竹茹) | **Phyllostachys nigra** | Bamboo shavings | Caulis Bambusae in Taeniis |
| 0246 Chu-li | 竹瀝 | **Phyllostachys nigra** | Bamboo juice | Succus Bambusae |
| 0247 Chu-ling | 豬苓(豬苓) | **Polyporus umbellatus** | *CHULING | Sclerotium Polypori |
| 0248 Chu-lung-ts'ao | 豬龍草 | **Nepenthes mirabilis** | PITCHER PLANT | Herba Nepenthitis |
| 0249 Chu-ma-kên | 苧麻根 | **Boehmeria nivea** | RAMIE (root) | Radix Boehmeriae |
| 0250 Chu-mao-ts'ai (Tz'ŭ-p'êng) | 豬毛菜(刺蓬) | **Salsola pestifera S. collina** | SALSOLA | Herba Salsolae |
| 0251 Chu-mu | 豬母 | **Anemarrhena asphodeloides** | ANEMARRHENA | Rhizoma Anemarrhenae |
| 0252 Chu-sha (Tan-sha, Ch'ên-sha) | 硃砂(丹砂，辰砂) | — | Cinnabar, Vermilion | Cinnabaris, Mercuric Sulfide |
| 0253 Chu-shih-tou | 豬屎豆 | **Crotalaria mucronata** | RATTLEBOX | Semen Crotalariae |
| 0254 Chu-yü (Chu-yü-jou) | 茱萸(茱萸肉) | **Cornus officinalis** | Asiatic Cornelian Cherry | Mesocarpium Corni III30.1998 officinalis |
| 0255 Ch'u-ch'un-chü | 除蟲菊 | **Chrysanthemum cinerariaefolium** | DALMATIAN PYRETHRUM | Flos Pyrethri |
| 0256 Ch'u-shih-tzŭ (Ch'u-tzŭ) | 楮實子(楮子) | **Broussonetia papyrifera** | PAPER MULBERRY | Fructus Broussonetiae |
| 0257 Chü-hêh | 橘核 | **Citrus sinensis** or **C. nobilis** | Orange seed, or Tangerine seed | Semen Citri |

| Transliteration | Chinese | Botanical Name | English | Pharmaceutical |
|---|---|---|---|---|
| 0259 Chü-hua | 菊花 | **Chrysanthemum morifolium** | CHRYSANTHEMUM | Flos Chrysanthemi Morifolii |
| Hang-chü-hua | 杭菊花 | ,, ,, | Hangchow ,, | ,, ,, ,, |
| Huang-chü-hua | 黃菊花 | ,, ,, | Yellow flower ,, | ,, ,, ,, |
| Kan-chü-hua | 甘菊花 | ,, ,, | Canton ,, | ,, ,, ,, |
| Pai-chü-hua | 白菊花 | ,, ,, | White flower ,, | ,, ,, ,, |
| 0260 Chü-hung (Chieh-hung) | 橘紅(桔紅) | **Citrus erythrocarpa** | RED TANGERINE (peel) | Pericarpium Citri Erythrocarpae |
| 0260A Chü-jo | 蒟蒻 | **Amorphophallus rivieri** | Devil's Tongue | Tuber Amorphophalli |
| 0261 Chü-kan (Chü-tzŭ-kan) | 橘甘(橘子乾) | **Citrus sinensis** | ORANGE (dried) | Fructus Citri Siccus |
| 0262 Chü-lo (Chieh-lo, Chü-pai,Chieh-pai) | 橘絡(桔絡,橘白,桔白) | **Citrus reticulata** | MANDARIN ORANGE (vascular bundles) | Fasciculus Vascularis Pericarpii Citri |
| 0263 Chü-p'i (Chieh-p'i) | 橘皮(桔皮) | **Citrus reticulata** | MANDARIN ORANGE (peel) | Pericarpium Aurantii |
| 0264 Chü-shên-tzŭ | 巨腎子 | **Dipsacus chinensis** | CHINESE TEASEL | Fructus Dipsaci |
| 0265 Chü-yeh (Chieh-yeh) | 橘葉(桔葉) | **Citrus sinensis** | ORANGE (leaves) | Folium Aurantii |
| 0266 Ch'ü-mai (Shih-Chu) | 瞿麥(石竹) | **Dianthus superbus** or **D. chinensis** | PINK | Herba Dianthi |
| 0267 Chuan-shên | 拳參 | **Polygonum bistorta** | ALPHINE KNOTWEED | Caudex Polygoni |
| 0268 Ch'uan-ch'i | 川芪 | See Huang-ch'i | — | — |
| 0269 Ch'uan-ch'iang (Ch'iang-huo) | 川羌(羌活) | See Ch'iang-huo | — | — |

| Transliteration | Chinese | Botanical Name | English | Pharmaceutical |
|---|---|---|---|---|
| 0270 Ch'uan-chiao | 川椒 | **Zanthoxylum simulans** | SZECHUAN PEPPER | Fructus Zanthoxyli |
| 0271 Ch'uan-chin-p'i | 川槿皮 | **Hibiscus syriacus** | ROSE-OF-SHARON | Cortex Hibisci |
| 0272 Ch'uan-chin-tzŭ | 川金子 | See Ch'ien-chin-tzŭ | — | — |
| 0273 Ch'uan-chü-chiu-pien (Chia-ying-chao) | 串珠酒餅(假鷹爪) | **Desmos cochinchinensis** | *DESMOS | Radix et Ramus Desmoris |
| 0274 Ch'uan-fu | 川附 | See Fu-tzŭ | — | — |
| 0275 Ch'uan-hou-p'o (Ch'uan-hou-p'u, Ch'uan-p'o) | 川厚朴(川厚樸,川朴) | **Magnolia officinalis** | MAGNOLIA (bark) | Cortex Magnoliae |
| 0276 Ch'uan-hsi (Ch'uan-niu-hsi) | 川膝(川牛膝) | **Cyathula officinalis** | *CYATHULA | Radix Cyathulae |
| 0277 Ch'uan-hsieh | 川瀉 | See Tsê-hsieh | — | — |
| 0278 Ch'uan-hsin-lien (K'u-tan-ts'ao) | 穿心蓮(苦膽草) | **Andrographis paniculata** | *ANDROGRAPHIS | Herba Andrographis |
| 0279 Ch'uan-hsiung (Ch'uan-chung, Hsi-hsiung) | 川芎(川藭,西芎) | **Ligusticum wallichii** | SZECHUAN LOVAGE | Rhizoma Ligustici |
| 0280 Ch'uan-hsü-tuan | 川續斷 | **Dipsacus asper** or **D. chinensis** | SZECHUAN TEASEL | Radix Dipsaci |
| 0281 Ch'uan-huo | 川活 | See Tu-huo | — | — |
| 0282 Ch'uan-kuei | 川桂 | **Cinnamomum wilsonii** | SZECHUAN CASSIA | Cortex Cinnamomi Wilsonii |
| 0283 Ch'uan-lien | 川連 | See Huang-lien | — | — |

23

| | Transliteration | Chinese | Botanical Name | English | Pharmaceutical |
|---|---|---|---|---|---|
| 0284 | Ch'uan-lien-tzǔ | 川練子(川楝子) | **Melia toosendan** | SZECHUAN PAGODA TREE | Fructus Toosendan |
| 0285 | Ch'uan-mu-hsiang | 川木香 | **Dolomiaea souliei** | *VLADIMIRIA | Radix Dolomiaeae |
| 0286 | Ch'uan-niu-hsi (Ch'uan-hsi) | 川牛膝(川膝) | **Cyathula officinalis** | CYATHULA | Radix Cyathulae |
| 0287 | Ch'uan-pa | 川巴(川芭) | See Pa-tou | — | — |
| 0288 | Ch'uan-pei (Pei-mu, Ch'uan-pei-mu) | 川貝(貝母,川貝母) | **Fritillaria cirrhosa** | SZECHUAN FRITILLARY | Bulbus Fritillariae Cirrhosae |
| 0289 | Ch'uan-p'o-hua (Hou-p'o-hua) | 川朴花(厚朴花) | **Magnolia officinalis** | MAGNOLIA (flower) | Flos Magnoliae Officinalis |
| 0290 | Ch'uan-p'o-shih (P'o-shih) | 穿破石(破石) | **Cudrania cochinchinensis** | *CUDRANIA (root) | Radix Cudraniae Cochinchinensis |
| 0291 | Ch'uan-shan-chia-p'ien (Shan-chia, Shan-chia-p'ien, Chia-p'ien) | 穿山甲片(山甲,山甲片,甲片) | — | Scales of Pangolin | Squama Manitis |
| 0292 | Ch'uan-tang | 川黨 | **Codonopsis tangshen** | SZECHUAN TANGSHEN | Radix Codonopsis Tangshen |
| 0293 | Ch'uan-tuan | 川斷 | **Dipsacus chinensis** or **D. asper** | SZECHUAN TEASEL | Radix Dipsaci |
| 0294 | Ch'uan-wu (Kuang-wu, Wu-t'ou, Hei-fu-tzǔ, T'ien-hsiung) | 川烏(光烏,烏頭,黑附子,天雄) | **Aconitum chinense** **A. carmichaelii** | *CHINESE ACONITE *SZECHUAN ACONITE | Radix Aconiti |
| 0295 | Chüan-pai | 卷柏 | **Selaginella tamariscina** | SPIKEMOSS | Herba Selaginellae |

| Transliteration | Chinese | Botanical Name | English | Pharmaceutical |
|---|---|---|---|---|
| 0296 Ch'üan-ch'ung (Ch'üan-hsieh) | 全虫(全蝎) | — | Scorpion | Buthus |
| 0297 Chüeh-ming (Chüeh-ming-tzǔ) | 决明(决明子) | **Cassia tora** | FOETID CASSIA | Semen Cassiae Torae |
| 0297A Chui-fêng-ch'i | 追風七 | **Geum aleppicum** | ALEPPO AVENS | Herba Gei |
| 0298 Ch'ui-p'êng-ts'ao | 垂盆草 | **Sedum sarmentosum** | *HANGING STONECROP | Herba Sedi Sarmentosi |
| 0299 Ch'ui-ssǔ-liu (Hsi-ho-liu) | 垂絲柳(西河柳) | **Tamarix chinensis** | TAMARISK | Ramus Tamaricis |
| 0300 Chün-kuei | 菌桂 | **Cinnamomum cassia** | CASSIA, CHINESE CINNAMON | Cortex Cinnamomi Cassiae |
| 0301 Ch'un-chin-p'i (Fu-sang-p'i) | 春槿皮(扶桑皮) | **Hibiscus rosa-sinensis** | CHINESE HIBISCUS (bark) | Cortex Hibisci Rosa-sinensis |
| 0302 Ch'un-hua (Hsin-i) | 春花(辛夷) | **Magnolia liliflora** | *RED MAGNOLIA | Flos Magnoliae Liliflorae |
| 0303 Ch'un-kên (Ch'un-kên-p'i, Ch'ung-kên-pai-p'i) | 椿根(椿根皮,椿根白皮) | **Ailanthus altissima** | TREE-OF-HEAVEN | Cortex Ailanthi |
| 0304 Ch'un-sha-hua (Sha-jên-hua) | 春砂花(砂仁花) | **Amomum villosum** | *Flower of Amomum | Flos Amomi Villosi |
| Ch'un-sha-jên (Yang-chun-sha) | 春砂仁(陽春砂) | ,, ,, | GRAIN-OF-PARADISE | Fructus Amomi Villosi |
| Ch'un-sha-k'o | 春砂殻 | ,, ,, | Husks of Amomum | Pericarpium Amomi Villosi |
| 0305 Chung-ju (Chung-ju-shih) | 鐘乳(鐘乳石) | — | Stalactite | Stalactitum |
| 0306 Chung-shu (Chung-pai-shu) | 種朮(種白朮) | See Pai-shu | — | — |

| Transliteration | Chinese | Botanical Name | English | Pharmaceutical | Ch'ung |
|---|---|---|---|---|---|
| 0307 Ch'ung-kuei-tzŭ (Ch'ung-wei-tzŭ, Ch'ung-wei, I-mu-ts'ao, Ch'ung-yü-tzŭ) | 沖貴子(沖桂子,茺蔚子,沖蔚,益母草,沖玉子) | **Leonurus artemisia L. tataricus** | CHINESE MOTHER-WORT | Semen Leonuri Artemisae | |
| 0308 Ch'ung-sha | 虫沙 | — | Cockroach excrete | Faeces Corydii | |
| 0309 Ch'ung-sha (Chia-chu-sha) | 沖砂(假硃砂) | — | Imitation cinnabar | Cinnabaris Artificialis | |
| 0310 Ch'ung-su | 虫酥 | Same as Ch'an-su | — | — | |
| 0311 Ch'ung-ts'ao (Hsia-ts'ao-tung-ch'ung, Tung-ch'ung-hsia-ts'ao) | 虫草(夏草冬虫,冬虫夏草) | **Cordyceps sinensis** | *CHUNTSAO, WINTER-WORM SUMMER-HERB | Sclerotium Cordycipitis Sinensis | |
| 0312 Ch'ung-wei-tzŭ (Ch'ung-wei, I-mu-ts'ao) | 茺蔚子(茺蔚,益母草) | **Leonurus artemisia L. tataricus** | CHINESE MOTHER-WORT | Fructus et Semen Leonuri | |
| 0313 Êrh-ch'a | 兒茶 | **Acacia catechu A. suma** | BLACK CUTCH, CATECHU | Catechu | |
| 0314 Êrh-ch'a-kao-t'êng | 兒茶鈎藤 | **Uncaria gambir** | GAMBIER, WHITE CUTCH | Ramus Uncariae | |
| 0315 Êrh-ch'ou (Hei-ch'ou, Pai-ch'ou, Ch'ou-niu, Hei-pai-ch'ou) | 二丑(黑丑,白丑,丑牛,黑白丑) | **Ipomoea hederacea I. nil** | *BLACK- and WHITE-seeded MORNING-GLORIES | Semen Ipomoeae | |
| 0316 Êrh-ts'ao (Hei-hsin-ts'ao) | 耳草(黑心草) | **Hedyotis auricularia (Oldenlandia auricularia)** | *AURICULAR HEDYOTIS | Herba Hedyotis Auriculatae | |

26

| Transliteration | Chinese | Botanical Name | English | Pharmaceutical |
|---|---|---|---|---|
| 0317 Fa-ts'ai | 髮荣 | **Nostoc flagelliforme** | *Nostoc | Herba Nostochis |
| 0318 Fan-hsieh-yeh | 番瀉葉 | **Cassia angustifolia**<br>**C. acutifolia** | Senna | Folium Sennae |
| 0319 Fan-hung-hua | 番紅花 | **Crocus sativus** | Saffron | Stigma et Stylus Croci |
| 0320 Fan-mu-kua | 番木瓜 | **Carica papaya** | Papaya | Fructus Caricae |
| 0321 Fan-mu-pieh<br>(Ma-chien-tzǔ) | 番木鼈(馬錢子) | **Strychnos nux-vomica** | Nux Vomica | Semen Strychnotis |
| 0322 Fan-pai-ts'ao | 翻白草 | **Potentilla discolor** | Silverweed | Radix Potentillae |
| 0323 Fan-shih-liu | 番石榴 | **Psidium guajava** | Guava | Folium Psidii |
| 0324 Fang-chi (Fang-ch'i) | 防己(防杞,方杞) | **Aristolochia** spp.<br>**Stephania tetrandra** | *Fangchi | See below |
| −a  Han-chung-fang-chi (Ch'ing-mu-hsiang, T'u-fang-chi) | 漢中防己(青木香,土防己) | **Aristolochia heterophylla** | Northern Fangchi | Radix Aristolochiae Heterophyllae |
| −b  Kuang-fang-chi (Mu-fang-chi, Shui-fang-chi) | 廣防己(木防己,水防己) | **Aristolochia westlandii**<br>**A. fangchi** | Southern Fangchi | Radix Aristolochiae Westlandii et Fangchi |
| −c  Fên-fang-chi | 粉防己 | **Stephania tetrandra** | Mealy Fangchi | Radix Stephaniae Tetrandrae |
| 0325 Fang-fêng (Fêng-jou, Fang-fêng-jou) | 防風(風肉,防風肉) | **Ledebouriella seseloides**<br>**(Saposhnikovia divaricata)** | *Fangfeng | Herba Ledebouriellae |

| Transliteration | Chinese | Botanical Name | English | Pharmaceutical |
|---|---|---|---|---|
| −a Ch'uan-fang-fêng | 川防風 | **Ligusticum brachylobum** | SZECHUAN FANGFENG | Radix Ligustici Brachylobi |
| 0326 Fang-fêng-ts'ao | 防風草 | **Anisomeles indica** | *ANISOMELES | Herba Anisomeletis |
| 0327 Fang-tang (Fang-tang-shên, Fang-fêng-tang-shên) | 防黨(防黨參, 防風黨參) | Same as Tang-shên (see 1484) | *TANGSHEN | — |
| 0328 Fang-t'ung (Fang-t'ung-ts'ao) | 方通(方通草) | See T'ung-ts'ao | T'ung-ts'ao of superior quality | — |
| 0329 Fei-lung-chang-hsüeh | 飛龍掌血 | **Toddalia asiatica** | LOPEZ ROOT | Cortex Toddaliae |
| 0330 Fei-shih (Fei-tzǔ, Hsiang-fei-tzǔ) | 榧實(榧子, 香榧子) | **Torreya grandis** | *TORREYA NUT | Semen Torreyae |
| 0331 Fei-tsao-tzǔ (Hsiao-tsao) | 肥皂子(小皂) | **Gymnocladus chinensis** | *CHINESE GYMNOCLADUS | Semen Gymnocladi |
| 0332 Fei-yang-ts'ao | 飛陽草 | **Euphorbia pilulifera** | HAIRY SPURGE | Herba Euphorbiae Piluliferae |
| 0333 Fên-chi-ma | 糞箕麻 | **Stephania longa** | LONG-LEAVED STEPHANIA | Herba et Radix Stephaniae longae |
| 0334 Fên-ko (Fên-ko-kan, Fên ko-t'êng) | 粉葛(粉葛乾, 粉葛藤) | **Pueraria thomsonii** | *SWEET PUERARIA | Radix Puerariae Thomsonii |
| 0335 Fêng-ch'ieh-hua (Yang-chin-hua) | 楓茄花(洋金花) | **Datura metel** | *UPRIGHT DATURA | Flos Daturae Metelis |
| 0336 Fêng-fang (Lu-fêng-fang) | 蜂房(露蜂房) | — | HORNET NEST | Nidus Vespae |

| | Transliteration | Chinese | Botanical Name | English | Pharmaceutical |
|---|---|---|---|---|---|
| 0337 | Fêng-ho-kuei (T'ien-o-fêng) | 楓荷桂(天鵝楓) | **Sassafras tsumu (Pseudosassafras laxiflora)** | CHINESE SASSAFRAS | Radix, Ramus et Folium Sassafratis |
| 0338 | Fêng-hsiang-chi-shêng | 楓香寄生 | **Viscum articulatum** | *CHINESE MISTLETOE | Caulis Visci Articulati |
| 0339 | Fêng-hsiang-chih | 楓香脂 | **Liquidambar formosana** | *CHINESE SWEET GUM | Resina Liquidambaris |
| 0340 | Fêng-hsiang-shu | 風箱樹 | **Cephalanthus occidentalis** | BUTTONBUSH | Radix et Flos Cephalanthi |
| 0341 | Fêng-hsien-hua | 鳳仙花 | **Impatiens balsamina** | GARDEN BALSAM, TOUCH-ME-NOT | Flos Impatientis |
| 0342 | Fêng-huang-ch'ang | 鳳凰腸 | **Caesalpina pulcherrima** | PEACOCK FLOWER | Radix Caesalpinae Pulcherrimae |
| 0343 | Fêng-huang-i (Fêng-huang-t'ai, Chi-tan-k'o, Fêng-t'i) | 鳳凰衣(鳳凰胎,鷄蛋殼,鳳退) | — | Inner shell of fowls' egg | Membrana Follicularis Ovi |
| 0344 | Fêng-jou | 風肉 | See Fang-fêng | — | — |
| 0345 | Fêng-la (Huang-la) | 蜂蜡(黃蠟) | — | Beeswax | Cera Flava |
| 0346 | Fêng-lung-yen | 鳳龍眼 | **Ailanthus altissima** | AILANTHUS (fruit) | Fructus Ailanthi |
| 0347 | Fêng-mao (Ta-fêng-mao, Fêng-mao-chü) | 風茅(大風茅,風茅菊) | **Saussurea japonica** | JAPANESE SAUSSUREA | Herba Saussureae |
| 0348 | Fêng-mi | 蜂蜜 | — | Honey | Mel |
| 0349 | Fêng-sha-t'êng | 風沙藤 | **Kadsura longipedunculata** | *LONG-STALKED KADSURA | Radix Kadsurae |

| | Transliteration | Chinese | Botanical Name | English | Pharmaceutical |
|---|---|---|---|---|---|
| 0350 | Fêng-shih | 楓實 | **Liquidambar formosana** | CHINESE SWEET GUM | Fructus Liquidambaris |
| 0351 | Fêng-shu-yeh | 楓樹葉 | **Liquidambar formosana** | CHINESE SWEET GUM | Folium Liquidambaris |
| 0352 | Fêng-t'êng (Hai-fêng-t'êng) | 風藤(海風藤) | **Ficus martinii,** or **Piper kadsura** | CREEPING FIG, FENGTENG | Ramus Fici Martinii Caulis Piperis Kadsurae |
| 0353 | Fêng-tou-ts'ai (Shê-t'ou-ts'ao) | 蜂斗荣(蛇頭草) | **Petasites japonicus** | COLTSFOOT | Rhizoma Petasitis |
| 0354 | Fêng-wei-chiao-yeh (Fêng-wei-sung, Su-t'ieh) | 鳳尾蕉葉(鳳尾松,蘇鉄) | **Cycas revoluta** | CYCAS, SAGE PALM | Folium Cycatis |
| 0355 | Fêng-wei-ts'ao (Chin-hsing-ts'ao) | 鳳尾草(金星草) | **Pteris multifida** | *PHOENIX-TAIL FERN | Herba Pteridis |
| 0356 | Fêng-wo-ts'ao | 蜂窩草 | **Leucas zeylanica** | *LEUCAS | Herba Leucasis |
| 0357 | Fêng-yang-yeh | 楓楊葉 | **Pterocarya stenoptera** | WING-NUT | Ramus et Folia Pterocaryae |
| 0358 | Fêng-yen-ts'ao (Fêng-yen-yeh) | 鳳眼草(鳳眼葉) | **Ailanthus altissima** | AILANTHUS (fruit) | Fructus Ailanthi |
| 0359 | Fo-chia-ts'ao | 佛甲草 | **Sedum lineare** | LINEAR STONECROP | Herba Sedi Linearis |
| 0360 | Fo-êrh-ts'ao (Shu-chü-ts'ao) | 佛耳草(鼠麴草) | **Gnaphalium affine** | CUDWEED | Herba Gnaphalii |
| 0361 | Fo-sang-hua (Fu-sang-hua, Ch'üan-hua) | 佛桑花(扶桑花,欓花) | **Hibiscus rosa-sinensis** | CHINESE HIBISCUS | Flos Hibisci Rosa-sinensis |
| 0362 | Fo-shou (Fo-shou-kan) | 佛手(佛手柑) | **Citrus medica** var. **sarcodactylis** | FINGER CITRON | Fructus Citri Sarcodactylis |

30

| Transliteration | Chinese | Botanical Name | English | Pharmaceutical |
|---|---|---|---|---|
| Fo-shou-hua | 佛手花 | | ,,  ,,  (flower) | Flos Citri Sarcodactylis |
| Fo-shou-kan | 佛手乾 | | ,,  ,,  (dried fruit) | Fructus Citri Sarcodactylis Exsiccati |
| Fo-shou-p'ien | 佛手片 | | ,,  ,,  (sliced) | |
| 0363 Fou-hai-shih (Fou-shih) | 浮海石(浮石) | — | Pumice | Pumex, Os Madreporariae |
| 0364 Fou-mai (Fou-hsiao-mai, Hsiao-mai) | 浮麥(浮小麥, 小麥) | **Triticum aestivum** | WHEAT (shriveled) | Semen Marcidum Tritici |
| 0365 Fou-p'ing | 浮萍 | **Lemna minor** | DUCKWEED | Herba Lemnae |
| 0366 Fou-p'ing-ts'ao (Ta-p'ing-yeh, Tzŭ-p'ing) | 浮萍草(大萍葉, 紫萍) | **Spirodela polyrhiza** | *SPIRODELA | Herba Spirodelae |
| 0367 Fu-hua | 覆花(福花, 茯花) | Same as Hsüan-fu-hua | — | — |
| 0368 Fu-jung-hua (Mu-fu-yung) | 芙蓉花(木芙蓉) | **Hibiscus mutabilis** | COTTON ROSE (flower) | Flos Hibisci Mutabilis |
| 0369 Fu-jung-yeh | 芙蓉葉 | ,,  ,, | COTTON ROSE (leaf) | Folium Hibisci Mutabilis |
| 0370 Fu-ling (Pai-fu-ling, Yün-fu-ling) | 茯苓(白茯苓, 雲茯苓) | **Poria cocos** | CHINA-ROOT | Sclerotium Poriae |
| 0371 Fu-lung-kan (Tsao-hsin-t'ou) | 伏龍肝(灶心土) | — | Furnace soil | Terra Flava Usta |
| 0372 Fu-p'ên-tzŭ (Fu-p'ên) | 覆盆子(覆盆) | **Rubus parvifolius** **R. palmatus** | CHINESE RASPBERRY | Fructus Rubi |
| 0373 Fu-shên | 茯神 | **Poria cocos** | CHINA-ROOT (host attached) | *Fushen |

| Transliteration | Chinese | Botanical Name | English | Pharmaceutical | Fu |
|---|---|---|---|---|---|
| 0374 Fu-shih | 伏虱 | **Carpesium abrotanoides** | *CRANE LICE | Fructus Carpesii | |
| 0375 Fu-shou-ts'ao | 福壽草 | **Adonis amurensis** | *ADONIS | Herba Adonidis | |
| 0376 Fu-t'ai | 腹胎 | **Areca catechu** | BETEL (fiber) | Pericarpium Arecae | |
| 0377 Fu-tzǔ (Ch'uan-fu, Fu-p'ien) | 附子(川附,附片) | **Aconitum carmichaelii** | SZECHUAN ACONITE | Radix Aconiti Carmichaelii | |
| 0378 Ha-ma (Ha-shih-ma) | 哈蟆(哈士蟆) | — | Dry frog | Rana | |
| 0379 Ha-ma-chi | 哈蟆七 | **Lobaria pulmonaria** var. **meridionalis** | LOBARIA | Herba Lobariae | |
| 0380 Hai-chin-sha (Chin-sha) | 海金砂(海金沙,金砂) | **Lygodium japonicum** | CLIMBING FERN | Herba et Spora Lygodii | |
| 0381 Hai-chou-ch'ang-shan | 海州常山 | **Clerodendrum trichotomum** | *HAIRY CLERODENDRUM | Folium Clerodendri | |
| 0382 Hai-fêng-t'êng (Fêng-t'êng) | 海楓藤(楓藤) | **Piper kadsura** **Ficus maritinii, Usnea diffracta, Akebia quinata** | *HAIFENGTENG | Caulis Piperis Kadsurae | |
| 0383 Hai-kou-shên (Hai-kou-p'ien) | 海狗腎(海狗鞭) | — | Testicles and penis of Seal | Testis et Penis Otariae | |
| 0384 Hai-lung | 海龍 | — | Pipe-fish | Syngnathus | |
| 0385 Hai-ma | 海馬 | — | Sea Horse | Hippocampus | |
| 0386 Hai-nan-chü | 海南菊 | **Piper hainanense** | HAINAN PEPPER | Herba Piperis Hainanense | |
| 0387 Hai-piao (Wu-tsei-ku, Hai-p'iao-shao, Tan-ku, Mo-yü-ku) | 海標(烏賊骨,海螵蛸, 淡骨,墨魚骨) | — | Cuttle-fish bone | Os Sepiae | |

| Transliteration | Chinese | Botanical Name | English | Pharmaceutical | Hai |
|---|---|---|---|---|---|
| 0388 Hai-tai | 海帶 | **Laminaria japonica** | KELP | Laminaria | |
| 0389 Hai-tan | 海膽 | — | Sea urchin | Corona Echinoideae | |
| 0389A Hai-ti-yeh | 海底椰 | **Lodoicea maldivica** | COCO-DE-MER | Endospermum Lodoiceae | |
| 0390 Hai-tsao | 海藻 | **Sargassium fusiforme S. pallidum** | Seaweed | Herba Sargassii | |
| 0391 Hai-ts'ung | 海葱 | **Urginea maritima** | *Sea-onion | Herba Urgineae | |
| 0392 Hai-t'ung-p'i (T'ung-p'i) | 海桐皮(桐皮) | **Kalopanax septemlobus** or **Erythrina indica** | *HAITUNGPI | Cortex Kalopanacis or Cortex Erythrinae | |
| 0393 Hai-yü (Kuang-tung-lang-tou, Lao-hu-yü, Tien-ho-yü) | 海芋(廣東狼毒, 老虎芋, 天河芋) | **Alocasia macrorhiza (A. odora)** | ALOCASIA | Caudex Alocasiae Macrorhizae | |
| 0394 Han-fang-chi (Shan-tou-kên) | 漢防己(山豆根) | **Menispermum dauricum** or **Aristolochia heterophylla** | *HANFANGCHI | Hanfangchi | |
| 0395 Han-hsin-ts'ao | 韓信草 | **Scutellaria indica** | SKULLCAP | Herba Scutellariae Indicae | |
| 0396 Han-hsiu-ts'ao | 含羞草 | **Mimosa pudica** | SENSITIVE PLANT | Herba Mimosae | |
| 0397 Han-lien-mu (Hsi-shu) | 旱蓮木(喜樹) | **Camptotheca acuminata** | *CAMPTOTHECA | Fructus Camptothecae | |
| 0398 Han-lien-ts'ao (Mai-t'ou-ts'ao) | 旱蓮草(黑頭草) See 0886 | **Eclipta prostrata** | ECLIPTA | Herba Ecliptae | |
| 0399 Han-shui-shih (Shui-shih) | 寒水石(水石) | — | Gypsum and Calcite | Gypsum Rubrum et Calcitum | |
| 0400 Hei-chih-ma (Chih-ma, Hu-ma, Chih-ma-k'o) | 黑脂麻(芝麻, 胡麻, 芝麻殼) | **Sesamum indicum** | SESAME (husk), BLACK SESAME | Pericarpium et Semen Sesami | |
| 0401 Hei-ch'ou | 黑丑 | See Êrh-ch'ou | — | — | |

| Transliteration | Chinese | Botanical Name | English | Pharmaceutical |
|---|---|---|---|---|
| 0402 Hei-fu-tzǔ | 黑附子 | **Aconitum chinense** | CHINESE ACONITE | Caudex Aconiti Chinensis |
| 0403 Hei-kou-chi | 黑狗脊 | **Blechnum orientale** | BLECHNUM | Rhizoma Blechni |
| 0404 Hei-ku-t'ou (Ta-fêng-t'êng, Ch'ing-fêng-t'êng, Hei-lung-ku) | 黑骨頭(達風藤,青風藤,黑龍骨) | **Periploca forrestii** | YUNNAN PERIPLOCA | Radix et Ramus Periplocae Forrestii |
| 0405 Hei-lao-hu (Chan-ti-fêng) | 黑老虎(鑽地風) | **Kadsura coccinea** | *SCARLET KADSURA | Radix Kadsurae Coccinae |
| 0406 Hei-mien-shên (Hei-mien-ch'ên) | 黑面神(黑面辰) | **Breynia fruticosa** | *BREYNIA | Radix et Ramus Breyniae |
| 0407 Hei-pai-ch'ou | 黑白丑 | See Êrh-ch'ou | — | |
| 0408 Hei-p'i-kên | 黑皮根 | **Polyalthia nemoralis** | *POLYALTHIA | Radix Polyalthiae |
| 0409 Hei-san-lêng | 黑三稜 | **Scirpus yagara** | *BLACK BULRUSH | Rhizoma Scirpi |
| 0410 Hei-tsao (Juan-tsao) | 黑棗(軟棗) | **Diospyros lotus** | WILD PERSIMMOM | Fructus Diospyroris Loti |
| 0411 Hêng-ching-hsi (Tê-ta-chiang-chun) | 橫經席(跌打將軍) | **Calophyllum membranaceum** | *CALOPHYLLUM | Radix et Folium Calophylli |
| 0412 Ho-ch'ê (Tzǔ-ho-ch'ê) | 河車(紫河車) | — | Human placenta | Placenta Hominis |
| 0413 Ho-hsiang (T'u-ho-hsiang) | 藿香(土藿香) | **Agastache rugosa** (see Huo-hsiang) | *AGASTACHE | Herba Agastachis |
| 0414 Ho-hsiang-yeh (Kuang-ho-hsiang) | 藿香葉(廣藿香) | **Pogostemon cablin** (see Huo-hsiang) | PATCHOULI | Herba Patchouli |

34

| Transliteration | Chinese | Botanical Name | English | Pharmaceutical |
|---|---|---|---|---|
| 0415 Ho-huan-hua | 合歡花 | **Albizzia julibrissin** | MIMOSA TREE (flower) | Flos et Cortex |
| Ho-huan-p'i | 合歡皮 | „ „ | „ „ (bark) | Albizziae |
| 0416 Ho-li-lê (Ho-tzǔ, Tsang-ch'ing-kuo) | 訶黎勒(訶子,藏青果) | **Terminalia chebula** | MYROBALANS | Fructus Chebulae |
| 0417 Ho-lien-hua (Lien-hua) | 河蓮花(蓮花) | **Nelumbo nucifera** | SACRED LOTUS | Flos Nelumbonis |
| 0418 Ho-shih (Huei-hao) | 鶴蝨(蛔蒿) | **Artemisia cina** **A. monogyna** (see Fu-shih) | WORMSEED | Santonin |
| 0419 Ho-shou-wu (Shou-wu, Ch'ao-wu) | 何首烏(首烏,潮烏) | **Polygonum multiflorum** | *CHINESE CORNBIND | Rhizoma Polygoni Multiflori |
| 0420 Ho-t'ao (Hêh-t'ao) | 合桃(核桃) | **Juglans regia** | WALNUT | Semen Juglandis Regiae |
| 0421 Ho-tzǔ (Ho-li-lê, Ko-tzǔ) | 訶子(訶黎勒,柯子) | **Terminalia chebula** | MYROBALANS | Fructus Chebulae |
| 0422 Ho-yeh (Lien-yeh) | 荷葉(蓮葉) | **Nelumbo nucifera** | LOTUS (leaves) | Folium Loti |
| 0423 Hou-k'o | 鱟殼 | — | King-crab shell | Limulus |
| 0424 Hou-p'o (Ch'uan-hou-p'o, Ch'uan-p'o) | 厚朴(川厚朴,川朴) | **Magnolia officinalis** | MAGNOLIA (bark) | Cortex Magnoliae Officinalis |
| 0425 Hou-p'o-hua (P'o-hua) | 厚朴花(朴花) | „ „ | „ (flower) | Flos Magnoliae Officinalis |
| 0426 Hou-p'o-kên (P'o-kên) | 厚朴根(朴根) | „ „ | „ (root) | Radix Magnoliae Officinalis |
| 0427 Hou-tsao | 猴棗 | — | Monkey Bezoar | Calculus Macacae |
| 0428 Hou-tzǔ-chieh | 猴子結 | — | Wens on monkey | — |

| Transliteration | Chinese | Botanical Name | English | Pharmaceutical |
|---|---|---|---|---|
| 0429 Hsi-chiao | 犀角 | — | Rhinoceros horn | Cornu Rhinocerotis |
| 0430 Hsi-hsien (Hsi-hsien-ts'ao, Nien-hu-ts'ao) | 豨薟(豨薟草,黏糊草) | **Siegesbeckia orientalis** | SIEGESBECKIA | Herba Siegesbeckiae |
| 0432 Hsi-hsin (Ma-hsin, Pei-hsin) | 細辛(馬辛,北辛) | **Asarum heterotropoides A. sieboldii** | *CHINESE WILD GINGER | Rhizoma Asari |
| 0433 Hsi-hsiung | 西芎 | **Ligusticum wallichii** | SHENSI LOVAGE | Radix Ligustici |
| 0434 Hsi-kua-shuang | 西瓜霜 | **Citrullus lanatus (C. vulgaris)** | WATERMELON (green, treated with tannin) | Mirabilitum Praeparatum Citrulli |
| 0435 Hsi-ming (Pai-chiang-ts'ao) | 菥蓂(敗醬草) | **Thlaspi arvense** | PENNY-CRESS | Herba Thlaspis |
| 0436 Hsi-pei-lang-tu | 西北狼毒 | **Stellera chamaejasme** | ARROW POISON | Radix Stellerae |
| 0437 Hsi-p'i (Pai-hsien-p'i) | 洗皮(白蘚皮) | **Dictamnus dasycarpus** | Chinese Dittany | Radix Dictamni |
| 0438 Hsi-shêng-t'êng | 錫生藤 | **Cissampelos pareira** | *CISSAMPELOS | Herba Cissampelos |
| 0439 Hsi-shu (Han-lien-mu) | 喜樹(旱蓮木) | **Camptotheca acuminata** | CAMPTOTHECA | Fructus Camptothecae |
| 0440 Hsi-shuo | 蟋蟀 | — | Crickets | Gryllodes |
| 0441 Hsi-tang | 西黨 | See Tang-shên | Tang-shên from Shensi | — |
| 0442 Hsi-tsang-hung-hua (Tsang-hung-hua, Fan-hung-hua, Hsi-hung-hua) | 西藏紅花(藏紅花,番紅花,西紅花) | **Crocus sativus** | SAFFRON (Introduced to China from India via Tibet) | Stigma Croci |
| 0443 Hsi-yang-shên (Hua-ch'i-shên) | 西洋參(花旗參) | **Panax quinquefolius** | AMERICAN GINSENG | Radix Panacis Quinquefolii |
| 0444 Hsi-yeh-t'êng | 錫葉藤 | **Tetracera asiatica** | *TETRACERA | Ramus Tetracerae |

36

| Transliteration | Chinese | Botanical Name | English | Pharmaceutical | Hsia |

| | Transliteration | Chinese | Botanical Name | English | Pharmaceutical |
|---|---|---|---|---|---|
| 0445 | Hsia-chien-ts'ao (Pai-hua-tzŭ) | 蝦鉗草(白花子) | **Alternanthera sessilis** | ALTERNANTHERA | Herba Alternantherae |
| 0446 | Hsia-k'u-ts'ao | 夏枯草 | **Prunella vulgaris** | Selfheal, Heal-all | Herba Prunellae |
| 0447 | Hsia-ma | 蝦蟆 | — | Dried frog | Rana |
| 0448 | Hsia-t'ien-wu (Hsia-wu-tsung) | 夏天無(夏無踪) | **Corydalis decumbens** | *Bending Corydalis | Tuber Corydalis Decumbentis |
| 0449 | Hsia-ts'ao-tung-ch'ung | 夏草冬虫 | See Ch'ung-ts'ao | — | — |
| 0450 | Hsiang-chia-p'i (Pei-wu-chia-p'i, Kang-liu-p'i) | 香加皮(北五加皮,杠柳皮) | **Periploca sepium** | *PURPLE-FLOWERED PERIPLOCA | Cortex Periplocae Sepii |
| 0451 | Hsiang-chü (Fu-jung-chü) | 香菊(芙蓉菊) | **Crossostephium chinense** | *FUJUNGCHU | Herba Crossostephii |
| 0452 | Hsiang-ch'un (Hsiang-ch'un-kên, Hsiang-ch'un-chih, Hsiang-ch'un-tzŭ) | 香椿(香椿根,香椿枝,香椿子) | **Toona sinensis (Cedrela sinensis)** | CHINESE CEDRELA | Cortex et Semen Toonae Sinensis |
| 0453 | Hsiang-chün (Hsiang-ku) | 香蕈(香菇) | **Lentinus edodes** | FRAGRANT MUSHROOM | Herba Lentini |
| 0454 | Hsiang-fei-tzŭ | 香榧子 | See Fei-shih | — | — |
| 0455 | Hsiang-fu-tzŭ (Hsiang-fu) | 香附子(香附) | **Cyperus rotundus** | NUT-GRASS | Rhizoma Cyperi |
| 0456 | Hsiang-ju (Hsiang-ju-ts'ao) | 香薷(香茹,香茹草) | **Elsholtzia haichowensis** or **E. splendens, E. ciliata** | AROMATIC MADDER | Herba Elsholtziae |

| | Transliteration | Chinese | Botanical Name | English | Pharmaceutical |
|---|---|---|---|---|---|
| 0457 | Hsiang-ku | 香菇 | See Hsiang-chün | — | — |
| 0458 | Hsiang-mao (Hsiang-mao-ts'ao) | 香茅(香茅草) | **Cymbopogon citratus** | LEMON-GRASS | Herba Cymbopogonis |
| 0459 | Hsiang-pai-chih | 香白芷 | **Angelica anomala** | CHINESE ANGELICA | Radix Angelicae |
| 0460 | Hsiang-pei (Chê-pei) | 象貝(浙貝) | See Chê-pei | FRITILLARY (from Hsiang-shan, 象山 ) | — |
| 0461 | Hsiang-p'i | 象皮 | — | Elephant hide | Corium Elephantis |
| 0462 | Hsiang-p'u (Hsiang-p'u-ts'ao) | 香蒲(香蒲草) | **Typha angustata** **T. angustifolia** **T. latifolia** | CAT-TAIL | Herba Typhae |
| 0463 | Hsiang-ssŭ-tzŭ (Hsiang-ssŭ-tou, Ma-liao-tou) | 相思草(相思豆,馬料豆) | **Abrus precatorius** | ROSARY PEA | Semen Abri |
| 0464 | Hsiang-yü-p'i (Yü-p'i) | 香榆皮(榆皮) | **Ulmus pumila** | CHINESE ELM | Cortex Ulmi |
| 0465 | Hsiang-yüan (Chü-yüan) | 香圓(枸櫞) | **Citrus medica** and **C. wilsonii** | CITRON | Fructus Citri Medicae |
| 0466 | Hsiao-chi (Chi-chi-ya) | 小薊(薊薊芽) | **Cephalanoplos segetum** | *FIELD THISTLE | Herba Cephalanoplosis |
| 0467 | Hsiao-fei-yang | 小飛揚 | **Euphorbia thymifolia** | THYME-LEAVED SPURGE | Herba Euphorbiae Thymifoliae |
| 0468 | Hsiao-hui-hsiang (Hsiao-hui) | 小茴香(小茴) | **Foeniculum vulgare** | FENNEL | Fructus Foeniculi |
| 0469 | Hsiao-hung-tou | 小紅豆 | **Phaseolus calcaratus** | SMALL RED-BEAN | Semen Phaseoli Calcarati |

38

| | Transliteration | Chinese | Botanical Name | English | Pharmaceutical |
|---|---|---|---|---|---|
| 0470 | Hsiao-lo-san | 小羅傘 | **Ardisia crispa** | SMALL ARDISIA | Radix et Ramus Ardisiae Crispae |
| 0471 | Hsiao-mi (Su-mi) | 小米(粟米) | **Setaria italica** | MILLET | Semen Setariae |
| 0472 | Hsiao-mu-t'ung | 小木通 | **Clematis armandii** | *ARMAND'S CLEMATIS | Ramus Clematis |
| 0473 | Hsiao-p'i (P'i-hsiao) | 硝皮(皮硝) | — | Sodium sulphate crude crystal | Natrium Sulfuricum, Sal Glauberis |
| 0474 | Hsiao-po-ku | 小駁骨 | **Gendarussa vulgaris** | SMALL GENDARUSSA | Herba Gendarussae |
| 0475 | Hsiao-tou-k'ou | 小豆蔻 | **Elettaria cardamomum** | CARDAMOM | Fructus Cardamomi |
| 0476 | Hsiao-yeh-mai-ma-t'êng (Chu-chieh-t'êng) | 小葉買麻藤(竹節藤) | **Gnetum parvifolium** | *SMALL GNETUM | Ramus Gneti Parvifolii |
| 0477 | Hsiao-yeh-p'i-pa | 小葉枇杷 | **Rhododendron anthopogonoides** | *ALPINE ROSEBAY | Folium Rhododendri |
| 0478 | Hsiao-yeh-shuang-yen-lung | 小葉雙眼龍 | **Croton lachnocarpus** | *SMALL CROTON | Radix Crotonis Lachnocarpi |
| 0479 | Hsieh (Chuan-hsieh) | 蝎(全蝎) | — | Scorpions | Buthus |
| 0480 | Hsieh-pai (Huo-ts'ung) | 薤白(火葱) | **Allium chinense** | CHINESE CHIVE | Bulbus Allii Chinensis |
| 0481 | Hsieh-ts'ao (Ou-hsieh-ts'ao) | 纈草(歐纈草) | **Valeriana officinalis** | VALERIAN | Rhizoma et Radix Valerianae |
| 0483 | Hsieh-yeh (Fan-hsieh-yeh) | 瀉葉(番瀉葉) | **Cassia angustifolia** and **C. acutifolia** | SENNA | Folium Sennae |
| 0484 | Hsien-ho-ts'ao (Lang-ya-ts'ao) | 仙鶴草(狼牙草) | **Agrimonia pilosa** | AGRIMONY | Herba Agrimoniae |

| Transliteration | Chinese | Botanical Name | English | Pharmaceutical |
|---|---|---|---|---|
| 0485 Hsien-hu | 鮮斛 | **Dendrobium nobile** **Dendrobium officinale** | (Fresh) DENDROBIUM | Herba Dendrobii Vivi |
| 0486 Hsien-mao (Tu-chüeh-hsien-mao) | 仙茅(獨脚仙茅) | **Curculigo orchioides** | GOLDEN EYE-GRASS | Rhizoma Curculiginis |
| 0487 Hsien-mi (Kêng-mi) | 籼米(粳米) | **Oryza sativa** | RICE | Semen Oryzae Sativae |
| 0488 Hsien-p'i (Pai-hsien-p'i) | 鮮皮(白鮮皮) | **Dictamnus dasycarpus** | CHINESE DATTANY | Radix Dictamni |
| 0489 Hsien-shuang-mei (Hua-mei) | 鹹霜梅(話梅) | **Prunus mume** | *(Medicated) MEI | Fructus Pruni Mume Praeparationis |
| 0490 Hsien-yên-chang | 仙人掌 | **Opuntia dillenii** | PRICKLY-PEAR | Herba Opuntiae |
| 0491 Hsin-ku-fêng | 尋骨風 | **Aristolochia mollissima** | HAIRY BIRTHWORT | Radix et Ramus Aristolochiae Mollissimae |
| 0492 Hsin-i (I-hua) | 辛夷(夷花) | **Magnolia liliflora** | *RED MAGNOLIA | Flos Magnoliae |
| 0493 Hsin-shih | 信石 | **—** | Arsenolite, Arsenopyrite | Arsenicum Rubrum, Arsenicum Album |
| 0494 Hsing-hsü-ts'ai | 星宿菜 | **Lysimachia fortunei** | *FORTUNE'S LYSIMACHIA | Herba Lysimachiae Fortunei |
| 0495 Hsing-jên | 杏仁 | **Prunus armeniaca** | APRICOT (kernel) | Semen Pruni Armeniacae |
| —a K'u-hsing-jên | 苦杏仁 | **brown, with seed coat** | wholesome, poisonous soaked, detoxified | |
| —b Tien-hsing-jên | 甜杏仁 | **white, seed coat removed** | | |
| 0496 Hsiung-ch'iung (Ch'uan-hsiung) | 芎藭(川芎) | **Ligusticum wallichii** | SZECHUAN LOVAGE | Radix Ligustici |
| 0497 Hsiung-huang (Ming-huang, K'uai-huang) | 雄黃(明黃,塊黃) | **—** | Realgar, Red arsenic sulphide | Realgar |

| | Transliteration | Chinese | Botanical Name | English | Pharmaceutical |
|---|---|---|---|---|---|
| 0498 | Hsiung-tan | 熊膽 | — | Bear's gall | Fel Ursi |
| 0499 | Hsü-ch'ang-ch'ing (Kuei-tu-yu, Liao-tiao-chu) | 徐長卿(鬼督郵,寮刁竹) | **Cynanchum paniculatum** | LIAOTIAOCHU | Radix Cynanchi Paniculati |
| 0500 | Hsü-sui-tzǔ (Ch'ien-chin-tzǔ) | 續隨子(千金子) | **Euphorbia lathyris** | LATHYROL SPURGE | Semen Euphorbiae Lathyris |
| 0501 | Hsü-tuan (Hsü-tuan-t'ou) | 續斷(續斷頭) | **Dipsacus japonicus** | JAPANESE TEASEL | Radix Dipsaci Japonici |
| 0502 | Hsüan-ching-shih | 玄精石 | — | Gypsum | Selenitum |
| 0503 | Hsüan-fu-hua (Fu-hua, Chin-fu-hua, Ch'üan-fu-hua) | 旋覆花(覆花,金茯花,全福花) | **Inula britannica** | *WILD ELECAMPANE | Flos Inulae |
| 0504 | Hsüan-ming-fên (Fêng-hua-hsiao) | 玄明粉(風化硝) | — | Weathered Sodium sulphate | Natrium Sulfuricum Exsiccatum |
| 0505 | Hsüan-shên (Hei-shên) | 玄參(黑參) | **Scrophularia ningpoensis** | NINGPO FIGWORT | Radix Scrophulariae |
| 0506 | Hsüan-ts'ao | 萱草 | **Hemerocallis fulva** | DAYLILY | Radis Hemerocallis |
| 0507 | Hsüeh-chieh | 血竭 | **Daemonorops draco** | DRAGON'S BLOOD | Sanguis Draconis |
| 0508 | Hsüeh-chien-ch'ou | 血見愁 | See the following | | |
| −a | North China Hsüeh-chien-ch'ou (= Mao-yen-ts'ai, T'ieh-hsien-ts'ai) | 華北血見愁 (=貓眼菜,鉄莧菜) | **Acalypha australis** | WILD COPPERLEAF | Herba Acalyphae |

| Transliteration | Chinese | Botanical Name | English | Pharmaceutical |
|---|---|---|---|---|
| −b South China Hsüeh-chieh-ch'ou (=Shan-huo-hsiang) | 華南血見愁（＝山藿香） | **Teucrium viscidum** | CHINESE GERMANDER | Herba Teucrii |
| 0509 Hsüeh-shan-lin (Fu-kuei-ts'ao) | 雪山林（富貴草） | **Pachysandra terminalis** | *PACHYSANDRA | Herba Pachysandrae |
| 0510 Hsüeh-shang-i-chih-hao | 雪上一枝蒿 | **Aconitum bullatifolium var. homotrichum** | *YUNNAN ALPINE ACONITE | Radix Aconiti Bullatifolii |
| 0511 Hsüeh-yü-t'an | 血餘炭 | — | Charred human hair | Crinis Carbonisatus |
| 0512 Hu-chang (Pan-kên, Ho-hsüeh-tan) | 虎杖（斑根，活血丹） | **Polygonum cuspidatum** | BUSHY KNOTWEED | Radix et Rhozoma Polygoni Cuspidati |
| 0513 Hu-chiao | 胡椒 | **Piper nigrum** | BLACK PEPPER | Fructus Piperis |
| 0514 Hu-chiao (Hu-ku-chiao) | 虎膠（虎骨膠） | — | Tiger bone glue | Gummi Tigris |
| 0515 Hu-êrh-ts'ao | 虎耳草 | **Saxifraga stolonifera** | SAXIFRAGE | Herba Saxifragae |
| 0516 Hu-huang-lien (Hu-lien) | 胡黃連（胡連） | **Picrorhiza kurrooa P. scrophulariaeflora** | *PICRORHIZA | Radix Picrorhizae |
| 0517 Hu-ku | 虎骨 | — | Tiger bone | Os Tigris |
| 0518 Hu-lu | 葫蘆 | **Lagenaria siceraria** | BOTTLE GOURD | Fructus Lagenariae |
| 0519 Hu-lu-ch'a | 葫蘆茶 | **Desmodium triquetrum (Pteroloma triquetrum)** | *BOTTLE-GOURD TEA | Herba Desmodii Triquetri |
| 0520 Hu-lu-pa (Lu-pa) | 胡盧巴（盧巴） | **Trigonella foenum-graecum** | FENUGREEK (seed) | Semen Foenumgraeci |

| Transliteration | Chinese | Botanical Name | English | Pharmaceutical |
|---|---|---|---|---|
| 0521 Hu-ma (Hu-ma-jên, Ya-ma) | 胡麻(胡麻仁,亞麻) | **Linum usitatissimum** | FLAX | Semen Lini |
| 0522 Hu-p'o (Hsüeh-p'o) | 琥珀(血珀) | — | Amber, fossilized resin | Succinum |
| 0523 Hu-shê-hung | 虎舌紅 | **Ardisia mamillata** | *PURPLE ARDISIA | Herba Ardisiae Mamillatae |
| 0524 Hu-sui (Yüan-sui) | 胡荽(芫荽) | **Coriandrum sativum** | CORIANDER | Herba et Fructus Coriandri |
| 0525 Hu-tan (Tan-kên) | 胡丹(丹根) | **Paeonia suffruticosa** | TREE PEONY | Radix Paeoniae Moutan |
| 0526 Hu-t'ung-lui (Wu-t'ung-lui) | 胡桐淚(梧桐淚) | **Populus diversifolia** P. euphratica | *TARTAR POPLAR (fossilized resin) | Resin Populi |
| 0527 Hu-tz'ŭ (Fu-niu-hua) | 虎刺(伏牛花) | **Damnacanthus indicus** | *DAMNACANTHUS | Ramus Damnacanthi |
| 0528 Hua-chiao (Chên-chiao, Ch'uan-chiao, Yao-chiao) | 花椒(秦椒,川椒,藥椒) | **Zanthoxylum simulans** **Z. bungeanum** | *SZECHUAN PEPPER | Fructus Zanthoxyli |
| 0529 Hua-chiao-yeh | 花椒葉 | **Zanthoxylum nitidum** | *SHINY BRAMBLE | Ramus Zanthoxyli Nitidi |
| 0530 Hua-fên | 花粉 | See T'ien-hua-fên | — | — |
| 0531 Hua-ju-shih (Hua-jui-shih) | 花乳石(花蕊石) | — | Ophicalcite | Ophicalcitum |
| 0532 Hua-mu-t'ung | 花木通 | **Clematis montana** | MONTANE CLEMATIS | Ramus Clematidis Montanae |
| 0533 Hua-p'i (Hua-mu-p'i, Ssŭ-pai-p'i) | 樺皮(樺木皮,絲白皮) | **Betula platyphylla** | CHINESE WHITE BIRCH (bark) | Cortex Betulae |

| Transliteration | Chinese | Botanical Name | English | Pharmaceutical |
|---|---|---|---|---|
| 0534 Hua-shih | 滑石 | — | Talc (soapstone) | Talcum |
| 0535 Hua-shih-fên | 滑石粉 | — | Powder of talc or Kaolinite | Kaolinum |
| 0536 Huai-chiao (Huai-shih, Huai-chiao-tzǔ, Huai-tzǔ) | 槐角(槐實, 槐角子, 槐子) | **Sophora japonica** | PAGODA TREE | Fructus et Semen Sophorae |
| 0537 Huai-hsiang (Hui-hsiang) | 懷香(茴香) | **Foeniculum vulgare** | FENNEL | Fructus Foeniculi |
| 0538 Huai-hua-mi (Huai-hua, Huai-mi, Huai-tzǔ) | 槐花米(槐花, 槐米, 槐子) | **Sophora japonica** | PAGODA TREE (flowers and buds) | Flos Sophorae |
| 0539 Huai-shan (Huai-shan-yao) | 淮山(淮山藥) | **Dioscorea opposita** | CHINESE YAM | Radix Dioscoreae |
| 0540 Huai-shu-chih | 槐樹枝 | **Sophora japonica** | PAGODA TREE | Ramus Sophorae |
| 0541 Huan-ch'ai (Yü-huan-ch'ai, Huan-ts'ao, Êrh-huan-shih-hu) | 環釵(玉環釵, 環草, 耳環石斛) | **Dendrobium lohohense** | *LOHOH DENDROBIUM | Herba Dendrobii Lohohensis |
| 0542 Huan-hun-ts'ao (Chüan-pai) | 還魂草(卷柏) | **Selaginella tamariscina** | Chinese Resurrection Plant | Herba Selaginellae Tamariscinae |
| 0543 Huang-ch'i | 黃芪 | **Astragalus membranaceus** | *HUANGCHI | Radix Astragali membranacei et mongholici |
| | | **A. mongholicus** | | |
| Hsi-ch'i | 西芪 | „ „ | Product from Shensi | |
| Mien-ch'i | 綿芪 | **A. membranaceus** **A. mongholicus** | Product from Shansi, Mien-shan | |
| Pei-ch'i | 北芪 | „ „ | | |

| Transliteration | Chinese | Botanical Name | English | Pharmaceutical | Huang |
|---|---|---|---|---|---|
| T'iao-ch'i | 條芪 | **A. mongholicus** | | | |
| —a Ch'uan-ch'i | 川芪 | **A. tongolensis** | SZECHUAN HUANGCHI | Radix Astragali tongolensis | |
| —b Hsiao-pai-ch'i | 小白芪 | **A. floridus** | SMALL WHITE HUANGCHI | Radix Astragali floridi | |
| —c Hung-ch'i | 紅芪 | **Hedysarum polybotrys** | KANSU HUANGCHI | Radix Hedysari polybotryis | |
| 0544 Huang-chih (Huang-chih-tzŭ, Chih-tzŭ, Shui-chih-tzŭ, Chien-chih) | 黃梔(黃枝, 黃梔子, 梔子, 水梔子, 建梔) | **Gardenia jasminoides** | GARDENIA | Fructus Gardeniae | |
| 0545 Huang-ch'in | 黃芩 | **Scutellaria baicalensis** | BAICAL SKULLCAP | Radix Scutellariae Baicalensis | |
| 0546 Huang-ching | 黃精 | **Polygonatum cirrhifolium** **P. sibiricum** **P. multiflorum** | SOLOMON'S SEAL | Rhizoma Polygonati | |
| 0547 Huang-ching-tzŭ | 黃荊子 | **Vitex cannabifolia** or **V. negundo** | HEMP-LEAVED VITEX | Fructus Viticis Cannabifoliae | |
| 0548 Huang-hao (Huang-hao-hua) | 黃蒿(黃蒿花) | **Artemisia annua** | ANNUAL ARTEMISIA | Herba Artemisiae Annuae | |
| 0549 Huang-hua-chia-chu-t'ao | 黃花夾竹桃 | **Thevetia peruviana** | Yellow Oleander | Folium et Semen Thevetiae | |
| 0550 Huang-hua-mu | 黃花母 | **Sida rhombifolia** | SIDA HEMP | Herba Sidae | |
| 0551 Huang-hua-ts'ai-kên (Hsüan-ts'ao-kên) | 黃花菜根(萱草根) | **Hemerocallis lilioasphodelus,** **H. citrina,** **H. minor** | YELLOW DAYLILY | Radix Hemerocallis | |

| | Transliteration | Chinese | Botanical Name | English | Pharmaceutical |
|---|---|---|---|---|---|
| 0552 | Huang-kou-shên | 黃狗腎 | — | Testicle & penis of dog | Testis et Penis Canis |
| 0553 | Huang-lien, Wei-lien (Chi-lien, Ch'uan-lien, Hsi-lien, Kuan-lien, Mu-lien, Shui-lien, Yün-lien) | 黃連, 味連(鷄連, 川連, 西連, 官連, 母連, 水連, 雲連) | **Coptis chinensis** | GOLDEN THREAD | Rhizoma Coptidis |
| —a | Ya-lien | 雅連 | **Coptis deltoides** | YALIEN | Rhizoma Yalien |
| —b | Yün-lien | 雲連 | **C. teetoides** | YUNLIEN | Rhizoma Yunlien |
| 0554 | Huang-lu | 黃櫨 | **Cotinus coggygria** | SMOKE-TREE | Radix et Ramus Cotini |
| 0555 | Huang-niu-ch'a | 黃牛茶 | **Cratoxylon ligustrinum amurense** | YOKE-WOOD TREE | Radix Cratoxylonis |
| 0557 | Huang-p'i-hêh (Huang-shih, Huang-p'i-yeh) | 黃皮核(黃實, 黃皮葉) | **Clausena lansium** | Wampee (seed, leaves) | Semen Wampee Folii Wampee |
| 0558 | Huang-t'êng (Huang-lien-t'êng, T'u-huang-lien) | 黃藤(黃連藤, 土黃連) | **Fibraurea tinctoria** | FIBRAUREA | Radix et Ramus Fibraureae |
| 0559 | Huang-t'u (Huang-yao, Huang-yao-tzǔ) | 黃獨(黃藥, 黃藥子) | **Dioscorea bulbifera** | *YELLOW-ROOT YAM | Radix Dioscoreae Bulbiferae |
| 0560 | Huang-yang-mu (Huang-yang-kên, Huang-yang-tzǔ) | 黃楊木(黃楊根, 黃楊子) | **Buxus microphylla** var. **sinica** | CHINESE BOX | Radix, Ramus, et Semen Buxi |
| 0561 | Huang-yen-ts'ai (Huan-yang-ts'ao) | 黃鵪菜(還陽草) | **Youngia japonica** | *YOUNGIA | Herba Youngiae |

46

| Transliteration | Chinese | Botanical Name | English | Pharmaceutical |
|---|---|---|---|---|
| 0562 Huang-yüan-hua | 黃芫花 | **Wikstroemia chamaedaphne** | WIKSTROEMIA | Radix et Ramus Wikstroemiae |
| 0563 Hui-hsiang (Hsiao-hui-hsiang) | 茴香(小茴香) | **Foeniculum vulgare** | FENNEL | Fructus Foeniculi |
| 0564 Hui-yeh (Hui-yeh-kên, Yeh-lan) | 灰葉(灰葉根,野藍) | **Tephrosia purpurea** | *TEPHROSIA | Radix et Ramus Tephrosiae |
| 0565 Hung-ch'iu-chiang | 紅球姜 | **Zingiber zerumbet** | *RED-BALL GINGER | Rhizoma Zingiberis Zerumbet |
| 0566 Hung-ch'ü-mi | 紅麯米 | **Oryza sativa** plus **Monascus purpureus** | *Fermented rice with red yeast | Semen Oryzae cum Monasco |
| 0567 Hung-fên (Hung-shêng) | 紅粉(紅昇·) | See Shêng-yao | Red oxide of Mercury | — |
| 0568 Hung-han-lien (Ta-han-ling-ts'ao) | 紅旱蓮(大汗淋草) | **Hypericum ascyron** | ST. JOHNSWORT | Herba Hyperici Ascyronis |
| 0569 Hung-hua (Yao-hua, Yao-hung-hua, Li-hung-hua, Li-hua) | 紅花(藥花,藥紅花,粒紅花,粒花) | **Carthamus tinctorius** | SAFFLOWER | Flos Carthami |
| 0570 Hung-k'ou | 紅蔻 | See Hung-tou-k'ou | — | — |
| 0571 Hung-niang-tzŭ | 紅娘子 | — | Red cicada | Huechys Sanguines |
| 0572 Hung-pi-san-chi (San-hsüeh-tan, T'u-san-chi) | 紅背三七(散血丹,土三七) | **Gynura segetum** | *CANTON TUSANCHI (Velvet Plant) | Herba Gynurae Segeti |
| 0573 Hung-szŭ-hsien | 紅絲綫 | **Peristrophe roxburghiana** | *RED SILK-THREAD | Herba Peristrophis Roxburghianae |

47

| | Transliteration | Chinese | Botanical Name | English | Pharmaceutical |
|---|---|---|---|---|---|
| 0574 | Hung-tou-k'ou (Hung-k'ou) | 紅豆蔻(紅叩) | **Alpinia galanga** | GREATER GALANGAL | Fructus Alpinae Galangae |
| 0575 | Hung-tsao (Ta-tsao) | 紅棗(大棗) | **Zizyphus jujuba** | CHINESE DATE, JUJUBE | Fructus Zizyphi Jujubae |
| 0576 | Hung-wu-chiu (Shan-wu-chiu) | 紅烏桕(山烏桕) | **Sapium discolor** | MOUNTAIN TALLOW-TREE | Radix et Ramus Sapii |
| 0577 | Hung-ya-ta-chi (Ya-chi) | 紅芽大戟(芽戟) | **Knoxia valerianoides** | *KNOXIA | Radix Knoxiae |
| 0578 | Hung-ya-tsao (Chu-ya-tsao) | 紅牙皂(豬牙皂) | **Gleditsia sinensis** | CHINESE HONEY-LOCUST | Fructus Gleditsiae |
| 0579 | Hung-yeh-tieh-shu (Chu-chiao) | 紅葉鐵樹(朱蕉) | **Cordyline fruticosa** | CORDYLINE | Radix, Ramus et Flos Cordylines |
| 0580 | Huo-chi-shêng (Liu-chi-shêng) | 槲寄生(柳寄生) | **Viscum coloratum** | ASIATIC MISTLETOE | Ramus Visci Colorati |
| 0581 | Huo-hsiang | 藿香 | See the following | — | — |
| −a | Kuang-huo-hsiang | 廣藿香 | **Pogostemon cablin** | PATCHOULI | Herba Patchouli |
| −b | T'u-huo-hsiang | 土藿香 | **Agastache rugosa** | *AGASTACHE | Herba Agastaches |
| 0582 | Huo-ma (Ta-ma, Huo-ma-jên) | 火麻(大麻,火麻仁) | **Cannabis sativa** | HEMP (seed), MARIJUANA | Semen Cannabis |
| 0583 | Huo-so-ma | 火索麻 | **Helicteres isora** | *HELICTERES | Radix Helicteridis Isorae |
| 0584 | Huo-t'an-mu | 火炭母 | **Polygonum chinense** | *CHINESE SMARTWEED | Herba Polygoni Chinense |
| 0585 | Huo-yang-lê | 火殃簕 | **Euphorbia antiquorum** | FLESHY SPURGE | Ramus Euphorbiae Antiquori |

| Transliteration | Chinese | Botanical Name | English | Pharmaceutical |
|---|---|---|---|---|
| 0586 I-chih (I-chih-jên, I-chih-tzǔ) | 益智(益智仁, 益智子) | **Alpinia oxyphylla** | *ICHIHJEN | Fructus Alpiniae Oxyphyllae |
| 0587 I-chih-chien | 一支箭 | **Ophioglossum vulgatum O. thermale** | ADDER'S TONGUE | Herba Ophioglossi |
| 0588 I-chih-huang-hua | 一支黃花 | **Solidago virgo-aurea** | GOLDEN ROD | Herba Solidaginis |
| 0589 I-i-jên (I-mi, I-jên-mi, I-mi-jên) | 薏苡仁(苡米, 苡仁米, 薏米仁) | **Coix lacryma-jobi** | JOB'S TEARS | Semen Coicis |
| 0590 I-mu-kao | 益母膏 | **Leonurus artemisia** | Concentrated infusion of Chinese motherwort | Extractus Leonuri Artemisiae |
| 0591 I-mu-ts'ao | 益母草 | **Leonurus artemisia L. tartarica** | CHINESE MOTHERWORT | Herba Leonuri Artemisiae vel Tartaricae |
| 0592 I-t'ang (Mai-ya-t'ang) | 飴糖(麥芽糖) | **Hordeum vulgare Sorghum bicolor** | Maltose | Saccharum Granorum |
| 0593 I-tien-hsüeh | 一點血 | **Begonia wilsonii** | WILSON'S BEGONIA | Herba Begoniae Wilsonii |
| 0594 I-tuo-yün (Wan-li-hsiang) | 一朵雲(萬里香) | **Pittosporum glabratum** | PITTOSPORUM | Radix Pittospori |
| 0594A I-yeh-ch'iu | 一葉萩 | See 2131 | | |
| 0595 Jan-shê-p'i | 蚺蛇皮 | — | Python skin | Cuticula Pythonis |
| 0596 Jê-fei-ts'ao | 熱痱草 | **Orthodon diantherus** | *PRICKLY-HEATWORT | Herba Orthodonis |
| 0597 Jên-chung-huang | 人中黃 | — | Human faeces preparation | — |
| 0598 Jên-chung-pai | 人中白 | — | Human urine sediment | — |
| 0599 Jên-shên | 人參 | **Panax ginseng** | GINSENG | Radix Ginseng |
| Chi-lin-shên | 吉林參 | ,,    ,, | Ginseng from Kirin | |
| Ch'ung-shan-shên | 中山參 | ,,    ,, | Imitation wild ginseng | |

**49**

| | Transliteration | Chinese | Botanical Name | English | Pharmaceutical |
|---|---|---|---|---|---|
| | Hung-shên | 紅參 | **Panax ginseng** | Red ginseng, processed with heat | |
| | Kao-li-shên | 高麗參 | ,,      ,, | Korean ginseng | |
| | Kuan-tung-shên | 關東參 | ,,      ,, | Ginseng from the North-east | |
| | Shan-shên | 山參 | ,,      ,, | Wild ginseng | |
| | Shên-hsü | 參鬚 | ,,      ,, | Ginseng rootlets | |
| | Shên-sui | 參碎 | ,,      ,, | Ginseng refuse | |
| | Shên-ting | 參丁 | ,,      ,, | Ginseng cuttings | |
| | T'ang-shên | 糖參 | ,,      ,, | Sugared ginseng, processed with sugar | |
| | Ts'ao-shên | 草參 | ,,      ,, | Cultivated ginseng | |
| | Yang-shên | 秧參 | ,,      ,, | Inferior ginseng | |
| | Yüan-shên | 圓參 | ,,      ,, | Cultivated ginseng | |
| 0600 | Jên-tung | 忍冬 | **Lonicera japonica** | HONEYSUCKLE | Ramus Lonicerae |
| 0601 | Jên-tzǔ-ts'ao (P'u-ti-chin, Ting-kuei-ts'ao) | 人字草(鋪地錦，丁癸草) | **Zornia diphylla** | *ZORNIA | Herba Zorniae |
| 0602 | Jou-kuei | 肉桂 | **Cinnamomum cassia** <br> **C. loureiroi** | CASSIA BARK <br> SAIGON CINNAMON | Cortex Cassiae <br> Cortex Cinnamomi Loureiroi |
| 0603 | Jou-tou-k'ou | 肉豆蔻 | **Myristica fragrans** | NUTMEG | Semen Myristicae |
| | Jou-tou-kên | 肉豆根 | **Myristica fragrans** | ,,     (root) | Flos Myristicae |
| | Jou-tou-hua | 肉豆花 | **Myristica fragrans** | ,,     (flower) | Radix Myristicae |
| 0604 | Jou-ts'ung-jung | 肉蓯蓉 | **Cistanche salsa** <br> **C. desertica** | MONGOLIAN BROOMRAPE | Herba Cistanches |
| 0605 | Ju-hsiang | 乳香(茹香) | **Boswellia carterii** <br> **B. neglecta** <br> **B. bhau-dajiana** | FRANKINCENSE | Gummi Olibanum |

50

| Transliteration | Chinese | Botanical Name | English | Pharmaceutical |
|---|---|---|---|---|
| 0606 Ju-t'i-lung (Suan-t'êng-kuo) | 入地龍(酸藤果) | **Embelia laeta** | *SOUR-LEAVED EMBELIA | Radix et Fructus Embeliae |
| 0607 Jui-jên | 蕤仁 | **Prinsepia uniflora** | PRINSEPIA (kernel) | Semen Prinsepiae |
| 0608 Jung-mo (Lu-jung-sui) | 茸末(鹿茸碎) | See Lu-jung | — | — |
| 0609 Kan-chê (Chu-chê) | 甘蔗(竹蔗) | **Saccharum sinense** | CHINESE SUGARCANE | Caulis Sacchari |
| 0610 Kan-ch'i | 乾漆 | **Rhus verniciflua** | Dried Lacquer | Lacca Sinica Exsiccatae |
| 0611 Kan-chiang | 乾姜(乾薑) | **Zingiber officinale** | Dried Ginger | Rhizoma Zingiberis Exsiccatae |
| 0612 Kan-hêh | 柑核 | **Citrus nobilis** | MANDARIN ORANGE (pips) | Semen Citri Nobilis |
| 0613 Kan-lan (Pai-lan, Ch'ing-kuo) | 橄欖(白欖, 青果) | **Canarium album** | CHINESE OLIVE | Fructus et Semen Canarii Albi |
| 0614 Kan-p'i | 柑皮 | **Citrus nobilis** | Orange peels | Pericarpium Citri |
| 0614A Kan-shan-ching-chieh | 甘陝荊芥 | **Nepeta cataria** | CATNIP | Herba Nepetae Catariae |
| 0615 Kan-sui | 甘遂 | **Euphorbia kansui** | *KANSUI | Semen Euphorbiae Kansui |
| 0616 Kan-sung (Ch'uan-sung) | 甘松(乾松, 川松) | **Nardostachys chinensis** | *CHINESE SPIKENARD | Rhizoma Nardostachydis |
| 0617 Kan-ts'ao (Mi-ts'ao, Fên-ts'ao, Kuo-lao) | 甘草(密草, 粉草, 國老) | **Glycyrrhiza uralensis** | LIQUORICE (UK) LICORICE (USA) | Radix Glycyrrhizae |
| 0618 Kang-chü (Chu-tsǔ-tou) | 崗菊(猪仔豆) | **Eriosma chinense** | *ERIOSMA | Radix Eriosmatis |
| 0619 Kang-lui-p'i (Hsiang-chia-p'i) | 杠柳皮(香加皮) | **Periploca sepium** | *PERIPLOCA | Cortex Periplocae |
| 0620 Kang-mei (Ch'êng-hsing-mu) | 崗梅(秤星木) | **Ilex asprella** | *KANGMEI | Radix et Ramus Ilicis Asprellae |

51

| Transliteration | Chinese | Botanical Name | English | Pharmaceutical |
|---|---|---|---|---|
| 0621 Kang-nien | 崗棯 | **Rhodomyrtus tomentosa** | ROSE MYRTLE | Radix, Ramus, et Fructus Rhodomyrti |
| 0622 Kang-pan-kuei | 杠板歸 | **Polygonum perfoliatum** | PRICKLY POLYGONUM | Herba Polygoni Perfoliatae |
| 0623 Kang-sung | 崗松 | **Baeckea frutescens** | *BAECKEA | Ramus Baeckeae |
| 0624 Kao-liang | 高粱 | **Sorghum bicolor (S. vulgare)** | SORGHUM, KAOLIANG | Fructus Sorghi |
| 0625 Kao-liang-chiang | 高良薑 | **Alpinia officinarum** | LESSER GALANGAL | Rhizoma Alpiniae Officinari |
| 0626 Kao-ling-shih (Juan-hua-shih) | 高嶺石(軟滑石) | — | KAOLINITE | Kaolinum |
| 0627 Kao-pên (Liao-kao-pên) | 藁本(遼藁本) | **Ligusticum sinense L. jeholense** | CHINESE LOVAGE | Radix Ligustici Sinensis |
| 0628 Kêng-mi | 粳米 | **Oryza sativa** | COMMON RICE | Semen Oryzae |
| 0629 Ko-chieh | 蛤蚧 | — | Red-spotted house lizard | Gecko |
| 0630 Ko-fên | 蛤粉 | — | Powdered clam shell | Concha Cyclinae |
| 0631 Ko-hsiang (Ju-hsiang) | 克香(乳香) | **Boswellia carteri** | FRANKINCENSE | Gummi Olibanum |
| 0632 Ko-hsien-mi | 葛仙米 | **Nostoc commune** | COMMON NOSTOC | Herba Nostochis |
| 0633 Ko-hua | 葛花 | **Pueraria lobata** | COMMON KUDZU | Flos Puerariae |
| 0634 Ko-kan (Fên-ko, Fên-ko-kan, Kan-ko) | 葛乾(粉葛,粉葛乾,甘葛) | **Pueraria thomsonii P. edulis** | *STARCH KUDZU | Radix Puerariae Edulis |

52

| | Transliteration | Chinese | Botanical Name | English | Pharmaceutical |
|---|---|---|---|---|---|
| 0635 | Ko-kên | 葛根 | **Pueraria lobata** | COMMON KUDZU | Radix Puerariae Lobatae |
| 0636 | Ko-k'o | 蛤殼 | — | Clam shell | Concha Cyclinae, or Concha Meretricis |
| 0637 | Ko-ma-yu | 蛤蟆油 | — | Oviduct of frog | Oviductus Ranae |
| 0638 | K'o-tzǔ (Ho-tzǔ) | 柯子(訶子) | **Terminalia chebula** | MYROBALAN | Fructus Chebulae |
| 0639 | Kou-chi (Kou-chi p'ien, Kou-chi-kuan-chung) | 狗脊(狗脊片, 狗脊貫眾) | **Woodwardia unigemmata W. japonica** | CHAIN-FERN | Rhizoma Woodwardiae |
| 0640 | Kou-ch'i-p'ien (Ti-ku-p'i) | 枸杞片(地骨皮) | **Lycium chinense** | (Sliced) MATRIMONY-VINE | Radix Lycii |
| 0641 | Kou-ch'i-t'ou (Kou-ch'i) | 枸杞頭(枸杞) | **Lycium chinense** | MATRIMONY-VINE (tender shoots) | Ramus et Folium Lycii |
| 0642 | Kou-ch'i-tzǔ (Kou-ch'i, Ch'i-tzǔ, Pên-ch'i, T'u-ch'i) | 枸杞子(枸杞, 杞子, 本杞, 土杞) | **Lycium chinense** | CHINESE MATRIMONY-VINE (fruit) | Fructus Lycii chinensis |
| —a | Ning-hsia-kou-ch'i | 寧夏枸杞 | **L. barbarum** | LYCIUM BERRY | Fructus Lycii barbari |
| 0643 | Kou-chü (Ch'ou-chieh-tzǔ) | 枸橘(臭桔子) | **Poncirus trifoliata** | TRIFOLIATE ORANGE | Fructus Ponciri |
| 0644 | Kou-chüeh-chi (Fan-t'ien-hua) | 狗腳跡(梵天花) | **Urena procumbens** | *URENA | Herba Urenae |
| 0645 | Kou-kan-ts'ai | 狗肝菜 | **Dicliptera chinensis** | *DICLIPTERA | Ramus Diclipterae |
| 0646 | Kou-pao | 狗寶 | — | Dog bezoar | Calculus Canis |

53

| | Transliteration | Chinese | Botanical Name | English | Pharmaceutical |
|---|---|---|---|---|---|
| 0647 | Kou-pien (Kou-shên) | 狗鞭(狗腎) | — | Dog's penis and testicle | Testis et Penis Canis |
| 0648 | Kou-t'êng (Kou-p'ien, Mi-kou) | 鈎藤(勾藤,鈎片,米鈎) | **Uncaria sinensis** **U. rhynchophylla** | GAMBIR VINE | Ramulus et Uncus Uncariae |
| 0649 | Kou-wên (Ta-ch'a-yao, Huang-yeh-ko, Huang-t'êng, Tu-kên) | 鈎吻(大茶藥,黃野葛,黃藤,毒根) | **Gelsemium elegans** | YELLOW JESSAMINE | Ramus et Folium Gelsemii |
| 0650 | K'ou-k'o | 蔻殼 | **Alpinia galanga** | GALANGAL (husk) | Pericarpium Alpiniae |
| 0651 | Ku-chih (P'o-ku-chih) | 故紙(故芷,破故紙) | (see 1103) | | |
| 0652 | Ku-ching ts'ao (Ku-ching-tzŭ, Ku-chu) | 穀精草(穀精子,穀珠) | **Ericaulon buergerianum** **E. wallichianum** | PIPEWORT | Scapus Eriocaulonis |
| 0653 | Ku-ch'ung (Wu-Ku-ch'ung, Ch'ü) | 穀虫(五穀虫,蛆) | — | Maggot | Larva Chrysomyiae |
| 0654 | Ku-ko-yeh | 古柯葉 | **Erythroxylon coca** | COCA (leaves) | Folium Cocae |
| 0655 | Ku-p'i (Ti-ku-p'i) | 骨皮(地骨皮) | **Lycium chinense** | MATRIMONY-VINE (root bark) | Cortex Radicis Lycii |
| 0656 | Ku-shan-lung | 古山龍 | **Arcangelisia loureiroi** | *MOUNTAIN DRAGON | Ramus Arcangelisiae |
| 0657 | Ku-sui-pu (Sui-pu) | 骨碎補(碎補) | **Drynaria fortunei** | *DRYNARIA | Rhizoma Drynariae |
| 0658 | Ku-tzŭ (Pu-ku-chih) | 故子(補骨脂) | (see 1103) | — | — |
| 0659 | Ku-ya | 穀芽 | **Oryza sativa** | RICE (sprout) | Fructus Oryzae Germinantis |

54

| Transliteration | Chinese | Botanical Name | English | Pharmaceutical |
|---|---|---|---|---|
| 0660 Ku-yang-t'êng (Nan-k'u-shên) | 古羊藤(南苦参) | **Streptocaulon griffithii** | *STREPTOCAULON | Radix Streptocaulonis |
| 0661 K'u-chü-yeh | 苦竹葉 | **Pleioblastus amarus** | *BITTER-BAMBOO (leaves) | Folium Pleioblasti |
| 0662 K'u-hsing-jên (Hsing-jên) | 苦杏仁(杏仁) | **Prunus armeniaca** | APRICOT (seed) | Semen Pruni Armeniacae |
| 0663 K'u-kua (K'u-kua-kên, K'u-kua-tzŭ) | 苦瓜(苦瓜根,苦瓜子) | **Momordica charantia** | BITTER MOMORDICA | Fructus Semen et Radix Momordicae Charantiae |
| 0664 K'u-kua-ti | 苦瓜蒂 | **Cucumis melo** | BITTER MELON | Pedicellus Cucumis |
| 0665 K'u-kuo | 苦果 | **Strychnos ignatii** | ST. IGNATIUS BEAN | Semen Strychnosis Ignatii |
| 0666 K'u-lang | 苦莨 | **Clerodendrum inerme** | GLORYBOWER | Cortex Clerodendri |
| 0667 K'u-lien-kên (K'u-lien-tzŭ, K'u-lien-p'i) | 苦楝根(苦楝子,苦楝皮) | **Melia azedarach** | CHINATREE (root, bark, seed) | Cortex et Semen Meliae Azedarachis |
| 0668 K'u-shên (K'u-shên-tzŭ, K'u-shên-kên) | 苦参(苦参子,苦参根) | **Sophora flavescens** | *SHRUBBY SOPHORA | Radix et Semen Sophora Flavescentis |
| 0669 K'u-têng-lung (Kuei-têng-lung) | 苦燈籠(鬼燈籠) | **Clerodendrum fortunatum** | *DEVIL'S LANTERN | Ramus Clerodendri Fortunati |
| 0670 Kua-chieh | 瓜杰(竭) | — | Imitation Dragon's Blood | — |
| 0671 Kua-lou (Kua-lou-jên, Lou-jên, Koa-lou-p'i) | 瓜蔞(瓜蔞仁,蔞仁,括蔞皮) | **Trichosanthes kirilowii** | *TRICHOSANTHES | Fructus et Semen Trichosanthis |

55

| Transliteration | Chinese | Botanical Name | English | Pharmaceutical |
|---|---|---|---|---|
| 0672 Kua-ti | 瓜蒂 | **Cucumis melo** | Young Melon stalk | Pedicellus Cucumis |
| 0673 Kuan-chung | 貫眾(管仲) | **Dryopteris crassirhizoma** **Cyrtomium fortunei** | SHIELD-FERN | Rhizoma Dryopteris |
| 0374 Kuan-kuei | 官桂 | **Cinnamomum loureiroi** | CINNAMON | Cortex Cinnamomi Loureiroi |
| 0675 Kuan-mu-t'ung (Ma-mu-t'ung) | 關木通(馬木通) | **Aristolochia mandshuriensis (Hocquartia mandshuriensis)** | *KUANMUTUNG | Ramus Aristolochiae Mandshuriensis |
| 0676 Kuan-pai-fu-tzŭ | 關白附子 | **Aconitum coreanum** | KOREAN ACONITE | Radix Aconiti Coreani |
| 0677 Kuan-yin-liu | 觀音柳 | **Tamarix chinensis** | TAMARISK | Ramus Tamaricis |
| 0678 K'uan-chin-t'êng | 寬筋藤 | **Tinospora sinensis** | CHINESE TINOSPORA | Ramus et Radix Tinosporae Sinensis |
| 0679 K'uan-tung-hua (Tung-hua, Chien-hua) | 款冬花(冬花,揀花) | **Tussilago farfara** | TUSSILAGO | Flos Farfarae |
| 0680 Kuang-ch'ên-p'i | 廣陳皮 | **Citrus reticulata** | MANDARIN ORANGE (peels) | Pericarpium Citri |
| 0681 Kuang-fang-chi | 廣防己 | **Aristolochia fangchi A. westlandii** | Southern Fangchi | Radix Kwang-fangchi |
| 0682 Kuang-ho-hsiang | 廣藿香 | **Pogostemon cablin P. patchouli** | PATCHOULI | Herba Patchouli |
| 0683 Kuang-ku (Shan-tz'u-ku) | 光菇(山慈菇) | **Tulipa edulis** | *CHINESE TULIP | Bulbus Tulipae Edulis |

56

| Transliteration | Chinese | Botanical Name | English | Pharmaceutical |
|---|---|---|---|---|
| 0684 Kuang-ming-tzǔ | 光明子 | **Ocimum basilicum** | SWEET BASIL | Semen Ocimi |
| 0685 Kuang-mu-hsiang | 廣木香 | **Saussurea lappa (Aucklandia lappa)** | COSTUS, PUCHOK | Radix Muhsiang |
| 0686 Kuang-tung-wan-nien-ch'ing | 廣東萬年青 | **Aglaonema modestum** | *AGLAONEMA | Herba Aglaonematis |
| 0687 Kuang-wu (Ch'uan-wu) | 光烏(川烏) | **Acontitum chinense** | CHINESE ACONITE | Rhizoma Aconiti |
| 0688 Kuei-chiao | 龜膠 | — | Tortoise-shell glue | *Kueichiao |
| 0689 Kuei-chien-yü | 鬼箭羽 | **Euonymus alatus** | WINGED SPINDLE TREE | Lignum Suberalatum Euonymi |
| 0690 Kuei-chih (Kuei-mu, Kuei-hsin) | 桂枝(桂木, 桂心) | **Cinnamomum cassia** | CASSIA (twigs) | Ramus Cinnamomi Cassiae |
| 0691 Kuei-chin-ts'ao | 鬼針草 | **Bidens pilosa** | HAIRY BEGGER-TICKS | Herba Bidentis |
| 0691A Kuei-chiu T'ao-erh-ch'i | 鬼臼, 桃兒七 | **Podophyllum hexandrum (P. emodi var. chinense)** | CHINESE MAY-APPLE | Rhizoma Podophylli |
| 0692 Kuei-hua | 桂花 | **Osmanthus fragrans** | *KUEIHUA | Flos Osmanthi |
| Kuei-hua-êrh | 桂花耳 | „ „ | Preparation of Kueihua | |
| Kuei-hua-yu | 桂花油 | „ „ | Oil from Kueihua | |
| 0693 Kuei-man-t'ou | 鬼饅頭 | **Ficus pumila** | *DEMON'S BREAD | Fructus Fici Pumilae |
| 0694 Kuei-mu (Pai-kuei-mu) | 鬼目, 桂木(白桂木) | **Artocarpus hypargyraeus** | ARTOCARPUS | Fructus Artocarpi Hypargyraei |
| 0695 Kuei-pan (Kuei-p'ien) | 龜板(龜片) | — | Land tortoise shell | Carapax Testudinis |
| 0696 Kuei-p'i | 桂皮 | **Cinnamomum cassia** | CASSIA (bark, oil) | Cortex Cinnamomi |
| Kuei-p'i-yu | 桂皮油 | | | |
| 0697 Kuei-têng-lung | 鬼燈籠 | **Clerodendrum fortunatum** | DEVIL'S LANTERN | Radix Clerodendri Fortunati |

| | Transliteration | Chinese | Botanical Name | English | Pharmaceutical | Kuei |
|---|---|---|---|---|---|---|
| 0698 | Kuei-t'i (Kuei-tzǔ) | 桂蒂(桂子) | **Cinnanmomum loureiroi** | CASSIA (buds on pedicels) | *Kueiti et Kueitzu | |
| 0699 | Kuei-wei | 歸尾 | **Angelica sinensis** | TANG-KUEI (end of lateral roots) | *Kueiwei | |
| 0700 | Kuei-yü-chien | 鬼羽箭 | **Euonymus alatus** See Yü-chien | WINGED SPINDLE TREE | Ramus Euonymi Alatae | |
| 0701 | K'uei (Tung-kuei, Tung-hsien-ts'ai, K'uei-yüan) | 葵(冬葵,冬莧菜,葵元) | **Malva verticillata** | MUSK MALLOW | Radix et Ramus Malvae Verticillatae | |
| 0702 | K'un-pu | 昆布 | See below | | Thallus Algae | |
| −a | Ch'un-tai-ts'ai | 裙帶菜 | **Undaria pinnatifida** | | | |
| −b | Hai-tai | 海帶 | **Laminaria japonica** | KELP | | |
| −c | O-chang-ts'ai | 鵝掌菜 | **Ecklonia kurome** | | | |
| 0703 | Kung-lao-tzǔ | 功勞子 | **Ilex cornuta** | CHINESE HOLLY | Fructus Ilicis Cornutae | |
| 0704 | Kung-lao-yeh | 功勞葉 | **Ilex cornuta** | CHINESE HOLLY | Folium Ilicis Cornutae | |
| 0705 | Kuo-chiang-lung | 過江龍 | **Entada phaseoloides** | *ENTADA | Radix et Semen Entadae | |
| 0706 | Kuo-lu-huang | 過路黃 | **Lysimachia christinae** | *CHRISTINA'S LYSIMACHIA | Herba Lysimachiae Christinae | |
| 0707 | Kuo-shan-lung | 過山龍 | **Vernonia andersonii** | *CLIMBING VERNONIA | Ramus Vernoniae Andersonii | |
| 0708 | Kuo-t'ang-lung | 過塘龍 | **Jussiaea repens** | *POND DRAGON | Herba Jussiaeae Repentis | |
| 0709 | La-chiao (La-chiao-kan) | 辣椒(辣椒乾) | **Capsicum annuum** | RED PEPPER, CHILI | Fructus Capsici | |
| 0710 | La-mei-hua | 蠟梅花 | **Chimonanthus praecox** | *LAMEI | Flos Chimonanthi | |

58

| Transliteration | Chinese | Botanical Name | English | Pharmaceutical | Lai |
|---|---|---|---|---|---|
| 0711 Lai-fu-tzǔ (Lai-fu, Lo-po-jên) | 萊菔子(萊菔, 蘿蔔仁) | **Raphanus sativus** | RADISH (seed) | Semen Raphani | |
| 0712 Lan-jên (Wu-lan-jên) | 欖仁(烏欖仁) | **Canarium pimela** | *BLACK CANARIUM (kernel) | Semen Canarii Pimelae | |
| 0713 Lang-tang | 莨菪 | **Hyoscyamus niger** | BLACK HENBANE | Folium Hyoscyami | |
| 0714 Lang-tu-t'ou (Lang-tu) | 狼毒頭(狼毒) | **Euphorbia fischeriana** | CHINESE WOLFSBANE | Radix Euphorbiae Fischerianae | |
| 0715 Lang-yü | 榔榆 | **Ulmus parvifolia** | CHINESE ELM | Cortex et Folium Ulmi Parvifoliae | |
| 0716 Lao-chun-hsü | 老君鬚 | **Usnea diffracta** | *OLD-MAN'S BEARD | Herba Usneae | |
| 0717 Lao-huan-ts'ao | 老鸛草 | **Geranium sibiricum G. wilfordii** | CRANESBILL | Herba Geranii | |
| 0718 Lao-lung-p'i | 老龍皮 | **Lobaria retigera L. isidiosa** | LICHENS | Herba Lobariae | |
| 0719 Lao-shu-la-tung-kua | 老鼠拉冬瓜 | **Zehneria indica** | ZEHNERIA | Radix Zehneriae | |
| 0720 Lao-shu-tz'ǔ | 老鼠刺 | **Acanthus ilicifolius** | *BEACH ACANTHUS | Radix Acanthi | |
| 0721 Lao-yeh (Chü-yeh, Chü-yeh-kan) | 蒟葉(蒟葉, 蒟葉乾) | **Piper betle** | Betel Pepper | Folium Piperis | |
| 0722 Lei-mo (Kou-mo) | 雷蘑(口蘑) | **Clitocybe gigantea** | Clitocybe | Fructificatio Clitocybes | |
| 0723 Lei-shih | 礧石 | — | Quartz | — | |
| 0724 Lei-wan | 雷丸 | **Polyporus mylittae (Omphalia lapidescens)** | *THUNDER BALL | Fructificatio Polypori | |
| 0725 Li | 藜 | **Chenopodium album** | PIGWEED | Herba Chenopodii | |

| | Transliteration | Chinese | Botanical Name | English | Pharmaceutical | Li |
|---|---|---|---|---|---|---|
| 0726 | Li-chih (Li-hêh, Li-chih-kên) | 荔枝(荔核，荔枝根) | **Litchi chinensis** | LICHEE | Fructus, Semen et Radix Litchis | |
| 0727 | Li-jên (Yü-li-jên) | 李仁(郁李仁) | **Prunus japonica** | JAPANESE PLUM | Semen Pruni Japonicae | |
| 0728 | Li-kan (Li-p'i) | 梨乾(梨皮) | **Pyrus serrulata P. betulaefolia** | CHINESE PEARS (dried, peels) | Fructus Pyri | |
| 0729 | Li-k'o (Pan-li) | 栗殼(板栗) | **Castanea mollissima** | CHESTNUT (husk) | Pericarpium Castaneae | |
| 0730 | Li-k'o (Mou-li, Li-k'o-fên) | 蠣殼(牡蠣，蠣殼粉) | — | Oyster shell | Concha Ostreae | |
| 0731 | Li-lu | 藜蘆 | **Veratrum nigrum V. maackii** | FALSE HELLEBORE | Rhizoma et Radix Veratri | |
| 0732 | Li-shu-p'i (Ch'ing-kang-p'i) | 櫟樹板(青剛皮) | **Quercus acutissima Q. mongolica** | Fibrous Oak | Cortex Querci Acutissimae et Mongolicae | |
| 0733 | Li-t'ou-chien | 犁頭尖 | **Typhonium divaricatum** | *LESSER TYPHONIUM | Rhizoma Typhonii | |
| 0734 | Liang-chiang (Kao-liang-chiang) | 良薑(高良薑) | **Alpinia officinarum** | LESSER GALANGAL | Rhizoma Alpiniae Officinari | |
| 0735 | Liang-fên-kuo | 涼粉果 | **Ficus pumila** | Jelly-seed | Fructus Fici Pumilae | |
| 0736 | Liang-fên-ts'ao | 涼粉草 | **Mesona chinensis** | *JELLYWORT | Herba Mesonae | |
| 0737 | Liang-hsien (Wei-liang-hsieh) | 靈仙(威靈仙) | **Clematis chinensis** | *CHINESE CLEMATIS | Radix Clematidis | |
| 0738 | Liang-mien-chin (Shan-chiao) | 兩面針(山椒) | **Zanthoxylum nitidum** | SHINY BRAMBLE | Radix et Ramus Zanthoxyli Nitidi | |
| 0738A | Liang-t'ien-ch'ih (Chien-hua) | 量天尺(劍花) | **Hylocereus undatus** | NIGHT-BLOOMING CEREUS | Flos Hylocerei | |
| 0739 | Liang-t'ou-chien | 兩頭尖 | **Anemone raddeana** | ANEMONE | Rhizoma Anemones Raddeanae | |

| Transliteration | Chinese | Botanical Name | English | Pharmaceutical | |
|---|---|---|---|---|---|
| 0740 Liao (La-liao) | 蓼(辣蓼) | **Polygonum hydropiper** | SMARTWEED | Herba Polygoni Hydropiperis | |
| 0741 Liao-ko-wang | 了哥王 | **Wikstroemia indica** | WIKSTROEMIA | Herba Wikstromiae | |
| 0742 Liao-shu (Pai-shu) | 料朮(白朮) | **Atractylodes macro-cephala** | *PAISHU | Radix Paishu | |
| 0743 Lien-ch'iao | 連翹 | **Forsythia suspensa** | FORSYTHIA | Fructus Forsythiae | |
| 0744 Lien-fang (Lien-p'êng) | 蓮房(蓮蓬) | **Nelumbo nucifeia** | LOTUS (receptacles) | Receptaculum Nelumbinis | |
| Lien-hsü | 蓮鬚 | ,,    ,, | ,,    (stamens) | Staminis Nelumbinis | |
| Lien-hua | 蓮花 | ,,    ,, | ,,    (flower) | Flos Nelumbinis | |
| Lien-tzǔ (Lien-shih) | 蓮子(蓮實) | ,,    ,, | ,,    (seed) | Semen Nelumbinis | |
| Lien-tzǔ-hsin | 蓮子心 | ,,    ,, | ,,    (embryonic shoot) | Embryon Nelumbinis | |
| 0745 Ling-chih (Chê-chih, Ling-chih-ts'ao) | 靈芝(赤芝,靈芝草) | **Ganoderma lucidum (Fomes japonicus)** | *LINGCHIH | *Lingchih | |
| 0746 Ling-chih (Wu-ling-chih) | 靈脂(五靈脂) | — | Bat dung | Excrementum Pteropi | |
| 0747 Ling-hsiang (Ling-hsiang-ts'ao, Ling-ling-hsiang) | 靈香(靈香草,靈陵香) | **Lysimachia foenum-graecum** | *LINGHSIANG, LOOSESTRIFE | Herba Lysimachiae | |
| 0748 Ling-hsiao-hua | 靈霄花(淩霄花) | **Campsis grandiflora** | TRUMPET FLOWER | Flos Campsitis | |

61

| | Transliteration | Chinese | Botanical Name | English | Pharmaceutical |
|---|---|---|---|---|---|
| 0749 | Ling-ts'ao | 苓草 | **Lysimachia foenum-graecum** | LINGHSIANG | Herba Lysimachiae |
| 0750 | Ling-yang-chio (Ling-yang, Sui-ling-yang) | 羚羊角(羚羊,碎羚羊) | — | Antelope horn | Cornu Antelopis |
| 0751 | Liu-chi-nu (Chi-nu) | 劉寄奴(寄奴) | **Artemisia anomala** | ARTEMISIA, MUGWORT | Herba Artemisiae Anomalae |
| 0752 | Liu-chi-shêng | 柳寄生 | **Viscum coloratum** | ASIATIC MISTLETOE | Herba Visci Colorati |
| 0753 | Liu-chih (Liu-yeh, Liu-kên) | 柳枝(柳葉,柳根) | **Salix babylonica** | WILLOW | Ramus Salicis |
| 0754 | Liu-hsin (Wang-pu-liu-hsing) | 留心(王不留行) | **Vaccaria segetalis** | *VACCARIA | Semen Vaccariae |
| 0755 | Liu-huang (T'ien-jan-liu-huang) | 硫黃(天然硫黃) | — | Sulfur | Sulfur |
| 0756 | Liu-lan | 柳蘭 | **Chamaenerion angustifolium** | *CHAMAENERION | Herba Chamaenerii |
| 0757 | Liu-p'i (Shih-liu-p'i) | 榴皮(石榴皮) | **Punica granatum** | POMEGRANATE (rind) | Pericarpium Granati |
| 0758 | Liu-yüeh-hsüeh (Liu-yüeh-shuang) | 六月雪(六月霜) | **Serissa foetida** | *SERISSA | Radix Serissae Foetidae |
| 0759 | Lo-fu-mu | 蘿芙木 | **Rauvolfia verticillata** | SNAKEROOT | Rauvolfia |
| 0760 | Lo-han-kuo | 羅漢果 | Siraitia grosvenori | *LOHANKUO | *Lohankuo |
| 0761 | Lo-hsin-fu | 落新婦 | **Astilbe chinensis** | *Chinese False Goat's Beard | Radix Astilbes Chinensis |

| Transliteration | Chinese | Botanical Name | English | Pharmaceutical | Lo |
|---|---|---|---|---|---|
| 0762 Lo-k'o | 螺殼 | — | Shells of spiral univalves | — | |
| 0763 Lo-lê | 羅勒 | **Ocimum basilicum** | SWEET BASIL | Herba Ocimi Basilici | |
| 0764 Lo-mo-chia (Lo-mo) | 蘿藦荚(蘿藦) | **Metaplexis japonica** | *METAPLEXIS | Fructus Metaplexis | |
| 0765 Lo-po-jên (Lo-po-kên) | 蘿蔔仁(蘿蔔根) | **Raphanus sativus** | CHINESE RADISH | Semen Raphani Radix ,, | |
| | | ,,       ,, | ,,       ,, | | |
| 0766 Lo-pu-ma (Ts'ê-ch'i-ma) | 羅布麻(澤漆麻) | **Apocynum venetum** | DOGBANE | Herba Apocyni | |
| 0767 Lo-shih | 絡石 | **Trachelospermum jasminoides** | STAR JASMINE | Ramus Trachelospermi | |
| 0768 Lo-ti-shêng-kên (Lo-ti) | 落地生根(羅地) | **Bryophyllum pinnatum** | AIRPLANT | Herba Bryophylli | |
| 0769 Lo-ti-ta (P'êng-ta-wan) | 落得打(崩大碗) | **Centella asiatica** | ASIATIC CENTELLA | Herba Centellae Asiaticae | |
| 0770 Lo-wang-tzǔ | 羅望子 | **Tamarindus indicus** | TAMARIND (see 1367) | Fructus Tamarindi | |
| 0771 Lou-jên | 蔞仁 | See Kua-lou-jên | — | — | |
| 0772 Lou-kên (Kua-lou-kên) | 蔞根(括蔞根) | See T'ien-hua-fên | — | — | |
| 0773 Lou-ku (Lou-ku-ch'ung) | 螻蛄(螻蛄虫) | — | Mole Cricket | Gryllotalpa | |
| 0774 Lou-lu | 漏蘆(蘆) | **Rhaponticum uniflorum** | *RHAPONTICUM | Radix Rhapontici | |
| 0775 Lu-chiao (Lu-chio-chiao) | 鹿膠(鹿角膠) | — | Deer horn glue | Colla Cornu Cervi | |
| 0776 Lu-chin | 鹿筋 | — | Deer sinew | Ligamentum Cervi | |

| Transliteration | Chinese | Botanical Name | English | Pharmaceutical | Lu |
|---|---|---|---|---|---|
| 0777 Lu-chio | 鹿角 | — | Deer horn | Cornu Cervi | |
| −a Lu-chio-shuang | 鹿角霜 | — | Refuse of deer horn glue | Cornu Cervi Degelatinatium | |
| 0778 Lu-chio-ying (Shu-wei-hung) | 六角英(鼠尾紅) | **Justicia procumbens** | *JUSTICIA | Herba Justiciae | |
| 0779 Lu-chu-ju | 綠竹茹 | **Phyllostachys nigra** | BAMBOO (shavings) | Caulis Bambusae Taeniam | |
| 0780 Lu-êrh-ling (Lu-êrh-ts'ao) | 鹿耳苓(鹿耳草) | **Laggera alata** | *LAGGERA | Herba Laggerae | |
| 0781 Lu-fan (Ch'ing-fan) | 綠矾(青矾) | — | Green vitriol, Ferrous sulfate | Melanteritum | |
| 0782 Lu-fêng-fang (Ma-fêng-wo) | 露蜂房(馬蜂窩) | — | Hornet nest | Nidus Vespae | |
| 0783 Lu-han-ts'ao (Lu-hsien-ts'ao) | 鹿含草(鹿衡草) | **Pyrola rotundifolia** | PYROLA | Herba Pyrolae | |
| 0784 Lu-hsüeh | 鹿血 | — | Deer blood | Sanguis Cervi | |
| 0785 Lu-hui | 蘆薈(會) | **Aloe barbadensis** or **A. ferox** | MEDICINAL ALOE | Herba Aloes | |
| 0786 Lu-jung | 鹿茸 | — | Young deer horn | Cornu Cervi Parvum | |
| −a Jung-t'ou | 茸頭 | — | Tips of young deer horn | | |
| −b Lu-jung-mo | 鹿茸末 | — | Deer horn powder | | |
| −c Lu-jung-p'ien | 鹿茸片 | — | Shavings of old deer horn | | |
| −d Lu-jung-sui | 鹿茸碎 | — | Broken deer horn | | |
| 0787 Lu-kan-shih (Kan-shih) | 爐甘石(甘石) | — | Calamine, Smithsonite | Calamina, Smithsonitum | |

64

| Transliteration | Chinese | Botanical Name | English | Pharmaceutical |
|---|---|---|---|---|
| 0788 Lu-kên (Lu-ti-kên, Lu-t'ou) | 蘆根(蘆荻根, 蘆頭) | **Phragmites communis P. karka** | REED | Rhizoma Phragmititis |
| 0789 Lu-lêng-chü | 六棱菊 | See Lu-êrh-ling | — | — |
| 0790 Lu-pa (Hu-lu-pa) | 蘆芭(巴)(胡蘆巴) | **Trigonella foenum-graecum** | FENUGREEK | Semen Foenumgraeci |
| 0791 Lu-pien | 鹿鞭 | — | Deer penis | — |
| 0792 Lu-sha | 磠砂 | — | Ammonium chloride | Sal Ammoniacum |
| 0793 Lu-t'ai | 鹿胎 | — | Deer fetus | Embryo Cervi |
| 0794 Lu-tang | 潞黨 | See Tang-shên | | |
| 0795 Lu-tao-kên (Lu-tou-lê) | 蘆刀根(露兜簕) | **Pandanus tectorius** | SCREW PINE | Radix Pandani |
| 0796 Lu-ti-chü (Huang-hua-p'un-chi) | 鹵地菊(黃花蟛蜞) | **Wedelia prostrata** | *WEDELIA | Herba Wedeliae |
| 0797 Lu-tou | 綠豆 | **Phaseolus mungo** | MUNGBEAN | Semen Phaseoli Munginis |
| 0798 Lu-tou-fên | 綠豆粉 | **Phaseolus mungo** | MUNGBEAN (flour) | Farina Phaseoli Munginis |
| 0799 Lu-tou-kên (Lu-tou-lê) | 露兜根(露兜簕) | **Pandanus tectorius** | SCREW PINE | Radix Pandani |
| 0800 Lu-tou-p'i (Tou-i) | 繪豆皮(豆衣) | **Glycine max** | SOYBEAN (husk) | Testa Glycines |
| 0801 Lu-tou-p'i (Lu-tou-i) | 綠豆皮(綠豆衣) | **Phaseolus mungo** | Mungbean (husk) | Testa Phaseoli Mungnis |
| 0802 Lu-wei | 鹿尾 | — | Deer tail | Cauda Cervi |
| 0803 Lü-p'i-chiao (Ah-chiao) | 驢皮膠(阿膠) | — | Donkey hide glue | Colla Asini |

| | Transliteration | Chinese | Botanical Name | English | Pharmaceutical |
|---|---|---|---|---|---|
| 0804 | Lü-pien | 驢鞭 | — | Donkey Penis | — |
| 0805 | Lü-ts'ao (La-la-yang) | 葎草(拉拉秧) | **Humulus scandens (H. japonicus)** | Japanese Hop | Herba Humuli Scandentis |
| 0806 | Luan-hua | 欒華 | **Koelreuteria paniculata** | China Tree | Flos Koelreuteriae |
| 0807 | Lui-kung-t'êng | 雷公藤 | **Tripterygium wilfordii** | *Tripterygium | Ramus Tripterygii wolfordii |
| 0808 | Lui-wan (Chu-ling) | 雷丸(竹苓) | **Polyporus mylittae (Omphalia lapidescens)** | *THUNDER BALL | Polyporus |
| 0809 | Lung-ch'ih | 龍齒 | — | Fossil teeth | Dens Draconis |
| 0810 | Lung-chuan-hua | 龍船花 | **Ixora chinensis** | *IXORA | Radix et Flos Ixorae |
| 0811 | Lung hsü-t'êng | 龍鬚藤 | **Bauhinia championii** | *Champion's Bauhinia | Ramus Bauhiniae Championii |
| —a | Lung-hsü-ts'ai | 龍鬚菜 | **Gracilaria verrucosa** | *DRAGON'S WHISKERS | Herba Gracilariae |
| 0812 | Lung-i | 龍衣 | — | Snake skin | — |
| 0813 | Lung-k'u | 龍骨 | — | Fossil bone | Os Draconis |
| 0814 | Lung-k'uei (K'u-k'uei) | 龍葵(苦葵) | **Solanum nigrum** | NIGHTSHADE | Herba Solani Nigri |
| 0815 | Lung-li-yeh | 龍脷葉 | **Sauropus spatulifolius (S. changiana)** | DRAGON'S TONGUE | Herba Sauropi |
| 0816 | Lung-nao-po-ho | 龍腦薄荷 | **Mentha arvensis** | FIELD MINT | Herba Menthae |
| 0817 | Lung-sê | 龍虱 | — | Giant Water Beetle | Cybister |
| 0818 | Lung-tan-ts'ao (Tan-ts'ao) | 龍膽草(膽草) | **Gentiana scabra** | GENTIAN | Radix Gentianae |
| 0819 | Lung-ya-ts'ao (Hsien-ho-ts'ao) | 龍牙草(仙鶴草) | **Agrimonia pilosa** | AGRIMONY | Herba Agrimoniae |
| 0820 | Lung-yen-hsiang | 龍涎香 | — | Ambergris, Whale spit | Ambra Grisea |

66

| Transliteration | Chinese | Botanical Name | English | Pharmaceutical |
|---|---|---|---|---|
| 0821 Lung-yen-hua | 龍眼花 | **Euphoria longan** | LONGAN (flower) | Flos Longanae |
| −a Lung-yen-jou | 龍眼肉 | ,, ,, | ,, (aril) | Arillus Longanae |
| −b Lung-yen-yeh | 龍眼葉 | ,, ,, | ,, (leaves) | Folium Longanae |
| 0822 Ma-an-t'êng (Ma-t'i-ts'ao, Pin-hai-chien-niu) | 馬鞍藤(馬蹄草, 濱海牽牛) | **Ipomoea pes-caprae** | BEACH MORNING-GLORY | Herba Ipomoeae Pes-capraes |
| 0823 Ma-chia-tzǔ | 馬甲子 | **Paliurus ramosissimus** | *PALIURUS | Radix et Semen Paliuri |
| 0824 Ma-ch'ien-tzǔ (Ma-ch'ien) | 馬錢子(馬前) | **Strychnos nux-vomica S. wallichiana** | NUX-VOMICA | Semen Strychnotis |
| 0825 Ma-ch'ih-hsien | 馬齒莧 | **Portulaca oleracea** | PURSLANE | Herba Portulacae |
| 0826 Ma-fên-pao | 馬糞包 | **Lycoperdon gemmatum** | PUFF-BALL | Fructificatio Lycoperdonis |
| 0827 Ma-hsien-hao (Hu-ma) | 馬先蒿(虎麻) | **Pedicularis resupinata** | *PEDICULARIS | Herba Pedicularis |
| 0828 Ma-huang | 麻黃 | **Ephedra sinica E. equisetina** | MA-HUANG | Herba Ephedrae |
| 0829 Ma-jên (Ta-ma-jên) | 麻仁(大麻仁) | **Cannabis sativa** | HEMP (seeds) | Semen Cannabis |
| 0830 Ma-lan (Ma-lan-t'ou) | 馬蘭(馬蘭頭) | **Kalimeris indica** | *MALAN | Herba Kalimeris |
| 0831 Ma-lin | 馬藺 | **Iris ensata (I. pallassii var. chinensis)** | NORTH CHINA IRIS | Flos et Semen Iridis Ensatae |
| −a Ma-lin-hua | 馬藺花 | **I. ensata** | ,, ,, ,, (flower) | |
| −b Ma-lin-tzǔ (Li-shih) | 馬藺子(蠡實) | ,, ,, | ,, ,, ,, (seed) | |

| Transliteration | Chinese | Botanical Name | English | Pharmaceutical |
|---|---|---|---|---|
| 0832 Ma-nao | 瑪瑙 | — | Agate | Achatum |
| 0833 Ma-pao | 馬寶 | — | Horse Bezoar | Calculus Equi |
| 0834 Ma-pien-ts'ao | 馬鞭草 | **Verbena officinalis** | VERVAIN | Herba Verbenae |
| 0835 Ma-p'o | 馬勃(馬浡) | **Lasiosphaera nipponica** **L. fenzlei** | PUFFBALL | Fructificatio Lasiosphaerae |
| –a  Hui-pao-ma-p'o | 灰包馬勃 | **Lycoperdon perlatum** | | Fructificatio Lycoperdontis |
| –b  Ta-ma-p'o | 大馬勃 | **Calvatia gigantea** | | Fructificatio Calvatiae |
| –c  Tz'ŭ-ma-p'o | 紫馬勃 | **C. lilacina** | | ”          ” |
| 0836 Ma-sang | 馬桑 | **Coriaria sinica** | *CORIARIA | Radix et Ramus Coriariae |
| 0837 Ma-t'ai (Tsou-ma-t'ai) | 馬胎(走馬胎) | **Ardisia gigantifolia** | LARGE-LEAVED ARDISIA | Radix Ardisiae Gigantifoliae |
| 0838 Ma-t'i (Ma-ti-fên, Pi-chi) | 馬蹄(馬蹄粉,荸薺) | **Eleocharis tuberosa** **(Heleocharis dulcis)** | WATER CHESTNUT | Tuber Eleocharitis |
| 0839 Ma-t'i-chin (Huang-tan-ts'ao) | 馬蹄金(黃膽草) | **Dichondra repens** | *DICHONDRA | Herba Dichondrae |
| 0840 Ma-t'i-chüeh (Ma-t'i-kên) | 馬蹄蕨(馬蹄根) | **Angiopteris fokiensis** **A. magna** | *ANGIOPTERIS | Rhizoma Angiopteridis |
| 0841 Ma-t'i-ts'ao (Lü-t'i-ts'ao) | 馬蹄草(驢蹄草) | **Caltha palustris** | MARSH MARIGOLD | Herba Calthae |
| 0842 Ma-tou-ling (Tou-ling) | 馬兜鈴(兜鈴) | **Aristolochia debilis** **A. contorta** | BIRTHWORT | Fructus Aristolochiae |
| 0843 Ma-wei-huang-lien (Tieh-ts'ai-hu) | 馬尾黃蓮(鉄柴胡) | **Thalictrum foliolosum** **T. delavayi** **T. baicalense** | MEADOW-RUE | Caudex Thalictri Foliolosi, Delavayi et Baicalensis |

68

| Transliteration | Chinese | Botanical Name | English | Pharmaceutical |
|---|---|---|---|---|
| 0844 Ma-wei-sung | 馬尾松 | **Pinus massoniana** | SOUTH CHINA PINE | Folium, Radix, Pollen et Resin Pini |
| 0845 Ma-ying-tan (Wu-sê-mei) | 馬纓丹(五色梅) | **Lantana camara** | *LANTANA | Ramus et Flos Lantanae |
| 0846 Mai-chio | 麥角 | **Claviceps purpurea** | ERGOT | Ergota |
| 0847 Mai-hu | 麥斛 | **Bulbophyllum inconspicuum** | *BULBOPHYLLUM | Herba Bulbophylli |
| 0848 Mai-tung (Mai-mên-tung, Mai-tung-su-mien, Su-mien) | 麥冬(麥門冬,麥冬蘇面,蘇面) | **Ophiopogon japonicus** **Liriope spicata** **L. gramifolia** | LILY-TURF | Radix Ophiopogonis, or Radix Liriopis |
| 0849 Mai-ya | 麥芽 | **Hordeum vulgare** or **Triticum aestivum** | BARLEY, or WHEAT (sprouts) | Fructus Hordei vel Tritici Germinantus |
| 0850 Mai-ya-t'ang | 麥芽糖 | — | Maltose | — |
| 0851 Man-ching (Man-ching-tzŭ, Ching-tzŭ) | 蔓荊(蔓荊子,荊子) | **Vitex trifolia,** or **V. rotundifolia** | *SEASHORE VITEx | Fructus Viticis |
| 0852 Man-hu-t'ui-tzŭ | 蔓胡頹子 | **Elaeagnus glabra** **E. pungens** **E. umbellata** | OLEASTER | Ramus et Fructus Elaeagni |
| 0853 Man-shan-hung | 滿山紅 | **Rhododendron dauricum** | DAURIAN RHODODENDRON | Radix et Ramus Rhododendri Daurici |
| 0854 Man-t'o-lo | 曼陀羅 | **Datura metel** | DATURA | Semen, Flos et Folium Daturae Metelis |

| | Transliteration | Chinese | Botanical Name | English | Pharmaceutical |
|---|---|---|---|---|---|
| 0855 | Mang-hsiao | 芒硝 | See P'i-hsiao, Pu-hsiao | Magnesium sulphate fine crystals | Magnesii Sulfuricum |
| 0856 | Mang-kuo-hêh | 芒果核 | **Mangifera indica** | MANGO (stone) | Semen Mangiferae |
| 0857 | Mao-chiang-chün (Mao-shê-hsiang) | 毛將軍(毛麝香) | **Adenosma glutinosum** | *ADENOSMA | Herba Adenosmatis Glutinosi |
| 0858 | Mao-chiang-huang | 毛薑黃 | **Curcuma aromatica** | *CURCUMA | Radix Curcumae |
| 0859 | Mao-hsü-ts'ao | 貓鬚草 | **Orthosiphon aristatus** | *ORTHOSIPHON | Herba Orthosiphonis |
| 0860 | Mao-kên (Pai-mao-kên) | 茅根(白茅根) | **Imperata cylindrica** | WOOLLY GRASS | Rhizoma Imperatae |
| 0861 | Mao-nien | 毛棯 | **Melastoma sanguineum** | *FOX-TONGUE MELASTOMA | Herba Melastomatis Sanguinei |
| 0862 | Mao-shan-shu (Mao-shu) | 毛山朮(毛朮) | See Ts'ang-shu | — | — |
| 0863 | Mao-shao | 毛芍 | See Pai-shao | — | — |
| 0864 | Mao-shê-hsiang | 毛麝香 | **Adenosma glutinosum** | *ADENOSMA | Herba Adenosmatis |
| −a | Mao-shê-hsiang-mo | 毛麝香末 | ,, ,, | ,, (powder) | Pulvis Adenosmatis |
| −b | Mao-shê-hsiang-yeh | 毛麝香葉 | ,, ,, | ,, (leaf) | Folium Adenosmatis |
| 0865 | Mao-tung-ch'ing (Mao-p'i-shu) | 毛冬青(毛披樹) | **Ilex pubescens** | HAIRY HOLLY | Radix et Folia Ilicis Pubescentis |
| 0866 | Mê-t'ou-ts'ao | 墨頭草 See 0398, 0886 | **Eclipta prostrata** | *ECLIPTA, YERBA-DE-TAGO | Herba Ecliptae |
| 0867 | Mei-hua | 梅花 | **Prunus mume** | *MEIHUA (flower) | Flos Pruni Mume |
| −a | Mei-p'i | 梅皮 | ,, ,, | ,, (bark) | Cortex Pruni Mume |
| −b | Mei-tz'ŭ | 梅莿 | ,, ,, | ,, (short shoot) | Spina Pruni Mume |
| 0868 | Mei-jên-chiao | 美人蕉 | **Canna indica** | INDIAN ROOT | Rhizoma Cannae |

| | Transliteration | Chinese | Botanical Name | English | Pharmaceutical |
|---|---|---|---|---|---|
| 0869 | Mei-kuei-hua | 玫瑰花 | **Rosa rugosa** | *MEIKUEI | Flos Rosae Rugosae |
| 0870 | Mên-tung (T'ien-mên-tung) | 門冬(天門冬) | **Asparagus cochin-chinensis or A. lucidus** | *CHINESE ASPARAGUS (root) | Radix Asparagi |
| 0871 | Mêng-ch'ung (Niu-mêng) | 虻虫(牛虻) | — | Gadfly | Tabanus |
| 0872 | Mêng-hua (Mi-mêng-hua) | 蒙花(密蒙花) | **Buddleia officinalis** | BUDDLEIA | Flos Buddleiae |
| 0873 | Mêng-shih | 礞石 | | | |
| | Chin-mêng-shih | 金礞石 | — | Mica-schist | Lapis Micae Aureum |
| | Ch'ing-mêng-shih | 青礞石 | — | Chlorite-schist | Lapis Chloriti |
| | Ming-shih= Ch'ing-mêng-shih | 明石＝青礞石 | | | |
| 0874 | Mi-mêng-hua (Mêng-hua) | 密蒙花(蒙花) | **Buddleia officinalis** | BUDDLEIA | Flos Buddleiae |
| 0875 | Mi-t'ang (Fêng-mi) | 蜜糖 (蜂蜜) | — | Honey | Mel |
| 0876 | Mi-t'o-sêng (T'o-sêng) | 密陀僧(佗僧) | — | Litharge, galena | Lithargyrum |
| 0877 | Mi-tsao | 蜜棗 | **Zizyphus jujuba** | JUJUBE (preserved) | Fructus Zizyphi |
| 0878 | Mi-yin-hua (Chin-yin-hua) | 蜜銀花(金銀花) | **Lonicera japonica** | HONEYSUCKLE (top grade flower) | Flos Lonicerae |
| 0879 | Mien-hua-jên (Mien-hua-tzǔ) | 棉花仁(棉花子) | **Gossypium herbaceum** | COTTON (seed) | Semen Gossypii |
| 0880 | Mien-tsao-êrh (Ti-tsao-tzǔ) | 綿棗兒(地棗子) | **Scilla sinensis** | *SCILLA | Bulbus Scillae |
| 0880A | Ming-cha | 榠樝 | **Chaenomeles, cathayensis** | FLOWERING QUINCE | Fructus Chaenomelis |
| 0881 | Ming (Ch'a) | 茗(茶) | **Camellia sinensis** | TEA | Folium Camelliae |

| | Transliteration | Chinese | Botanical Name | English | Pharmaceutical |
|---|---|---|---|---|---|
| 0882 | Ming-hsiung | 明雄 | — | High grade Realgar | — |
| 0883 | Ming-i (Wu-ming-i, Ming-i-fên) | 名異(無名異，名異粉) | — | Pyrolusite | Pyrolusitum |
| 0884 | Ming-tang (Ming-tang-shên) | 明黨(明黨參) | **Changium smyrnioides** | *MINGTANGSENG | *Radix Mingtangseng |
| 0885 | Mo-chiang (Hou-chiang, Shên-chiang, Hu-chüeh) | 磨薑(猴薑，申薑，槲蕨) | **Drynaria fortunei** | *DRYNARIA | Rhizoma Drynariae |
| 0886 | Mo-han-lien (Li-ch'ang-ts'ao) | 墨旱蓮(鱧腸草) | **Eclipta prostrata** | ECLIPTA | Herba Ecliptae |
| 0887 | Mo-ku | 蘑菇 | **Agaricus bisporus** | *MOKU | Fructificatio Agarici Bispori |
| 0888 | Mo-li-hua | 茉莉花 | **Jasminum sambac** | SAMBAC | Flos Jasmini Sambac |
| 0889 | Mo-p'an-ts'ao (Ch'ing-ma) | 磨盤草(茼麻) | **Abutilon indicum A. theophrastii** | *ABUTILON | Herba et Semen Abutilonis |
| 0890 | Mo-yü-ku (Hai-p'iao-shao) | 墨魚骨(海螵蛸) | — | Bone of squid | Os Sepiae |
| 0891 | Mou-ching | 牡荊 | **Vitex negundo** | VITEX | Semen Viticis Negundinis |
| 0892 | Mou-li (Mou-li-k'o, Hao-k'o) | 牡蠣(牡蠣殼，蠔殼) | — | Oyster shell | Concha Ostreae |
| 0893 | Mou-tan-p'i (Tan-p'i) | 牡丹皮(丹皮) | **Paeonia suffruticosa** | TREE PEONY, MOUTAN | Cortex Moutan |
| 0894 | Mu-chin-hua) (Mu-chin-tzŭ) | 木槿花(木槿子) | **Hibiscus syriacus** | ROSR-OF-SHARON | Flos et semen Hibisci Syriaci |
| 0894A | Mu-erh, (Yün-erh) | 木耳(雲耳) | **Auricularia aricula-judas** | AURICULARIA, WOOD-EAR | Fructificatio Auriculariae |
| 0895 | Mu-fang-chi | 木防己 | **Cocculus orbiculatus** | *COCCULUS | Radix Cocculi |

| | Transliteration | Chinese | Botanical Name | English | Pharmaceutical | Mu |
|---|---|---|---|---|---|---|
| 0896 | Mu-fu-jung (Fu-jung) | 木芙蓉(芙蓉) | **Hibiscus mutibilis** | Cotton Rose | Ramus et Flos Hibisci Mutabilis | |
| 0897 | Mu-hsiang | 木香 | See the following | *MUHSIANG, COSTUS | Radix Muhsiang | |
| —a | Ch'uan-mu-hsiang | 川木香 | **Dolomiaea souliei** | CHUANMUHSIANG, | Radix Dolomiaeae | |
| —b | Kuang-mu-hsiang | 廣木香 | **Aucklandia lappa (Saussurea lappa)** | KUANGMUHSIANG | Radix Aucklandiae | |
| 0898 | Mu-hu (Shui-hu, Kan-mu-hu) | 木斛(水斛, 乾木斛) | **Dendrobium nobile D. aduncum, D. chrysanthum,** and others growing on trees | *MUHU | Ramus Dendrobii | |
| 0899 | Mu-hu-tieh (Ch'ien-chang-chih) | 木蝴蝶(千張紙) | **Oroxylum indicum** | *OROXYLUM | Semen Oroxyli | |
| 0900 | Mu-huan-tzŭ (Mu-yüan-tzŭ, Wu-huan-tzŭ) | 木槵子(木圓子, 無槵子) | **Sapindus mukorosii** | SOAPBERRY | Fructus Sapindi | |
| | Mu-huan-jou | 木槵肉 | ,,    ,, | ,,    (pericarp) | Pericarpium Sapindi | |
| | Mu-huan-kên | 木槵根 | ,,    ,, | ,,    (root) | Radix Sapindi | |
| 0901 | Mu-kua | 木瓜 | **Chaenomeles cathayensis (C. sinensis)** | CHINESE QUINCE | Fructus Chaenomelis | |
| | Mu-kua-chiu | 木瓜酒 | ,,    ,, | (tincture) of Chinese quince | — | |
| | Mu-kua-kan | 木瓜乾 | ,,    ,, | (dried) Chinese quince | — | |
| 0902 | Mu-mien-hua (Mu-mien-kên) | 木棉花(木棉根) | **Bombax ceiba** | TREE COTTON | Radix et Flos Bombacis | |
| 0903 | Mu-pieh-tzŭ | 木鼈子(木鱉子) | **Momordica cochinchinensis** | *VEGETABLE TURTLE (seeds) | Semen Momordicae | |

| Transliteration | Chinese | Botanical Name | English | Pharmaceutical |
|---|---|---|---|---|
| 0904 Mu-shih-tzŭ (Mu-shih-tzŭ, Mo-shih-tzŭ, Wu-shih-tzŭ) | 沒石子(沒食子,墨石子,無食子) | **Quercus infectoria** | OAK (insect gall) | Galla Turcica |
| 0905 Mu-ting-hsiang | 母丁香 | **Syzygium aromaticum (Eugenia caryophyllata)** | CLOVE (fruit) | Fructus Caryophylli |
| 0906 Mu-tou-hui | 墓頭回 | **Ixeris denticulata** | *IXERIS | Herba Ixeris |
| 0907 Mu-ts'ao (P'u-ti-lien) | 母草(鋪地蓮) | **Lindernia crustacea** | *CRUSTACEOUS PIMPERNEL | Herba Linderniae |
| 0908 Mu-tsei (Mu-tsei-ts'ao) | 木賊(木賊草) | **Equisetum hiemale** | SCOURING RUSH | Herba Equiseti |
| 0909 Mu-t'ung (Huai-t'ung) | 木通(淮通) | **Akebia quinata** and **Aristolochia mandshuriensis** | *MUTUNG | Caulis Mutung |
| 0910 Mu-yao | 沒藥 | **Commiphora myrrha** | MYRRH | Myrrha |
| 0911 Nai-jên (Nei-jên, Nai-jên-jou) | 奈仁(內仁,奈仁肉) | **Prinsepia uniflora** | *PRINSEPIA | Semen Princepiae |
| 0912 Nan-chu-tzŭ | 南竹子 | **Vaccinium bracteatum** | *ASIATIC BILBERRY | Fructus Vaccinii |
| 0913 Nan-hsing (T'ien-nan-hsing) | 南星(天南星) | **Arisaema consanguineum** **A. heterophyllum** and many other species | JACK-IN-THE-PULPIT | Rhizoma Arisaematis |
| 0914 Nan-huo-hsiang | 南藿香 | **Agastache rugosa** | AGASTACHE | Nanhuohsiang |
| 0915 Nan-kua-t'i (Kua-t'i) | 南瓜蒂(瓜蒂) | **Cucurbita moschata** | SQUASH (stalk) | Pedicellus Cucurbitae |

| Transliteration | Chinese | Botanical Name | English | Pharmaceutical |
|---|---|---|---|---|
| 0916 Nan-kua-tzǔ | 南瓜子 | **Cucurbita moschata** | SQUASH (seed) | Semen Cucurbitae |
| 0917 Nan-sha-shên | 南沙参 | **Adenophora tetraphylla** | ADENOPHORA | Radix Adenophorae |
| —a Ch'uan-tsang-sha shên | 川藏沙参 | **A. lilifolioides** | | |
| —b Hsien-ch'ih-sha-shên | 縫齒沙参 | **A. capillaris** | | |
| —c Hsing-yeh-sha-shên | 杏葉沙参 | **A. axilliflora** | | |
| —d K'uo-yeh-sha-shên | 濶葉沙参 | **A. pereskiaefolia** | | |
| —e Lun-yeh-sha-shên | 輪葉沙参 | **A. tetraphylla (A. verticillata)** | | |
| —f P'ao-sha-shên | 泡沙参 | **A. potaninii** | | |
| —g T'êng-chih-sha-shên | 挺枝沙参 | **A. stricta** | | |
| —h Tsao-yeh-sha-shên | 糙葉沙参 | **A. polyantha** | | |
| —i Yunnan-sha-shên | 雲南沙参 | **A. bulleyana** | | |
| 0918 Nan-shê-lê | 南蛇籬 | **Caesalpinia minax** | *SNAKE BRAMBLE | Radix Caesalpiniae Minacis |
| 0919 Nan-shê-t'êng | 南蛇藤 | **Celastrus orbiculatus** | BITTERSWEET | Ramus Celastris |
| 0919A Nan-tan-shên | 南丹参 | **Salvia bowleygna** | SOUTHERN SAGE | Radix Salviae Bowleygnae |
| 0920 Nan-t'êng (Ting-kung-t'êng, Fêng-t'êng) | 南藤（丁公藤，風藤） | **Piper wallichii** **P. puberulum** | SHIHNANTENG | Herba Piperis |
| 0921 Nan-t'ien-chu | 南天竺 | **Nandina domestica** | NANDINA | Fructus Nandinae |
| 0922 Nao-sha (Lu-sha) | 硇砂（磠砂） | | Halite or Sal ammoniac | Halitum Violaceum Sal Ammoniacum |

| Transliteration | Chinese | Botanical Name | English | Pharmaceutical |
|---|---|---|---|---|
| —a Tzǔ-nao-sha | 紫硇砂 | | Purple Halite | |
| —b Pai-nao-sha | 白硇砂 | | White Sal ammoniac | |
| 0923 Nao-yang-hua | 鬧羊花 | **Rhododendron molle** | *YELLOW AZALEA (flower) | Flos et fructus |
| —a Nao-yang-hua-shih | 鬧羊花實 | ,,　　　,, | | Rhododendri mollis |
| 0924 Nei-chin (Chi-nei-chin) | 內金(鷄內金) | — | Chicken gizzard lining | Corium Stomachichum Galli |
| 0925 Ngo-shu | 莪朮 | **Curcuma zedoaria** | ZEDOARY | Rhizoma Curcumae |
| 0926 Niao-pu-su (Hai-tung-p'i, Niao-pu-ta) | 鳥不宿(海桐皮，鳥不踏) | **Kalopanax septemlobus (K. pictus)** | *KALOPANAX | Ramus Kalopanacis |
| 0927 Nien-chien (Ch'ien-nien-chien) | 年健(千年健) | **Homalomena occulta** | *HOMALOMENA | Rhizoma Homalomenae |
| 0928 Niu-chiao-sui (Niu-chiao-sai) | 牛角碎(牛角腮) | — | Broken ox horn | Os in Cornu Bovis |
| 0929 Niu-êrh-fêng | 牛耳楓 | **Daphniphyllum calycinum** | *DAPHNIPHYLLUM | Radix et Folium Daphniphylli |
| 0930 Niu-fang (Niu-p'ang-tzǔ) | 牛房(牛蒡子) | **Arctium lappa** | BURDOCK | Fructus Bardanae |
| 0931 Niu-hsi | 牛膝 | **Achyranthes bidentata** | *ACHYRANTHES | Radix Achyranthis |
| —a Ch'uan-niu-hsi | 川牛膝 | **Cyathula capitata** | *CYATHULA | Radix Caythulae |
| —b T'u-niu-hsi | 土牛膝 | **Achyranthes aspera** | *TUNIUHSI | Radix Achyranthis Asperae |
| 0932 Niu-huang | 牛黃 | — | Ox or buffalo gall stone | Bezoar, Calculus Bovis |
| 0933 Niu-ku-sui | 牛骨碎 | — | Broken buffalo bone | — |
| 0934 Niu-mêng (Fei-mêng) | 牛虻(蜚虻) | — | Gadfly | Tabanus |

| | Transliteration | Chinese | Botanical Name | English | Pharmaceutical | Niu |
|---|---|---|---|---|---|---|
| 0935 | Niu-niu-t'êng | 扭扭藤 | **Jasminum amplexicaule** | HAIRY JASMINE | Herba Jasmini Amplexi-caulis | |
| 0936 | Niu-p'ang-tzŭ (Niu-tzŭ, Ta-li-tzŭ) | 牛蒡子(牛旁子, 牛子, 大力子) | **Arctium lappa** | BURDOCK | Fructus Bardanae | |
| 0937 | Niu-p'i-hsiao (Kê-shan-hsiao) | 牛皮消(隔山消) | **Cynanchum wilfordii (C. caudatum)** | *CYNANCHUM | Radix Cynanchi Wilfordii | |
| 0938 | Niu-pien | 牛鞭 | — | Ox or buffalo penis | Testis et Penis Bovis vel Bubali | |
| 0939 | Niu-ta-li | 牛大力 | **Millettia speciosa** | *NIUTALI | Radix Millettiae Speciosae | |
| 0940 | Niu-tan | 牛膽 | — | Ox gall | Fel Bovis | |
| 0941 | No-tao-kên | 糯稻根 | **Oryza glutinosa** | Glutinous Rice (root) | Radix Oryzae Glutinosae | |
| 0942 | Nü-chên (Nü-chên-tzŭ) | 女貞(女貞子) | **Ligustrum lucidum L. japonicum** | PRIVET | Fructus Ligustri | |
| 0943 | O-chiao (Ching-chiao) | 阿膠(京膠) | — | Ass hide glue | Gelatinum Asini | |
| 0944 | O-chüeh-pan | 鵝腳板 | **Pimpinella diversifolia** | CHINESE ANISE | Herba Pimpinellae | |
| 0945 | O-kuan-shih (Chung-ju-shih) | 鵝管石(鐘乳石) | — | Tubular stalactites | Stalactitum | |
| 0946 | O-ling (T'u-san-lêng) | 莪苓(土三稜) | **Curcuma kwangsiensis C. zedoaria** | *OLING | Tuber Curcumae | |
| 0947 | O-pu-shih-ts'ao | 鵝不食草(不食草) | **Centipeda minima** | *CENTIPEDA | Herba Centipedae | |
| 0947A | O-shên, (Chin-shan-t'ien-ch'i) | 峨參(金山田七) | **Anthriscus, sylvestris** | COW PARSLEY | Radix Anthrisci | |
| 0948 | O-shu (O-ling, Kuang-o-shu) | 莪朮(莪苓, 廣莪朮) | **Curcuma zedoaria C. kwangsiensis** | ZEDOARY | Rhizoma Zedoariae | |

77

| | Transliteration | Chinese | Botanical Name | English | Pharmaceutical |
|---|---|---|---|---|---|
| 0949 | Ou-chieh (Ou-fên, Ou-p'ien) | 藕節(藕粉, 藕片) | **Nelumbo nucifera** | SACRED LOTUS | Rhizoma et Farina Nelumbinis |
| 0950 | Pa-chi (Pa-chi-t'ien, Chi-ch'ang-fêng, Pa-chi-jou, Chi-jou) | 巴戟(巴戟天, 鷄腸楓, 巴戟肉, 戟肉) | **Morinda officinalis** | *MORINDA | Radix Morindae |
| 0951 | Pa-chio (Ta-hui-hsiang) | 八角(大茴香) | **Illicium verum** | STAR ANISE | Fructus Anisi Stellati |
| 0952 | Pa-chio-fêng | 八角楓 | **Alangium chinense** | *ALANGIUM | Radix et Ramus Alangii |
| 0953 | Pa-chio-lien (Pa-chio-chin-p'an-yeh, Pa-chio-yeh) | 八角蓮(八角金盤葉, 八角葉) | **Dysosma pleiantha** | *DYSOSMA | Radix Dysosmatis |
| 0954 | Pa-tan (Tan-p'i) | 杷丹(丹皮) | **Paeonia suffruticosa** | TREE PEONY | Cortex Moutan |
| 0955 | Pa-tou (Ch'uan-pa, Chiang-tzŭ, Tou-jên) | 巴豆(川巴, 江子, 豆仁) | **Croton tiglium** | CROTON | Semen Tiglii |
| 0955A | Pa-tou-shuang | 巴豆霜 | **Croton tiglium** | DETOXIFIED-CRACKED CROTON | Semen Tiglii Detoxicati |
| 0955B | Pa-wang-pien | 霸王鞭 | **Hylocereus undatus** | NIGHT-BLOOMING CEREUS | Flos Hylocerei |
| 0956 | Pa-yeh (P'i-pa-yeh) | 杷葉(枇杷葉) | **Eriobotrya japonica** | LOQUAT (leaves) | Folium Eriobotryae |
| 0957 | Pa-yüeh-cha (Mu-tung-shih) | 八月扎(木通實) | **Akebia quinata** | *AKEBIA | Fructus Akebiae |
| 0958 | Pai-ch'ang (Ch'ang-p'u) | 白菖(菖蒲) | **Acorus calamus** | CALAMUS | Rhizoma Calami |
| 0959 | Pai-chi (Pai-chi-êrh) | 白芨(白鷄兒) | **Bletilla striata** | BLETILLA | Rhizoma Bletillae |
| 0960 | Pai-chi-li (Pai-chi) | 白蒺藜(白蒺) | **Tribulus terrestris** | CALTROP | Fructus Tribuli |

| | Transliteration | Chinese | Botanical Name | English | Pharmaceutical |
|---|---|---|---|---|---|
| 0961 | Pai-ch'i (Huang-ch'i) | 白芪(黃芪) | **Astragalus membrana-ceus** | MILK-VETCH | Radix Astragali |
| 0962 | Pai-chiang-ts'ao | 敗醬草 | **Sonchus brachyotus** **Thlaspi arvense** | SNOW-THISTLE PENNY CRESS | *Herba Sonchi Brachyot Herba Thlaspi |
| 0963 | Pai-chiao-hsiang (Fêng-hsiang-chih) | 白膠香(楓香脂) | **Liquidambar formosana** | CHINESE SWEET-GUM | Resina Liquidambaris |
| 0964 | Pai-chieh-tzŭ | 白芥子 | **Brassica hirta** | WHITE MUSTARD | Semen Sinapis |
| 0965 | Pai-ch'ien | 白前 | **Cynanchum stauntonii** | *PAICHIEN | Radix Cynanchi Stauntonii |
| 0966 | Pai-ch'ien-ts'êng | 白千層 | **Melaleuca leucadendron** | *MELALEUCA | Ramus Melaleucae |
| 0967 | Pai-chih (Hsiang-pai-chih, Hang-pai-chih, Ch'uan-pai-chih) | 白芷(香白芷,杭白芷, 川白芷) | **Angelica anomala** or **A. dahurica** | FRAGRANT ANGELICA | Radix Angelicae |
| 0968 | Pai-chih-shan | 白紙扇 | **Mussaenda pubescens** | *MUSSAENDA | Ramux Mussaendae |
| 0969 | Pai-ch'ou | 白丑 | See Êrh-ch'ou | — | |
| 0970 | Pai-ch'ü-ts'ai | 白屈菜 | **Chelidonium majus** | CELANDINE | Herba Chelidonii |
| 0971 | Pai-fan (Ming-fan) | 白礬(明矾) | — | Common alum, White vitriol | Alumen, Alunitum |
| 0972 | Pai-fu (Pai-fu-tzŭ, Yü-pai-fu) | 白附(白附子,禹白附) | **Typhonium giganteum** | *GIANT TYPHONIUM | Rhizoma Typhonii |
| −a | Kuan-pai-fu | 關白附 | **Aconitum coreanum** | *KOREAN ACONITE | Rhizoma Coreani |
| 0973 | Pai-ho (Pai-ho-fên) | 百合(百合粉) | **Lilium brownii** **L. concolor** **L. pumilum** | LILY (bulbs) | Bulbus et Farina Lilii |

| | Transliteration | Chinese | Botanical Name | English | Pharmaceutical |
|---|---|---|---|---|---|
| 0974 | Pai-ho-ling-chih (Hsüan-ts'ao) | 白鶴靈芝(癬草) | **Rhinacanthus nasutus** | *RHINACANTHUS | Herba Rhinacanthi |
| 0975 | Pai-ho-t'êng | 白鶴藤 | **Argyreia acuta** | ARGYREIA | Herba Argyreiae |
| 0976 | Pai-hsien (Pai-hsien-p'i, Hsien-p'i, Hsi-p'i) | 白蘚(白蘚皮,鮮皮,洗皮) | **Dictamnus dasycarpus** | Chinese Dittany | Radix Dictamni |
| 0977 | Pai-hua-hao (Ya-chüeh-ai) | 白花蒿(鴨腳艾) | **Artemisia lactiflora** | *DUCK-FOOT MUGWORT | Herba Artemisiae Lactiflorae |
| 0978 | Pai-hua-shê | 白花蛇 | — | Agkistrodon or *White band krait | Bungarus Parvus |
| 0979 | Pai-hua-shê-shê-ts'ao | 白花蛇舌草 | **Hedyotis diffusa (Oldenlandia diffusa)** | *SPREADING HEDYOTIS | Herba Hedyotis Diffusae |
| 0980 | Pai-hua-tan | 白花丹 | **Plumbago zeylanica** | *PLUMBAGO | Radix et Folium Plumbaginis |
| 0981 | Pai-hua-ts'ai (Yang-chiao-ts'ai) | 白花菜(羊角菜) | **Cleome gynandra** | *CLEOME | Herba Cleomes |
| 0982 | Pai-jên (Pai-tzǔ-jên, Pien-pai-tzǔ) | 柏仁(柏子仁,扁柏子) | **Thuja orientalis (Biota orientalis)** | ARBOR-VITAE | Semen Thujae |
| 0983 | Pai-jui-ts'ao | 百蕊草 | **Thesium chinensis** | *THESIUM | Herba Thesii |
| 0984 | Pai-kuei-mu | 白桂木 | **Artocarpus hypargyraeus** | ARTOCARPUS | Radis et Fructus Artocarpi |
| 0985 | Pai-kuo | 白果 | **Ginkgo biloba** | PAIKUO, GINKGO | Semen Ginkginis |
| 0986 | Pai-la (Ch'ung-pai-la) | 白蠟(虫白腊) | — | Insect white wax | Cera Chinensis |

| | Transliteration | Chinese | Botanical Name | English | Pharmaceutical |
|---|---|---|---|---|---|
| 0987 | Pai-la-shu-p'i | 白蠟樹皮 | **Fraxinus chinensis** | CHINESE ASH (bark) | Cortex Frazini Chinensis |
| 0988 | Pai-lan-hua | 白蘭花 | **Michelia alba** | *MICHELIA | Flos Micheliae |
| 0989 | Pai-lien | 白蘞 | **Ampelopsis japonica** | AMPELOPSIS | Radix Ampelopsis |
| 0990 | Pai-ma-ku (Man-t'ien-hsing) | 白馬骨(滿天星) | **Serissa serissoides** | *SERISSA | Ramus Serissae |
| 0991 | Pai-mao-hsia-k'u-ts'ao (Chin-ku-ts'ao) | 白毛夏枯草(筋骨草) | **Ajuga decumbens** | BUGLEWEED | Herba Ajugae |
| 0992 | Pai-mao-kên | 白茅根 | **Imperata cylindrica** | WOOLLY GRASS | Rhizoma Imperatae |
| 0993 | Pai-mei (Yên-mei, Shuang-mei) | 白梅(鹽梅,霜梅) | **Prunus mume** | MEI FRUIT (salted) | *Paimei vel Shuangmei |
| 0994 | Pai-mei-hua | 白梅花 | **Prunus mume** | MAIHUA (white) | Flos Pruni Mumes |
| 0995 | Pai-mo (K'ou-mo) | 白磨(口蘑) | **Tricholoma mongolicum** | *PAIMO | Fructificatio Tricholomatis |
| 0996 | Pai-mu (Chi-luan-huang) | 白木(鷄卵黃) | **Micromelum falcatum** | *MICROMELUM | Radix et Cortex Micromeli |
| 0997 | Pai-mu-êrh (Yin-êrh) | 白木耳(銀耳) | **Tremella fuciformis** | *SILVER EAR | Fructificatio Tremellae |
| 0998 | Pai-mu-t'ung | 白木通 | **Akebia trifoliata** | AKEBIA | Ramus Akebiae |
| 0999 | Pai-niu-tan (Shan-pai-chih, Mao-ch'a) | 白牛膽(山白芷,毛茶) | **Inula cappa** | *GOAT-EAR ELECAMPANE | Ramus Inula Cappae |
| 1000 | Pai-niu-t'êng | 白牛藤 | **Hedyotis hedyotidea (Oldenlandia hedyotidea)** | WHITE OX-CREEPER | Radix et Ramus Hedyotis Hedyotideae |

| Transliteration | Chinese | Botanical Name | English | Pharmaceutical |
|---|---|---|---|---|
| 1001 Pai-pan-fêng-ho | 白半楓荷 | **Dendropanax proteus** | *Dendropanax | Radix Dentropanacis |
| 1002 Pai-p'i-san-ch'i | 白背三七 | **Gynura divaricata** | *Gynura | Herba Gynurae Divaricatae |
| 1003 Pai-p'i-yeh | 白背葉 | **Mallotus apelta** | *Mallotus | Radix et Ramus Malloti |
| 1004 Pai-pien-tou | 白扁豆(白藊豆) | **Dolichos lablab** | Hyacinth Bean | Semen Dolichoris |
| 1005 Pai-pu | 百部 | **Stemona japonica, S. sessilifolia, S. tuberosa** | Stemona | Radix Stemonae |
| 1006 Pai-pu-shê | 百步蛇 | — | Paipu Snake | Agkistrodon |
| 1007 Pai-shao (Pai-shao-yao) | 白芍(白芍藥) | **Paeonia lactiflora** | Peony | Radix Paeoniae Lactiflorae |
| 1008 Pai-shih-ying | 白石英 | — | Quartz | Quartz Album |
| 1009 Pai-shou-wu Ke-shan-hsiao | 白首烏,隔山消 | **Cynanchum auriculatum, C. bungei** | *Paishouwu | Radix Cynanchi Auriculati |
| 1010 Pai-shu | 白朮 | **Atractylodes macro-cephala** | *Paichu | Rhizoma Atractylodis Macrocephalae |
| Chun-shu | 種朮 ⎫ | | | |
| P'ing-shu | 平朮 ⎪ | | | |
| Shêng-shu | 生朮 ⎪ | | | |
| Tung-shu | 冬朮 ⎬ | | | |
| T'u-shu | 土朮 ⎪ | | Common market forms | |
| Wu-shu | 吳朮 ⎪ | | | |
| Yüan-shu | 元朮 ⎪ | | | |
| Yün-shu | 雲朮 ⎭ | | | |

| Transliteration | Chinese | Botanical Name | English | Pharmaceutical |
|---|---|---|---|---|
| Pai-shu (*cont.*) | | | | |
|   Yü-shu | 於术 | | Superior form from Yü-chien, Chekiang | |
|   Liao-shu | 料术 | | Inferior form | |
| 1011 Pai-shu-liang (Shu-liang) | 日薯莨 (薯莨) | **Dioscorea hispida** | *SHULIANG | Tuber Dioscoreae Hispidae |
| 1012 Pai-su-tzǔ | 白蘇子 | **Perilla frutescens** | *PERILLA | Semen Perillae |
| 1012A Pai-t'ang, Ping-t'ang | 白糖, 冰糖 | **Saccharum officinarum** | SUGAR, ROCK SUGAR | Saccharum |
| 1013 Pai-ting-hsiang | 白丁香 | — | Sparrow excrement | Faeces Passerum |
| 1014 Pai-tou (Fan-tou, Mei-tou) | 白豆 (飯豆, 眉豆) | **Vigna cylindrica** | COWPEA | Semen Vignae Cylindricae |
| 1015 Pai-tou-k'ou, | 白豆蔻 | **Amomum krervanh** | KRERVANH | Fructus Amomi Krervanh |
| —a Hsiao-tou-k'ou | 小豆蔻 See 475 | **Elettaria cardamomum** | CARDAMOM | Fructus Elettariae |
| 1016 Pai-t'ou-wêng | 白頭翁 | **Pulsatilla chinensis** | CHINESE ANEMONE | Radix Pulsatillae |
| 1017 Pai-ts'ao-shuang (Kuo-ti-hui) | 百草霜 (鍋底灰) | — | Soot from the bottom of a boiler | Pulvis Fumi Carbonisatus |
| 1018 Pai-tsu (Wu-kung) | 百足 (蜈蚣) | — | Centipede | Scolopendra |
| 1019 Pai-tzǔ-jên | 柏子仁 | **Thuja orientalis (Biota orientalis)** | ARBOR-VITAE | Semen Thujae |
| 1020 Pai-wei | 白薇 | **Cynanchum atratum** | *CYNANCHUM | Radix Cynanchi Atrati |
| 1021 Pai-yang-chih (Pai-yang-p'i, Pai-yang-yeh) | 白楊枝 (白楊皮, 白楊葉) | **Populus davidiana** | DAVID'S POPLAR | Cortex, Ramus et Folium Populi Davidianae |
| 1022 Pai-yao | 白藥 | **Millettia lasiopetala** | *PAIYAO | Radix Millettiae Lasiopetalae |
| 1023 Pai-yao-tzǔ (Chin-hsien-tao-wu-kuei) | 白藥子 (金線吊烏龜) | **Stephania cepharantha** | *STEPHANIA | Radix Stephaniae Cepharanthae |

| | Transliteration | Chinese | Botanical Name | English | Pharmaceutical |
|---|---|---|---|---|---|
| 1024 | Pai-ying (Shu-yang-ch'üan) | 白英(蜀羊泉) | **Solanum lyratum** | CLIMBING NIGHTSHADE | Herba Solani Lyrati |
| 1025 | Pai-ying-shih (Pai-shih-ying) | 白英石(白石英) | — | Common quartz | Quartz Album |
| 1026 | Pai-yu-wei (Po-k'u-tan) | 白魚尾(駁骨丹) | **Buddleia asiatica** | BUDDLEIA | Radix Buddleiae Asiaticae |
| 1027 | Pai-yün-hsiang (Ta-yün-hsiang, Fêng-hsiang-chih) | 白芸香(大芸香,楓香脂) | **Liquidambar formosana** | CHINESE SWEET GUM | Resina Liquidambaris |
| 1028 | P'ai-chien-ts'ao | 排錢草 | **Desmodium pulchellum** | *STRING-OF-COIN | Radix Desmodii Pulchelli |
| 1029 | Pan-chih-lien (Ping-t'ou-ts'ao) | 半枝蓮(并頭草) | **Scutellaria barbata** | *PANCHIHLIEN | Herba Scutellariae barbatae |
| 1030 | Pan-fêng-ho | 半楓荷 | **Pterospermum heterophyllum** | *PANFENGHO | Radix Pterospermi |
| 1031 | Pan-hsia | 半夏 | **Pinellia ternata** | *PANHSIA | Rhizoma Pinelliae |
| | Pan-hsia-ch'ü | 半夏麴 | „ „ | *Panhsia preparation | „ „ |
| | Pan-hsia-mo | 半夏末 | „ „ | Powdered Panhsia | „ „ |
| | Pan-hsia-p'ien | 半夏片 | „ „ | Sliced Panhsia | „ „ |
| 1032 | Pan-kên | 斑根 | **Polygonum cuspidatum** | BUSHY KNOTWEED | Radix Polygoni Cuspidati |
| 1033 | Pan-lan-kên | 板藍根 | **Isatis tinctoria** I. indigotica | WOAD | Radix Isatidis |
| 1034 | Pan-mao | 斑蝥 | — | Cantharides | Mylabris |
| 1035 | Pan-pien-ch'i | 半邊旗 | **Pteris semipinnata** | *PANPIENCHI | Herba Pteridis Semipinnatae |

84

| Transliteration | Chinese | Botanical Name | English | Pharmaceutical |
|---|---|---|---|---|
| 1036 Pan-pien-lien | 半邊蓮 | **Lobelia chinensis** | CHINESE LOBELIA | Herba Lobeliae chinensis |
| 1037 Pan-p'o (Ch'ai-p'o, Hou-p'o, Tzŭ-p'o) | 板朴(柴朴,厚朴,紫朴) | **Magnolia officinalis** | MAGNOLIA (bark) | Cortex Magnoliae |
| 1038 P'an-lung-shên | 盤龍參 | **Spiranthes sinensis** | SPIRANTHES | Radix Spiranthis |
| 1039 Pang-hua | 蚌花 | **Rhoeo discolor** | RHOEO | Herba et Flos Rhoeinis |
| 1040 Pang-k'o | 蚌殼 | — | Clam shell | Concha Anodontae |
| 1041 Pang-pang-mu (Pang-tzŭ-shu) | 棒棒木(棒子樹) | **Celtis bungeana** | *BUNGE'S HACKBERRY | Ramus Celtis Bungeanae |
| 1042 Pang-ta-hai (P'êng-ta-hai) | 胖大海(蓬大海) | **Scaphium affines** (Sterculia scaphigera S. lunchnophera) | *PANGTAHAI, BUNGTALAI (Siamese) | Semen Scaphii |
| 1043 Pao-ku | 豹骨 | — | Leopard bone | Os Leopardi |
| 1044 Pao-ma-tzŭ (Pai-ting-ch'ing) | 暴馬子(白丁青) | **Syringa reticulata** (S. amurensis) | AMUR LILAC | Cortex et Ramus Syringae Reticulatae |
| 1045 Pei-ch'i (Huang-ch'i) | 北芪(黃芪) | **Astragalus mongholicus** | Northern Huangchi | Radix Huangchi |
| 1046 Pei-fu (Ch'ao-fu-p'ien) | 焙附(炒附片) | See Fu-tzŭ | — | — |
| 1047 Pei-ho-sê | 北鶴虱 | **Daucus carota** | CARROT (fruit) | Fructus Carotae |
| 1048 Pei-hsieh (Shan-pei-hsieh, Pei-kai) | 萆薢(山萆薢,萆荄) | **Dioscorea tokoro** **D. futschauensis** | FISH-POISON YAM | *Rhizoma Peihsieh |
| Ch'uan-pei-hsieh | 川萆薢 | | From Szechuan | |
| Ch'uan-t'ai-p'ien | 川太片 | | „    „ | |
| T'u-pei-hsieh (T'u-p'ien) | 土萆薢(土片) | | Local product | |

| | Transliteration | Chinese | Botanical Name | English | Pharmaceutical |
|---|---|---|---|---|---|
| 1049 | Pei-hsin (Hsi-hsin) | 北辛(細辛) | **Asarum sieboldii** | WILD GINGER | Rhizoma Asari |
| 1050 | Pei-ma (Pei-ma-tzŭ, Pei-ma-yeh, Pei-ma-yu) | 萆麻(萆麻子,萆麻葉,萆麻油) | **Ricinus communis** | CASTOR-OIL PLANT (seed, oil) | Herba, Semen, et Oleum Ricini |
| 1051 | Pei-mu | 貝母 | **Fritillaria** spp. | FRITILLARY | Bulbus Fritillariae |
| —a | Chê-pei (Chia-pei-mu, Hsiang-pei, T'u-pei) | 浙貝(假貝母,象貝,土貝) | **F. thunbergii** | Chekiang Fritillary | |
| —b | Ch'uan-pei (Chên-pei-mu) | 川貝(眞貝母) | **F. cirrhosa** **F. roylei** | West China Fritillary | |
| —c | I-pei | 伊貝 | **F. walujewii** **F. pallidiflora** | | |
| —d | P'ing-pei | 平貝 | **F. ussuriensis** | North China Fritillary | |
| —e | Lu-pei | 蘆貝 | **F. przewalskii** **F. delavayi** | | |
| 1052 | Pei-sha-shên | 北沙參 | **Glehnia littoralis** | BEACH SILVER-TOP | Radix Glehniae |
| 1053 | Pei-shan-tou-kên (Shan-tou-kên, Pien-fu-ko-kên) | 北山豆根(山豆根,蝙蝠葛根) | **Menispermum dauricum** | SIBERIAN MOONSEED | Radix Menispermi |
| 1054 | Pei-tzŭ | 倍子 | See Wu-pei-tzŭ | — | — |
| 1056 | Pei-tz'ŭ | 貝齒 | — | Cowry | Concha Cypraeae |
| 1057 | Pei-wei (Pei-wu-wei, Pei-wu-wei-tzŭ) | 北味(北五味,北五味子) | **Schisandra chinensis** | *SCHISANDRA (fruit) | Fructus Schisandrae Chinensis |

86

| | Transliteration | Chinese | Botanical Name | English | Pharmaceutical |
|---|---|---|---|---|---|
| 1058 | Pei-wu-chia-p'i (Kang-liu-p'i) | 北五加皮(杠柳皮) | **Periploca sepium** | *PERIPLOCA | Cortex Periplocae |
| 1059 | P'ei-lan (P'ei-lan-yeh, Tsê-lan) | 佩蘭(佩蘭葉,澤蘭) | **Eupatorium japonicum E. fortunei** | *EUPATORIUM | Herba Eupatorii |
| 1060 | Pên-ch'i (Kou-ch'i-tzŭ) | 本杞(枸杞子) | **Lycium chinense** | MATRIMONY VINE | Herba Lycii |
| 1061 | P'ên-shang-yüan-sui (T'ien-hu-sui) | 盆上芫荽(天胡荽) | **Hydrocotyle sibthorpi-oides** | PENNYWORT | Herba Hydrocotylis |
| 1062 | P'êng-chi-ts'ao | 蟛蜞草 | **Wedelia chinensis** | *WEDELIA | Herba Wedelia |
| 1063 | P'êng-o-shu (P'êng-shu, O-shu) | 蓬莪述(蓬朮,莪朮) | **Curcuma zedoaria** | ZEDOARY | Rhizoma Zedoariae |
| 1064 | P'êng-sha | 硼沙 | — | Borax | Borax |
| 1065 | P'êng-ta-hai (P'ang-ta-hai) | 蓬大海(胖大海) | **(Scaphium affine)** (see 1042) | PANGTAHAI | Semen Scaphii |
| 1066 | P'êng-ta-wan | 崩大碗 | **Centella asiatica** | *CENTELLA | Herba Centellae |
| 1067 | Pi-ch'êng-ch'ieh (Ch'êng-ch'ieh) | 畢澄茄(澄茄) | **Piper cubeba** | CUBEBS | Fructus Cubebae |
| 1068 | Pi-chi-ts'ao (T'ung-t'ien-ts'ao) | 荸薺草(通天草) | **Eleocharis tuberosa (Heleocharis dulcis)** | WATER CHESTNUT | Cormus Eleocharitis |
| 1069 | Pi-chien (Pi-hsi) | 壁錢(壁蟢) | — | Wall spider egg mass | — |
| 1070 | Pi-ma-tzŭ | 蓖麻子 | **Ricinus communis** | CASTOR BEAN | Semen Ricini |
| 1071 | Pi-po | 畢茇(蓽茇) | **Piper longum** | LONG PEPPER | Fructus Piperis Longi |
| 1072 | Pi-tao-kan | 碧桃乾 | **Prunus persica** | (Unripe) PEACH | Fructus Persicae Immaturi |
| 1073 | P'i-chiao | 皮膠 | — | Glue from hide | Colla Asini |

| --- | --- | --- | --- | --- | --- |
| 1074 P'i-hsiao (P'o-hsiao) | 皮硝(朴硝) | — | Sulfate of soda (Mirabilita) | Sal Glauberis (Natrium Sulfuricum) | |
| 1075 P'i-li-shih (Liang-fên-kuo) | 薜荔實(涼粉果) | **Ficus pumila** | JELLY-SEED | Fructus Fici Pumilae | |
| 1076 P'i-p'a-yeh (P'a-yeh) | 枇杷葉(杷葉) | **Eriobotrya japonica** | LOQUAT (leaves) | Folium Eriobotryae | |
| 1077 P'i-shuang | 砒霜 | — | Arsenic | Arsenicum | |
| 1078 P'i-yen (Shêng-p'i-yen) | 皮烟(生皮烟) | — | Soot from tanning factory | *Piyen | |
| 1079 P'iao-ch'ung | 瓢虫 | — | Lady-Bird Beetle | — | |
| 1080 Pieh-chia | 鼈(鱉)甲 | — | Fresh-water turtle shell | Carapax Amydae | |
| 1081 Pieh-ch'ün | 鼈裙 | — | Rim of fresh-water turtle shell | — | |
| 1082 Pieh-ch'ung (Ti-pieh-ch'ung, T'u-pieh-tzǔ) | 鼈虫(地鼈虫,土鼈子) | — | Wingless cockroach | Eupolyphaga | |
| 1083 Pien-hsing (T'ien-nan-hsing) | 邊星(天南星) | **Arisaema ambiguum** **A. amurense** **A. consanguineum** | JACK-IN-THE-PULPIT | Cormus Arisaematis | |
| 1084 Pien-hsü (Pien-yü) | 萹蓄(扁郁) | **Polygonum aviculare** | KNOTWEED | Herba Polygoni Avicularis | |
| 1085 Pien-pai (Pai-yeh) | 扁柏(柏葉) | **Thuja orientalis** | ARBOR-VITAE | Ramus Thujae | |
| 1086 Pien-shu (Shê-kan) | 扁束(蛇乾) | — | dried snake | *Pienshu | |
| 1087 Pien-t'êng (Pien-tan-t'êng) | 扁藤(扁擔藤) | **Tetrastigma planicaule** | *TETRASTIGMA | Ramus Tetrastigmatis | |

88

| | Transliteration | Chinese | Botanical Name | English | Pharmaceutical |
|---|---|---|---|---|---|
| 1088 | Pien-tou (Nan-pien-tou, Pai-pien-tou, Chüeh-tou) | 藊豆(南藊豆,白藊豆,鵲豆) | **Dolichos lablab** | HYACINTH BEAN | Semen Lablab |
| 1089 | Pien-tou-hua | 藊豆花 | **Dolichos lablab** | HYACINTH BEAN (flower) | Flos Lablab |
| 1090 | P'ien-chiao (A-chiao) | 片膠(阿膠) | — | Glue from Ass hide | Colla Asini (Gelatinum Asini) |
| 1091 | P'ien-tzŭ-ts'ao (Tzŭ-ts'ao-jung) | 片紫草(紫草茸或蓉) | **Lithospermum erythro-rhizon** | *ASIATIC GROOMWELL (sliced) | Radix Lithospermi |
| 1092 | Pin-lang (Pin-lang-hsin) | 檳榔(檳榔心) | **Areca catechu** | BETEL (nut) | Semen Arecae |
| 1093 | Pin-lang-p'i (Ta-fu-p'i, Pin-lang-i) | 檳榔皮(大腹皮,檳榔衣) | **Areca catechu** | BETEL (husk) | Pericarpium Arecae |
| 1094 | Ping-p'ien | 冰片 | See the following | BORNEOL CAMPHOR | Borneol |
| | Shang-ping-p'ien | 上冰片 | **Dryobalanops aromatica** | | |
| | Hsia-ping-p'ien | 下冰片 | **Blumea balsamifera** | | |
| 1095 | P'ing (T'ien-tzŭ-ts'ao) | 蘋(田字草) | **Marsilea quadrifolia** | CLOVER-FERN | Herba Marsileae |
| 1096 | Po-ho | 薄荷 | **Mentha arvensis M. haplocalyx** | FIELD MINT | Herba Menthae |
| | Poho-ping | 薄荷餅 | „          „ | Mint cake | |
| | Poho-ping | 薄荷冰 | „          „ | Menthol | |
| | Poho-yeh | 薄荷葉 | „          „ | Mint shoots | |
| | Poho-yu | 薄荷油 | „          „ | Mint oil | |

| Transliteration | Chinese | Botanical Name | English | Pharmaceutical |
|---|---|---|---|---|
| 1098 Po-lo-hui (Shan-huo-t'ung) | 博落回(山火筒) | **Macleaya cordata** | PLUME POPPY | Cordex et Herba Macleayae |
| 1099 Po-shao (Pai-shao) | 薄芍(白芍) | **Paeonia lactiflora** | PEONY (root) | Radix Paeoniae Lactiflorae |
| 1100 Po-tzǔ (Lo-po-tzǔ) | 蔔子(蘿蔔子) | **Raphanus sativus** | CHINESE RADISH | Semen Raphani Sativi |
| 1101 P'o (Hou-p'o) | 朴(厚樸) | **Magnolia officinalis** | MAGNOLIA (bark) | Cortex Magnoliae |
| Hou-p'o-kên (P'o-kên) | 厚朴根 | | From Wênchow & Fukien | |
| Nao-p'o (T'ung-p'o) | 腦朴(筒朴) | | From Wênchow | |
| Pan-p'o (P'o-pan, Chai-p'o, Tzǔ-po) | 板朴(朴板,柴朴,紫朴) | | From Kwangsi & Wênchow | |
| T'u-p'o (Liao-p'o) | 土朴(料朴) | | From Kiangsu, Chekiang | |
| T'u-p'o-p'i | 土朴皮 | | From Fukien | |
| Tz'u-p'o | 次朴 | | From Kiangsu | |
| 1102 P'o-hsiao (P'i-hsiao, Hsiao-p'i) | 朴硝(皮硝,硝皮) | — | Sulphate of Soda containing $MgSO_4$ (Glauber's salt) | Sal Glauberis |
| 1103 P'o-ku-chih (Ku-chih, Pu-ku-chih) | 破故紙(故紙,補骨脂,補骨紙) | **Cullen corylifolia** (Psoralea corylifolia) | BAUCHEE SEED, SCURFY PEA | Semen Cullinis |
| 1104 P'o-pu-yeh (Pu-cha-yeh) | 破布葉(布渣葉) | **Microcos paniculata** | *MICROCOS | Ramus Microcoris |
| 1105 Pu-ku-sui (Ku-sui-pu, Sui-pu) | 補骨碎(骨碎補,碎補) | **Drynaria fortunei** | *DRYNARIA | Rhizoma Drynariae |

| Transliteration | Chinese | Botanical Name | English | Pharmaceutical | **Pu** |
|---|---|---|---|---|---|
| 1106 Pu-liu-tzǔ | 不留子 | **Vaccaria segetalis** | COW COCKLE (seed), VACCARIA | Semen Vaccariae | |
| 1107 Pu-shih-ts'ao | 不食草 | See O-pu-shih-ts'ao | — | — | |
| 1108 Pu-ti-wu-kung | 鋪地蜈蚣 | **Lycopodium cernuum** | *NODDING CLUB-MOSS | Herba Lycopodii Cernui | |
| 1109 P'u-hua | 樸花 | **Magnolia officinalis** | Magnolia (flower) | Flos Magnolia Officinalis | |
| 1110 P'u-huang (P'u-kên) | 蒲黃(蒲根) | **Typha orientalis** **T. angustifolia** | Cat-tail (pollen and root) | Radix et Pollen Typhae | |
| 1111 P'u-k'uei | 蒲葵 | **Livistona chinensis** | FAN-PALM | Semen Livistonae | |
| 1112 P'u-kung-ying | 蒲公英 | **Taraxacum officinale** **T. mongolicum** | DANDELION | Herba Taraxaci | |
| 1113 P'u-t'ao-kan | 葡萄乾 | Vitis vinifera | RAISIN | Fructus Vitis Viniferae | |
| 1114 San-chang-yeh (T'u-yüan-chih) | 三張葉(土遠志) | **Lysimachia insignis** | *LYSIMACHIA | Herba et Radix Lysimachiae | |
| 1115 San-ch'i (Shan-ch'i, Shên-san-ch'i) | 三七(山漆,參三七) | **Panax notoginseng** | *SANCHI | Radix, Folium et Flos Sanchis | |
| 1116 San-ch'i-ts'ao (T'u-san-ch'i, T'ien-ch'i, T'ien-ch'ing-ti-hung) | 三七草(土三七,田七,天青地紅) | **Gynura segetum** | CANTON TUSANCHI (Velvet Plant) | Radix Gynurae Segeti | |
| 1117 San-chia-p'i | 三加皮 | **Eleutherococcus trifoliatus** | *ELEUTHERO | Radix Eleutherococci | |
| 1118 San-chio-fêng | 三角楓 | **Parthenocissus heterophylla** | *CHINA CREEPER | Ramus Parthenocissi | |
| 1119 San-chio-ts'ao | 三角草 | **Chlorophytum laxum** | *CHLOROPHYTUM | Herba Chlorophyti | |

91

| Transliteration | Chinese | Botanical Name | English | Pharmaceutical | San-c |
|---|---|---|---|---|---|
| 1120 San-chuan-fêng (San-ya-wu-yao) | 三鑽風(三丫烏藥) | **Lindera obtusiloba** | *LINDERA | Cortex Linderae | |
| 1121 San-fên-san (Shan-yeh-yen) | 三分三(山野烟) | **Scopolia acutangula Anisodus luridus** | *SANFENGSAN | Herba et Semen Scopoliae | |
| 1122 San-hsiao-ts'ao | 三消草 | **Trifolium repens** | WHITE CLOVER | Herba Trifolii | |
| 1123 San-hsien (San-hsien-tan) | 三仙(三仙丹) | — | Red oxide of mercury | Hydrargyrum Oxydatum Crudum | |
| 1124 San-hu (Hung-san) | 珊瑚(紅珊) | — | Coral | Os Coralli | |
| 1125 San-jên-hua | 三稔花 | **Averrhoa carambola** | CARAMBOLA | Flos Averrhoae | |
| 1126 San-k'o-chin | 三顆針 | **Berberis sargentiana B. brachypoda** & others | CHINESE BARBERRY | Cortex Berberidis | |
| 1127 San-lêng (Shan-lêng, San-ling, Hei-san-lêng) | 三稜(山稜,三苓,黑三稜) | **Sparganium stoloniferum S. simplex, S. stenophyllum** | BUR-REED | Rhizoma Sparganii | |
| 1128 San-mien-tao (Ch'a-ch'i) | 三面刀(茶七) | **Cimicifuga acerina** | BUGBANE | Herba et Radix Cimicifugae | |
| 1129 San-mu | 杉木 | **Cunninghamia lanceolata** | CHINA FIR | Cortex et Lignum Cunninghamiae | |
| 1130 San-nai (Shan-nai, San-lai,Sha-chiang) | 三奈(山奈,三賴,沙薑) | **Kaempferia galanga** | *KAEMPFERIA | Rhizoma Kaempferiae | |
| 1131 San-pai-ts'ao (San-pai-ts'ao-kên) | 三白草(三白草根) | **Saururus chinensis** | *SAURURUS | Rhizoma Saururi | |

| Transliteration | Chinese | Botanical Name | English | Pharmaceutical |
|---|---|---|---|---|
| 1132 San-pien-fêng (Ti-fêng-tzǔ, San-yeh-wei-ling-ts'ai) | 三片風(地蜂子, 三葉委陵菜) | **Potentilla freyniana** | CHINESE CINQUEFOIL | Herba Potentillae |
| 1133 San-sê-chin | 三色菫 | **Viola tricolor** | PANSY | Herba Violae Tricoloris |
| 1134 San-shêng-mi | 三升米 | **Ribes tenue** | SLENDER GOOSEBERRY | Radix Ribetis |
| 1135 San-shih-lu-kên (San-shih-lu-tan, Shuang-fei-hu-tieh) | 三十六根(三十六蕩, 雙飛蝴蝶) | **Tylophora ovata** | *TYLOPHORA | Radix Tylophorae |
| 1136 San-t'ai-hung-hua (San-t'ai-hua) | 三台紅花(三台花) | **Clerodendrum serratum** | *THREE-TIERED PAGODA FLOWER | Herba Clerodendri Serrati |
| 1137 San-t'iao-chin (Ts'ai-chang) | 三條筋(柴樟) | **Cinnamomum tamala** | *TAMALA | Cortex et Ramus Cinnamomi Tamulae |
| 1138 San-ya-k'u (San-ya-hu, San-chih-ch'iang) | 三椏苦(三丫虎, 三枝槍) | **Evodia lepta** | *BITTER EVODIA | Radix et Ramus Evodiae Leptae |
| 1139 Sang-chên-tzǔ (Sang-chên-kao) | 桑椹子 桑椹膏 | **Morus alba** „   „ | MULBERRY (Mulberry jam) | Fructus Mori Albae |
| 1140 Sang-chi-shêng | 桑寄生 | **Taxillis chinensis T. sutchuenensis** | MEDICINAL MISTLETOC | Ramus Taxillis |
| —a Pei-chi-shêng | 北寄生 | **Viscum coloratum** | RED MISTLETOE | Ramus Visci |
| —b Kuang-chi-shêng | 廣寄生 | **Scurrula parasiticus** | SOUITERN MISTLETOE | Ramus Scurrulae |
| 1141 Sang-chih (Sang-yeh) | 桑枝(桑葉) | **Morus alba** | MULBERRY | Ramus et Folium Mori Albae |
| 1142 Sang-ch'ung (Sang-tu-chung, Chu-chung) | 桑蟲(桑蠹蟲, 蛀蟲) | — | Longhorn Beetle larva growing in mulberry | Apriona Germari |

93

| Transliteration | Chinese | Botanical Name | English | Pharmaceutical |
|---|---|---|---|---|
| 1143 Sang-hsiao (Sang-p'iao, Sang-p'iao-shao) | 桑蛸(桑螵, 桑螵蛸) | — | Praying Mantis egg case on Mulberry branch | Oötheca Mantidis |
| 1144 Sang-pai-p'i (Sang-pai, Sang-kên-pai-p'i) | 桑白皮(桑白, 桑根白皮) | **Morus alba** | Mulberry (root bark) | Cortex Mori Albae |
| 1144A Sha-chi (Ts'u-liu-kuo) | 沙棘(醋柳果) | **Hippophae rhamnoides** | SAND THORNS | Fructus Hippophois |
| 1145 Sha-chiang | 沙薑 | **Kaempferia galanga** | KAEMPFERIA | Rhizoma Kaempferiae |
| 1146 Sha-chien-hu | 沙前胡 | **Ferula borealis** | *BOREAL ASAFETIDA | Radix Ferulae Borealis |
| 1147 Sha-jên (Sha-jên-k'o, Sha-k'o) | 沙仁(砂仁, 砂仁殼, 沙殼) | **Amomum villosum** | GRAINS-OF-PARADISE | Semen et Pericarpium Amomi |
| —a Shu-sha-jên | 縮沙仁 | **A. xanthioides** | | |
| 1148 Sha-kuai-tsao | 沙拐棗 | **Calligonum mongolicum** | *CALLIGONUM | Fructus Calligoni |
| 1149 Sha-lou-lu | 沙漏蘆 | **Echinops gmelinii** | *ECHINOPS | Radix Echinopis |
| 1150 Sha-shên | 沙參 | **Adenophora polymorpha** **A. tetraphylla (A. verticillata)** | *ADENOPHORA | Radix Adenophorae |
| 1151 Sha-tsao (Sha-tsao-chiao, Sha-tsao-p'i, Sha-tsao-hua) | 沙棗(沙棗膠, 沙棗皮, 沙棗花) | **Elaeagnus angustifolia** | OLEASTER | Flos, Fructus et Gummi Elaeagni |
| 1152 Sha-yüan-tzǔ (Sha-yüan, T'ung-chi, T'ung-chi-li) | 砂苑子(砂苑, 潼蒺, 潼蒺藜) | **Astragalus complanatus** **A. adsurgens** **A. chinensis** | CHINESE MILK VETCH | Semen Astragali |

94

| | Transliteration | Chinese | Botanical Name | English | Pharmaceutical |
|---|---|---|---|---|---|
| 1153 | Shan-cha (Shan-cha-jou, Shan-cha-kan, Shan-cha-kao, Shan-cha-p'ien) | 山楂(山楂肉，山楂乾，山楂糕，楂片) | **Crataegus pinnatifida C. cuneata** | CHINESE HAWTHORN | Fructus Crataegi et Praeparatum |
| 1154 | Shan-ch'a-hua | 山茶花 | **Camellia japonica** | CAMELLIA | Flos Camelliae |
| 1155 | Shan-ch'êng | 山橙 | **Melodinus suaveolens** | *MELODINUS | Fructus Melodini |
| 1156 | Shan-chi-tan | 山鷄蛋 | **Codonopsis convolvulacea** | *TWINING CODONOPSIS | Radix Codonopsis Convolvulaceae |
| 1157 | Shan-chia (Ch'uan-shan-chia) | 山甲(穿山甲) | — | Pangolin carapace | Squama Manidis |
| 1158 | Shan-chia-p'i | 山甲皮 | — | Pangolin skin | Pellis Manidis |
| 1159 | Shan-chiang-tzŭ (Hung-tou-k'ou) | 山薑子(紅豆蔻) | **Alpinia officinarum** | LESSER GALANGAL | Fructus Alpiniae Officinari |
| 1160 | Shan-chih-jên (Shan-chih-kên, Shan-chih-cha) | 山枝仁(山枝根，山枝茶) | **Pittosporum glabratum** | *PITTOSPORUM | Radix et Semen Pittospori |
| 1161 | Shan-chih-ma | 山枳麻 | **Helicteres angustifolia** | *HELICTERES | Radix Helicteris |
| 1162 | Shan-chih-tzŭ | 山栀子 | **Gardenia jasminoides** | GARDENIA | Fructus Gardeniae |
| 1163 | Shan-chu-tan | 山猪膽 | — | Wild boar gallbladder | Fel Verris |
| 1164 | Shan-chu-tzŭ (Shan-chu-kên) | 山竹子(山竹根) | **Garcinia multiflora** | *GARCINIA | Cortex et Fructus Garciniae |
| 1165 | Shan-chu-yü (Chu-yü, Yü-jou) | 山茱萸(茱萸，萸肉) | **Cornus officinalis** | ASIATIC CORNELIAN CHERRY | Fructus Corni Officinalis |
| 1166 | Shan-chü | 山蒟 | **Piper hancei** | *HANCE'S PEPPER | Herba Piperis Hancei |

| | Transliteration | Chinese | Botanical Name | English | Pharmaceutical |
|---|---|---|---|---|---|
| 1167 | Shan-chü (Shan-hsiao-chü) | 山橘(山小橘) | **Glycosmis parviflora** (**G. citrifolia**) | *GLYCOSMIS | Radix et Folium Glycosmidis |
| 1168 | Shan-fan-hua (Shan-fan-kên, Shan-fan-yeh) | 山礬花(山礬根,山礬葉) | **Symplocos caudata** **S. racemosa** | *SYMPLOCOS | Radix, Folium et Flos Symplocoris |
| 1169 | Shan-hai-lo (T'u-tang-shên) | 山海螺(土黨參) | **Codonopsis lanceolata** | *CODONOPSIS | Radix Codonopsis Lanceolatae |
| 1170 | Shan-hêh-t'ao | 山核桃 | **Carya cathayensis** | CHINESE HICKORY | Fructus Caryae |
| 1171 | Shan-ho-yeh (Wo-êrh-ch'i) | 山荷葉(窩兒七) | **Diphylleia grayi** **D. sinensis** | *DIPHYLLEIA | Caudex Diphylleiae |
| 1172 | Shan-hsiai (Shih-hsiai) | 山蟹(石蟹) | **Geastrum hygrometricum** | *GEASTRUM | Geastrum |
| 1173 | Shan-hu-chiao | 山胡椒 | **Lindera glauca** | *GLAUCOUS ALLSPICE | Fructus Litseae |
| 1174 | Shan-hua (Kuan-shan) | 蟬花(冠蟬) | **Cordyceps scotianus** | Fungus sclerotia on Cicada | Cordyceps Cicadae |
| 1175 | Shan-hung-chih-jên | 山紅梔仁 | **Gardenia jasminoides** | WILD GARDENIA | Semen Gardeniae |
| 1176 | Shan-huo-hsiang (Hsüeh-chien-ch'ou, Fei-hsing-ts'ao) | 山藿香(血見愁,肺形草) | **Teucrium viscidum** | CHINESE GERMANDER | Herba Teucrii |
| 1177 | Shan-kan-ts'ao (Pai-chih-shan) | 山甘草(白紙扇) | **Mussaenda pubescens** | *MUSSAENDA | Radix et Ramus Mussaendae |
| 1178 | Shan-k'u-mai | 山苦蕒 | **Ixeris chinensis** | *CHINESE IXERIS | Herba Ixeridis |
| 1179 | Shan-li-chih | 山荔枝 | **Cudrania cochinchinensis** | CUDRANIA | Fructus Cudraniae |

96

| | Transliteration | Chinese | Botanical Name | English | Pharmaceutical |
|---|---|---|---|---|---|
| 1180 | Shan-ma-chio-p'ien | 山馬角片 | — | Shaving of red deer horn | — |
| 1181 | Shan-ma-huang | 山螞蝗 | **Desmodium racemosum** | *CHINESE DESMODIUM | Herba Desmodii Racemosi |
| 1182 | Shan-mei-kên | 山梅根 | **Philadelphus sericanthus** | *PHILADELPHUS | Radix Philadelphi |
| 1183 | Shan-mou-tan | 山牡丹 | **Argyreia seguinii** | *ARGYREIA | Cortex et Ramus Argyreiae |
| 1184 | Shan-nai (San-nai) | 山奈(三奈) | **Kaempferia galanga** | KAEMPFERIA | Rhizoma Kaempferiae |
| 1185 | Shan-pai-chü | 山白菊 | **Aster ageratoides** | *WHITE ASTER | Herba Asteris |
| 1186 | Shan-p'i-pa | 山枇杷 | **Ilex franchetiana** | *SHANPIPA | Ramus Ilicis Franchetiana |
| 1187 | Shan-pien-t'ou | 山扁豆 | **Cassia mimosoides** | *DWARF CASSIA | Herba Cassiae Mimosoidis |
| 1188 | Shan-suan (Chê-suan) | 山蒜(澤蒜) | **Allium nipponicum** | *WILD CHIVE | Herba Allii Nipponici |
| 1189 | Shan-ta-yen (Shan-ta-tao) | 山大顏(山大刀) | **Psychotria rubra** | *RED PSYCHOTRIA | Herba Phychotriae Rubrae |
| 1190 | Shan-tan (Hung-pai-ho) | 山丹(紅百合) | **Lilium** spp. | LILIES | Bulbus Shantan |
| −a | Chuan-tan | 捲丹 | **L. lancifolium** | | |
| −b | Shan-tan | 山丹 | **L. pumilum** | | |
| −c | Wu-tan | 渥丹 | **L. concolor** | | |
| 1191 | Shan-tao-nien-hao | 山道年蒿 | **Artemisia cina** | SANTONIN | Herba Artemisiae Cinae |

| | Transliteration | Chinese | Botanical Name | English | Pharmaceutical |
|---|---|---|---|---|---|
| 1192 | Shan-tou-kên (Tou-kên, Kuang-tou-kên) | 山豆根(豆根, 廣豆根) | **Sophora tonkinensis (S. subprostrata)** | *BUSHY SOPHORA | Radix Sophorae Tonkinensis |
| —a | Pei-shan-tou-ken | 北山豆根 | (see 1053) | | |
| 1193 | Shan-ts'ang-tzǔ | 山蒼子 | **Litsea cubeba** | FRAGRANT LITSEA | Fructus Litseae Cubebae |
| 1194 | Shan-t'ung-tzǔ | 山桐子 | **Mallotus nepalensis** | *NEPALESE MALLOTUS | Cortex Malloti |
| 1195 | Shan-tz'ǔ-ku (Shan-ku) | 山慈菇(山菰) | **Tulipa edulis** | CHINESE TULIP | *Rhizoma vel Bulbus Shantzuku |
| | | | **Asarum sagittarioides** | *ARROW-LEAVED WILD GINGER | |
| | | | **Cremastra variabilis** | *CREMASTRA | |
| | | | **Pleione** spp. and others | *PLEIONE | |
| 1196 | Shan-tz'ǔ-pai | 山刺柏 | **Juniperus formosana** | SPINY JUNIPER | Fructus et Radix Juniperi Formosanae |
| 1197 | Shan-wu-chiu-kên | 山烏桕根 | **Sapium discolor** | MOUNTAIN TALLOW TREE | Radix Sapii Discoloris |
| 1198 | Shan-yang-chin Shan-yang-chio Shan-yang-hsüeh | 山羊筋 山羊角 山羊血 | — | Goat sinew, horn, and blood | Naemorhedus |
| 1199 | Shan-yao (Huai-shan, Shan-yao-t'ou) | 山藥(淮山, 山藥頭) | **Dioscorea opposita** | CHINESE YAM | Radix Dioscoreae Oppositae |
| 1200 | Shan-yin-hua | 山銀花 | **Lonicera japonica** | HONEYSUCKLE | Flos Lonicerae |
| 1201 | Shan-ying-t'ao | 山櫻桃 | **Prunus tomentosa** | NANKING CHERRY | Fructus et Semen Pruni Tomentosae |
| 1202 | Shan-yu-kan | 山油柑 | **Acronychia pedunculata** | *ACRONYCHIA | Fructus Acronychiae |
| 1203 | Shang-lu (Shan-lo-po, Pai-ch'ang) | 商陸(山蘿蔔, 白昌) | **Phytolacca acinosa** | POKE ROOT | Radix Phytolaccae |

98

| | Transliteration | Chinese | Botanical Name | English | Pharmaceutical |
|---|---|---|---|---|---|
| 1204 | Shao-yao | 芍藥 | **Paeonia lactiflora** | PEONY | Radix Paeoniae Lactiflorae |
| 1205 | Shê-ch'uang-tzŭ | 蛇床子 | **Cnidium monnieri** | *CNIDIUM | Fructus Cnidii |
| 1206 | Shê-han-shih (Shê-huang) | 蛇含石(蛇黃) | — | Limonite | Limonitum Globuloforme |
| 1207 | Shê-hsiang | 麝香 | — | Musk deer (navel gland secretion) | Secretio Moschi |
| 1208 | Shê-hsiang-ts'ao | 麝香草 | **Thymus vulgaris** | THYME | Herba Thymi |
| 1209 | Shê-hu-tzŭ (Pi-hu) | 蛇虎子(壁虎) | — | House lizard, Gecko | Gecko Chinensis |
| 1210 | Shê-i (Shê-p'i, Shê-t'ui) | 蛇衣(蛇皮,蛇退) | — | Snake slough | Periostachum Serpentis |
| 1211 | Shê-kan | 射干 | **Belamcanda chinensis** | *BELAMCANDA | Rhizoma Belamcandae |
| 1212 | Shê-mei | 蛇莓 | **Duchesnea indica** | *SNAKE STRAWBERRY | Herba Duchesneae |
| 1213 | Shê-p'ao-lê | 蛇泡竻 | **Rubus parvifolius** | CHINESE RASPBERRY | Radix Rubi Parvifolii |
| 1214 | Shê-p'u-t'ao | 蛇葡萄 | **Ampelopsis brevipedunculata** | SNAKE-GRAPE | Radix et Ramus Ampelopsis |
| 1215 | Shê-shih (Tz'ŭ-shih) | 攝石(磁石) | — | Magnetic oxide of Iron | Magnetitum |
| 1216 | Shê-shui (Shê-k'o, Lung-i) | 蛇蛻(蛇殼,龍衣) | See Shê-i | — | — |
| 1217 | Shê-wang-t'êng | 蛇王藤 | **Passiflora cochinchinensis** | PASSION FLOWER | Herba Passiflorae |
| 1218 | Shên-chiang (Mao-chiang, Mo-chiang) | 申薑(毛薑,磨薑) | **Drynaria fortunei** | *DRYNARIA | Rhizoma Drynariae |

| Transliteration | Chinese | Botanical Name | English | Pharmaceutical |
|---|---|---|---|---|
| 1219 Shên-chin-ts'ao | 伸筋草 | **Lycopodium clavatum L. cernuum** | Lycopods CLUB-MOSS | Herba Lycopodii |
| 1220 Shên-ch'ü (Shên-ch'ü-ch'a) | 神糲(神糲茶) | **Six source species See introduction** | Fermented herb mixture | Massa Medicata Fermentata |
| 1221 Shên-huang-tou | 神黃豆 | **Cassia nodosa** | PINK-WHITE SHOWER | Semen Cassiae Nodosae |
| 1222 Shên-yeh | 參葉 | **Panax japonicus** | JAPANESE GINSENG (leaves) | Folium Panacis Japonici |
| 1223 Shêng-ma (Shêng-ma-jou, Shêng-ma-tou) | 升麻(升麻肉,升麻頭) | **Cimicifuga foetida C. dahurica C. heracleifolia** | CHINESE BUGBANE | Rhizoma Cimicifugae |
| 1224 Shêng-shu (Pai-shu) | 生朮(白朮) | **Atractylodes macrocephala** | PAISHU (raw) | Radix Atractylodis |
| 1225 Shêng-ti (Hsiao-shêng-ti, Ti-huang) | 生地(小生地,地黃) | **Rehmannia glutinosa** | CHINESE FOX-GLOVE (raw) | Radix Rehmanniae Crudae |
| 1226 Shêng-yao (San-hsien-tan) | 昇藥(三仙丹) | — | Mercuric oxide | Hydrargyrum Oxydatum Crudum |
| 1227 Shih | 蓍 | **Achillea alpina** | ALPINE YARROW | Herba Achilleae |
| 1228 Shih-ch'ang-p'u | 石菖蒲 | **Acorus gramineus** | ROCK SWEET-FLAG | Herba Acori Graminei |
| 1229 Shih-chi-chia (Fo-chi-chia) | 石指甲(佛指甲) | **Sedum sarmentosum** | STONEWORT | Herba Sedi Sarmentosi |
| 1230 Shih-chi-ning (Kuei-hsiang-ts'ao) | 石薺薴(鬼香草) | **Mosla scabra** | *ROUGH MOSLA | Herba Moslae Scabrae |

100

| | Transliteration | Chinese | Botanical Name | English | Pharmaceutical | Shih-c |
|---|---|---|---|---|---|---|
| 1231 | Shih-chi-shêng | 石寄生 | **Stereocaulon paschale** | *DENDROID LICHEN | Herba Stereocaulonis | |
| 1232 | Shih-chiang-tou | 石豇豆 | **Lepisorus eilophyllus** | LEPISORUS, ROCK COWPEA | Herba Lepisori | |
| 1233 | Shih-chien-ch'uan (Hei-mien-fêng, Tzǔ-shên) | 石見穿(黑面風,紫參) | **Salvia chinensis** | *CHINESE SAGE | Herba Salviae Chinensis | |
| 1234 | Shih-chih (Ch'ih-shih-chih) | 石脂(赤石脂) | — | Halloysite | Halloysitum Rubrum | |
| 1235 | Shih-chu | 石竹 | **Dianthus superbus** | PINK | Herba Dianthi Superbi | |
| 1236 | Shih-chüeh-ming | 石決明 | — | Abalone shell | Concha Haliotidis | |
| 1237 | Shih-ch'un | 石蓴 | **Ulva lactuca** | SEA-LETTACE | Herba Ulvae Lactucae | |
| 1238 | Shih-chün-tzǔ (Shui-chün-tzǔ) | 使君子(水君子) | **Quisqualis indica** | RANGOON CREEPER | Fructus Quisqualis | |
| 1239 | Shih-êrh (Shih-mu-êrh) | 石耳(石木耳) | **Umbilicaria esculenta** | UMBILICARIA (fruiting body) | Fructificatio Umbilicariae | |
| 1240 | Shih-fang-fêng | 石防風 | **Peucedanum terebinthaceum** | *CHINESE MASTER-WORT | Radix Peucedani | |
| 1241 | Shih-fêng-tan | 石風丹 | **Goodyera procera** | BOTTLEBRUSH ORCHID | Herba Goodyerae Procerae | |
| 1242 | Shih-hsiang-jou (Ch'ing-hsiang-ju) | 石香菜(青香薷) | **Mosla chinensis** | *CHINESE MOSLA | Herba Moslae Chinensis | |
| 1243 | Shih-hsieh | 石蟹(蠏) | — | Fossil crab | Fossilia Brachyurae | |
| 1244 | Shih-hsien-t'ao | 石仙桃 | **Pholidota chinensis** | RATTLESNAKE ORCHID | Herba Pholidotae | |
| 1245 | Shih-hu (Shih-huo) | 石斛(石活) | **Dendrobium** spp. | DENDROBIUM | Herba Dendrobii | |
| -a | Chin-ch'a shih-hu | 金釵石斛 | **D. nobile** | GOLDEN HAIRPIN DENDROBIUM | | |

| Transliteration | Chinese | Botanical Name | English | Pharmaceutical |
|---|---|---|---|---|
| Shih-hu (*cont.*) | | | | |
| —b Fên-hua-shih-hu | 粉花石斛 | **D. loddigesii** | LODDIGES DENDROBIUM | |
| —c Hsi-yeh-shih-hu | 細葉石斛 | **D. hancockii** | HANCOCK'S  ,, | |
| —d Lo-ho-shih-hu | 羅河石斛 | **D. lohohense** | LOHOH  ,, | |
| —e T'ieh-p'i-shih-hu | 鐵皮石斛 | **D. officinale** | OFFICINAL  ,, | |
| —f T'ung-p'i-shih-hu | 銅皮石斛 | **D. crispulum** | COPPER  ,, | |
| —g Wang-mei-ch'un-shih-hu | 網脉唇石斛 | **D. hercoglossum** | POUCH-LIPPED  ,, | |
| 1246 Shih-hu-sui | 石胡荽 | **Hydrocotyle sibthorpioides** | PENNYWORT | Herba Hydrocotylis |
| 1247 Shih-hua | 石花 | **Parmelia saxatilis** | BOULDER LICHEN | Herba Parmeliae |
| 1248 Shih-hua-ts'ai | 石花菜 | **Eucheuma gelatina** | SEAWEED | Herba Eucheumata |
| 1249 Shih-huang-p'i | 石黃皮 | **Nephrolepis cordifolia** | SWORD-FERN (tuber) | Tuber Nephrolepis |
| 1250 Shih-hui | 石灰 | — | Lime | Calcium Oxide |
| 1251 Shih-kan-tzŭ | 石柑子 | **Pothos chinensis** | *POTHOS | Herba Pothoris |
| 1252 Shih-kao | 石膏 | — | Gypsum | Calcium Sulphate |
| 1253 Shih-kên (Shih-mu-p'i) | 柿根(柿木皮) | **Diospyros kaki** | PERSIMMON (root & bark) | Radix et Cortex Diospyroris |
| 1254 Shih-kuo (Shih-tzŭ) | 柿果(柿子) | **Diospyros kaki** | PERSIMMON (fruit) | Fructus Diospyroris |
| Shih-ping | 柿餅 | ,,  ,, | PERSIMMON fruit cake | Fructus Diospyroris |
| Shih-shuang | 柿霜 | ,,  ,, | PERSIMMON frost | *Shihshuang |
| Shih-t'i | 柿蒂 | ,,  ,, | PERSIMMON calyx | Calyx Diospyroris |
| 1255 Shih-la-hung | 石臘紅 | **Pelargonium graveolens** | GARDEN GERANIUM | Flos Pelargonii |
| 1256 Shih-lan-t'êng (Shih-nan-t'êng) | 石蘭藤(石南藤) | **Piper wallichii** <br> **P. puberulum** | *WILD PEPPER | Herba Piperis |
| 1257 Shih-li (Shih-li-tzŭ) | 石栗(石栗子) | **Aleurites moluccana** | CANDLENUT TREE | Semen Aleurititis |

102

| Transliteration | Chinese | Botanical Name | English | Pharmaceutical |
|---|---|---|---|---|
| 1258 Shih-lien (Shih-lien-tzŭ) | 石蓮(石蓮子) | **Caesalpinia minax** | SNAKE BRAMBLE (Seed) | Semen Caesalpiniae |
| 1259 Shih-liu-hua (Shih-liu-p'i) | 石榴花(石榴皮) | **Punica granatum** | POMEGRANATE | Flos et Pericarpium Granati |
| Shih-liu-shu-p'i | 石榴樹皮 | **Punica granatum** | POMEGRANATE (bark) | Cortex Granati |
| 1260 Shih-lo-t'êng | 石羅藤 | **Berchemia hypochrysa** | *BERCHIEMIA, SUPPLE-JACK | Radix et Ramus Berchemiae |
| 1261 Shih-lo-tzŭ | 蒔蘿子 | **Anethum graveolens (Peucedanum graveolens)** | DILL | Fructus Anethi |
| 1262 Shih-lung-ch'u | 石龍芻 | **Juncus decipiens** | BOG-RUSH | Herba et Rhizoma Junci |
| 1263 Shih-lung-jui | 石龍芮 | **Ranunculus sceleratus** | BUTTERCUP | Herba Ranunculi Scelerati |
| 1264 Shih-lung-tzŭ (Hsi-i) | 石龍子(蜥蜴) | — | Lizard | *Shihlungtzu |
| 1265 Shih-nan (Shih-nan-yeh) | 石楠(石楠葉) | **Photinia serrulata** | *PHOTINIA | Ramus Photiniae |
| 1266 Shih-nan-t'êng | 石南藤 | **Piper wallichii var. hupehense** | *WALLICH'S PEPPER | Ramus Piperis Wallichii |
| 1267 Shih-nao-yu (Yang-yu) | 石腦油(洋油) | — | Petroleum | Petroleum |
| 1268 Shih-p'ung-tzŭ | 石澎子 | **Ficus sarmentosa** | *CREEPING-FIG | Fructus Fici Sarmentosae |
| 1269 Shih-shan-shu | 石蟾蜍 | **Stephania tetrandra** | *FOUR-ANTHERED STEPHANIA | Radix Stephaniae Tetrandrae |
| 1270 Shih-shan-ts'ao | 石蟬草 | **Peperomia dindygulensis** | *PEPEROMIA | Herba Peperomiae |

| Transliteration | Chinese | Botanical Name | English | Pharmaceutical |
|---|---|---|---|---|
| 1271 Shih-shang-pai | 石上柏 | **Selaginella doederleinii** | *GREATER SELAGINELLA | Herba Selaginellae Doederleinii |
| 1272 Shih-shua-pa | 石刷把 | **Psilotum nudum** | PSILOTUM | Herba Psiloti |
| 1273 Shih-shuang | 柿霜 | See Shih-kuo | — | — |
| 1274 Shih-suan | 石蒜 | **Lycoris radiata** & related species | *LYCORIS (bulb) | Bulbus Lycoris |
| 1275 Shih-sung | 石松 | **Lycopodium clavatum** | CLUB-MOSS | Herba Lycopodii |
| 1276 Shih-ta-kung-lao (Kung-lao-yeh, Kung-lao-mu) | 十大功勞(功勞葉,功勞木) | **Mahonia beali** **M. japonica,** **M. fortunei** | *MAHONIA | Radix, Ramus et Folium Mahoniae |
| 1277 Shih-t'i | 柿蒂 | See Shih-kuo | — | — |
| 1278 Shih-tiao-lan | 石吊蘭 | **Lysionotus pauciflora** | *LYSIONOTUS | Herba Lysionoti |
| 1279 Shih-ts'an (Shih-shang-ngou) | 石蠶(石上藕) | **Ludisia discolor (Haemaria discolor)** | *BLOOD-LEAVED ORCHID | Herba Ludisiae |
| 1280 Shih-tsao | 石棗 | **Bulbophyllum radiatum** | *RADIATE BULBOPHYLLUM | Herba Bulbophylli |
| 1281 Shih-wei (Shih-wei-yeh) | 石葦(石葦葉) | **Pyrrosia lingua** (South) **P. sheareri** (Central) **P. davidii** (North) | *PYRROSIA | Herba Pyrrosiae |
| 1282 Shih-yen | 石燕 | — | Fossil shell of Spirifer | Fossilia Spirifera |
| 1283 Shih-ying | 石英 | — | Crystallized quartz | Quartz |
| 1284 Shou-p'ien | 手片 | **Citrus medica** var. **sarcodactylis** (see Fo-shou) | FINGER CITRON (sliced) | Fructus Citri Medicae |
| 1285 Shou-wu | 首烏 | See Ho-shou-wu | — | — |

| Transliteration | Chinese | Botanical Name | English | Pharmaceutical | Shu |
|---|---|---|---|---|---|
| 1286 Shu | 朮 | See the following | | | |
| −a O-shu | 莪朮 | **Curcuma zedoaria** | ZEDOARY | Rhizoma Curcumatis | |
| −b Pai-shu | 白朮 | **Atractylodes macrocephala** | PAISHU | *Radix Paishu | |
| −c Ts'ang-shu | 蒼朮 | **Atractylodes chinensis A. japonica, A. lancea** | TSANGSHU | *Radix Tsangshu | |
| 1287 Shu-chü-ts'ao | 鼠麴草 | **Gnaphalium multiceps** | MANY-HEAD CUDWEED | Herba Gnaphalii | |
| 1288 Shu-fu | 鼠婦(負) | — | Wood louse | Porcellio | |
| 1289 Shu-liang | 薯莨 | **Dioscorea cirrhosa** | *DYEING YAM | *Radix Shuliang | |
| 1290 Shu-pai-p'i (Ch'ung-kên-pai-p'i) | 樗白皮(椿根白皮) | **Ailanthus altissima** | CHINESE AILANTHUS (bark) | Cortex Ailanthi | |
| 1291 Shu-ti (Shu-ti-huang) | 熟地(熟地黃) | **Rehmannia glutinosa** See Ti-huang | CHINESE FOXGLOVE (Steam-dried) | Radix Rehmanniae Glutinosae Conquitae | |
| 1292 Shu-t'ou (Ts'ang-shu) | 朮頭(蒼朮) | **Atractylodes chinensis A. lancea, A. japonica** | *TSANGSHU | Radix Tsangshu | |
| 1293 Shui-an-pan | 水案板 | **Potamogeton natans** | PONDWEED | Herba Potamogetonis | |
| 1294 Shui-chê-êrh | 水折耳 | **Gymnotheca involucrata** | *GYMNOTHECA | Herba Gymnothecae | |
| 1295 Shui-chê-ts'ao | 水蔗草 | **Apluda mutica** | *APLUDA | Herba Apludae | |
| 1296 Shui-ch'ieh | 水茄 | **Solanum torvum** | WILD TOMATO | Radix Solani Torvi | |
| 1297 Shui-chih (Ma-huang) | 水蛭(螞蟥) | — | Leech | Hirudo | |
| 1298 Shui-chih-kên Shui-chih-yeh | 水梔根 水梔葉 | **Gardenia jasminoides** **Gardenia jasminoides** | GARDENIA (root) GARDENIA (leaves) | Radix Gardeniae Folium Gardeniae | |

| Transliteration | Chinese | Botanical Name | English | Pharmaceutical |
|---|---|---|---|---|
| 1299 Shui-chin-fêng | 水金鳳 | **Impatiens uliginosa** | JEWELWEED | Herba Impatientis Uliginosae |
| 1300 Shui-ch'in | 水芹 | **Oenanthe javanica** | *OENANTHE, WATER-CELERY | Herba Oenanthis |
| 1301 Shui-ching-lan | 水晶蘭 | **Monotropa uniflora** | FITS-ROOT | Caudix Monotropae |
| 1302 Shui-chün-tzǔ | 水君子 | See Shih-chün-tzǔ | — | — |
| 1302A Shui-fei-lien | 水飛廉 | **Symphytum officinale** | COMMON CAMFREY | Herba Symphyti |
| 1303 Shui-fên | 水粉 | — | White lead | — |
| 1304 Shui-fu-jung | 水芙蓉 | **Limnophila aromatica** | *LIMNOPHILA | Herba Limnophilae |
| 1305 Shui-hsia-tzǔ-ts'ao (Ya-li-ts'ao, Ni-hua-ts'ao) | 水蝦子草(鴨㖫草, 泥花草) | **Lindernia antipoda** | *DUCK'S TONGUE PIMPERNEL | Herba Linderniae Antipodae |
| 1306 Shui-hsien-hua (Shui-hsien-kên) | 水仙花(水仙根) | **Narcissus tazetta** | CHINESE SACRED LILY | Herba et Flos Narcissi |
| 1307 Shui-hsien-t'ao (Mao-ts'ao-lung) | 水仙桃(毛草龍) | **Jussiaea suffruticosa** | PRIMROSE WILLOW | Herba Jussiaeae |
| 1308 Shui-hsien-ts'ai | 水莧荣 | **Ammannia baccifera** | *AMMANNIA | Herba Ammanniae |
| 1309 Shui-hsien-ts'ao | 水綾草 | **Hedyotis corymbosa** | *CORYMBOSE HEDYOTIS | Herba Hedyotis Corymbosae |
| 1310 Shui-hsien-tzǔ | 水仙子 | — | Maggots | Vermiculus |
| 1311 Shui-hu-lu (Yang-shui-hsien) | 水葫蘆(洋水仙) | **Eichhornia crassipes** | WATER HYACINTH | Herba Eichhorniae |
| 1312 Shui-hu-man (K'u-lang-shu, Ch'ou-k'u-lang) | 水胡滿(苦朗樹, 臭苦朗) | **Clerodendrum inerme** | GLORYBOWER | Ramus Clerodendri Inermis |

106

| Transliteration | Chinese | Botanical Name | English | Pharmaceutical |
|---|---|---|---|---|
| 1313 Shui-huang-lien | 水黃蓮 | **Thalictrum ramosum T. angustifolium, T. contortum** | *WATER-MEADOWRUE | Herba Thalictri Ramosi, Angustifolii et Contorti |
| 1314 Shui-hung-hua-tzǔ | 水紅花子 | **Polygonum lapathifolium** | WATER PEPPER | Fructus Polygoni Lapathifolii |
| 1315 Shui-huo (Ch'iang-huo) | 水活(羌活) | See Ch'iang-huo | — | — |
| 1316 Shui-k'u-mai | 水苦蕒 | **Veronica anagallis-aquatica** | SPEEDWELL | Herba Veronicae |
| 1317 Shui-k'uei | 水葵 | **Nymphoides peltatum (Limnanthemum nymphoides)** | *FLOATING HEART | Herba Shuikuei |
| 1318 Shui-li-t'êng | 水梨藤 | **Actinidia callosa** | *ACTINIDIA | Ramus Actinidiae |
| 1319 Shui-liao (La-liao) | 水蓼(辣蓼) | **Polygonum hydropiper** | SMARTWEED | Herba Polygoni Hydropiperis |
| 1320 Shui-lien-sha (Hsun-tz'ǔ-mu) | 水蓮沙(枸刺木) | **Cotoneaster horizontalis** | COTONEASTER | Radix et Ramus Cotoneastri |
| 1321 Shui-liu-tou (Shui-lo-tou) | 水流豆(水羅豆) | **Pongamia pinnata** | *PONGAMIA | Semen Pongamiae |
| 1322 Shui-lung-k'u (Shui-lung) | 水龍骨(水龍) | **Polypodium nipponicum** | *JAPANESE POLYPODY | Rhizoma Polypodii |
| 1323 Shui-mu-ts'ao | 水木草 | **Mnium cuspidata** | *MNIUM | Herba Mnii |
| 1324 Shui-niu-chio | 水牛角 | — | Water Buffalo horn | Cornu Bubali |
| 1325 Shui-pai-chih | 水柏枝 | **Myricaria germanica** | *MYRICARIA | Ramus Myricariae |
| 1326 Shui-pai-ho | 水百合 | **Cardiocrinum cathayanum** | *CARDIOCRINUM | Herba Cardiocrini |

| | Transliteration | Chinese | Botanical Name | English | Pharmaceutical |
|---|---|---|---|---|---|
| 1327 | Shui-pai-la | 水白腊 | **Ligustrum quihuoi** (North) **L. sinense** var. **nitidum** | *LESSER PRIVET | Radix, Cortex, et Folium Ligustri Quihuoi vel L. Sinensi Nitidi |
| 1328 | Shui-p'i-pa | 水枇杷 | **Saurauia tristyla** | *SAURAUIA | Radix Saurauiae |
| 1329 | Shui-shih | 水石 | See Han-shui-shih | — | — |
| 1330 | Shui-shih-liu-yeh-ts'ai (Tu-mu-niu) | 水濕柳葉荣(獨木牛) | **Epilobium palustre** | WILLOW-HERB | Herba Epilobii |
| 1331 | Shui-su (Shui-chi-su, Chi-su) | 水蘇(水鷄蘇,鷄蘇) | **Stachys recta** **S. baicalensis** **S. neglecta** | CHINESE FIELDNETTLE | Herba Stachydis |
| 1332 | Shui-sung (Tz'ŭ-hai-sung) | 水松(刺海松) | **Codium fragile** | SEAWEED | Herba Codii Fragilis |
| 1333 | Shui-sung-hsü (Shui-sung-p'i) | 水松鬚(水松皮) | **Glyptostrobus pensilis** | *GLYPTOSTROBUS | Ramus et Cortex Glyptostrobi |
| 1334 | Shui-t'a-kan | 水獺肝 | — | Otter liver | Iecur Lutrae |
| 1335 | Shui-t'ien-ch'i (Shui-chi-t'ou) | 水田七(水鷄頭) | **Schizocapsa plantaginea** (**Tacca plantaginea**) | *SCHIZOCAPSA | Herba Schizocapsae |
| 1336 | Shui-t'ing-hsiang | 水丁香 | **Ludwigia prostrata** | *LUDWIGIA | Herba Ludwigiae |
| 1337 | Shui-tsao-chia | 水皂荚 | **Cassia nomame** | *ANNUAL CASSIA | Herba Cassiae Nomamis |
| 1338 | Shui-tsê-lan | 水澤蘭 | **Penthorum chinense** | *PENTHORUM | Herba Penthori |
| 1339 | Shui-ts'ung | 水葱 | **Scirpus lacustris** **S. validus** | *LAKE BULRUSH *ROBUST BULRUSH | Herba et Rhizoma Scirpi |

| | Transliteration | Chinese | Botanical Name | English | Pharmaceutical |
|---|---|---|---|---|---|
| 1340 | Shui-t'uan-hua (Shui-yang-mei, Ch'uan-yü-liu) | 水團花(水楊莓,穿魚柳) | **Adina pilulifera** | *ADINA | Ramus Adinae |
| 1341 | Shui-wêng-p'i, Shui-wêng-hua | 水翁皮,水翁花 | **Cleistocalyx operculata** | *CLEISTOCALYX | Cortex et Flos Cleistocalicis |
| 1342 | Shui-wu-kung | 水蜈蚣 | **Kyllinga brevifolia** | KYLLINGA | Herba Kyllingae |
| 1343 | Shui-yang-chih (Shui-yang-kên, Shui-yang-mu-pai-p'i) | 水楊枝(水楊根,水楊木白皮) | **Salix purpurea** | BASKET WILLOW | Ramus, Radix, et Cortex Salicis |
| 1344 | Shui-yang-mei | 水楊莓 | **Geum japonicum** | AVENS | Herba Gei |
| 1345 | Shui-yin | 水銀 | — | Quicksilver or Mercury | Hydrargyrum |
| 1346 | Shui-yü-kuo | 水榆果 | **Sorbus alnifolia** | *ALDER-LEAVED MOUNTAIN ASH | Fructus Sorbi |
| 1347 | So-yang | 鎖陽 | **Cynomorium coccineum C. songaricum** | *CYNOMORIUM | Herba Cynomorii |
| 1348 | Ssŭ-kua | 絲瓜 | **Luffa cylindrica L. acutangula** | *LUFFA | Parts used see below |
| | Ssŭ-kua-hua | 絲瓜花 | ,, ,, | ,, (flower) | Flos Luffae |
| | Ssŭ-kua-kên | 絲瓜根 | ,, ,, | ,, (root) | Radix Luffae |
| | Ssŭ-kua-lo | 絲瓜絡 | ,, ,, | ,, (vegetable sponge) | Fasciculus Vascularis Luffae |
| | Ssŭ-kua-p'i | 絲瓜皮 | ,, ,, | ,, (peel) | Pericarpium Luffae |
| | Ssŭ-kua-t'i | 絲瓜蒂 | ,, ,, | ,, (pedicel) | Pedicellus Luffae |
| | Ssŭ-kua-tzŭ | 絲瓜子 | ,, ,, | ,, (seed) | Semen Luffae |
| | Ssŭ-kua-yeh | 絲瓜葉 | ,, ,, | ,, (leaf) | Folium Luffae |
| | Ssŭ-kua-t'êng | 絲瓜藤 | ,, ,, | ,, (vine) | Ramus Luffae |

109

| Transliteration | Chinese | Botanical Name | English | Pharmaceutical |
|---|---|---|---|---|
| 1349 Ssŭ-mien | 絲綿 | — | Silk-wool | — |
| 1350 Ssŭ-mien-mu (Pai-t'ao-shu, Pai-tu, Yeh-tu-chung) | 絲棉木（白桃樹，白杜，野杜仲） | **Euonymus bungeanus** | *PEKING EUONYMUS | Radix, Cortex et Fructus Euonymi Bungeani |
| 1351 Ssŭ-pai-p'i (Hua-p'i) | 絲白皮（樺皮） | **Betula platyphylla** | BIRCH (bark) | Cortex Betulae |
| 1352 Ssŭ-tai-chüeh | 絲帶蕨 | **Drymotaenium miyoshianum** | *DRYMOTAENIUM | Herba Drymotaenii |
| 1353 Ssŭ-t'ung (T'ung-ts'ao) | 絲通（通草） | See T'ung-ts'ao | Ricepaper (shred) | — |
| 1354 Su-ch'ing (Su-mien) | 蘇青（蘇面） | **Ophiopogon japonicus** | *OPHIOPGON | Radix Ophiopogonis |
| 1355 Su-ho-hsiang (Su-ho-yu) | 蘇合香（蘇合油） | **Liquidambar orientalis** | ROSE MALOES | Styrax Liquidus (Storax) |
| 1356 Su-hsia (Pan-hsia) | 蘇夏（半夏） | **Pinellia ternata** | *PINELLIA | Rhizoma Pinelliae |
| 1357 Su-hsin-hua | 素馨花 | **Jasminum officinale** | *WHITE JASMINE | Flos Jasmini Officinalis |
| 1358 Su-huang-ch'i (T'u-huang-ch'i) | 蘇黃耆（土黃耆） | **Malva neglecta** | CHEESEWEED | Herba Malvae Neglectae |
| 1359 Su-kêng | 蘇梗 | **Perilla ocymoides** | PERILLA | Caulis Perillae |
| 1360 Su-k'o | 粟殼 | **Papaver somniferum** | OPIUM POPPY (pod) | Fructus Papaveris |
| 1361 Su-mu (Su-mu-k'ang) | 蘇木（蘇木糠） | **Caesalpinia sappan** **Haematoxylon campechianum** | SAPPAN WOOD LOG WOOD | Lignum Sappan Lignum Haematoxylonis |

110

| Transliteration | Chinese | Botanical Name | English | Pharmaceutical |
|---|---|---|---|---|
| 1362 Su-tzǔ (Pai-su-tzǔ) | 蘇子（白蘇子） | **Perilla ocymoides** | PERILLA (seed) | Semen Perillae |
| 1363 Su-yeh | 蘇葉 | **Perilla ocymoides** | PERILLA (leaves) | Folium Perillae |
| 1364 Suan-chiang-kên | 酸漿根 | **Physalis alkekengi** | CHINESE LANTERN-PLANT (root) | Radix Physalis |
| 1365 Suan-chiang-shih | 酸漿實 | **Physalis alkekengi** | CHINESE LATERN-PLANT (fruit) | Fructus Physalis |
| 1366 Suan-chiang-ts'ai | 酸漿荣 | **Oxyria digyna** | MOUNTAIN-SORREL | Herba Oxyriae |
| 1367 Suan-chio (Suan-tou, Lo-wang-tzǔ) | 酸角（酸豆，羅望子） | **Tamarindus indica** | TAMARIND | Fructus Tamarindi |
| 1368 Suan-lou-kên (Suan-wei-ts'ao) | 酸蔞根（酸味草） | **Oxalis corniculata** | WOOD-SORREL | Herba Oxalidis |
| 1369 Suan-mu | 酸模 | **Rumex acetosa** | DOCK, or SORREL | Radix et Folium Rumicis |
| 1370 Suan-p'an-tzǔ | 算盤子 | **Glochidion puberum** | *GLOCHIDION | Radix Glochidionis |
| 1371 Suan-pu-liu | 酸不溜 | **Polygonum divaricatum** | KNOTWEED | Herba Polygoni Divaricati |
| 1372 Suan-shui-ts'ao | 酸水草 | **Potamogeton perfoliatus** | PONDWEED | Herba Potamogetonis |
| 1373 Suan-t'êng-tzǔ (Suan-t'êng-kuo) | 酸藤子（酸藤果） | **Embelia laeta** | *EMBELIA | Ramus et Fructus Embeliae Laetae |
| 1374 Suan-tsao-jên | 酸棗仁 | **Zizyphus jupuba** var. **spinosa** | SOUR JUJUBE | Semen Ziziphi Spinosae |
| 1375 Sui-jên (Jui-jên, Nai-jên, Nei-jên) | 遂仁（芮仁，蕤仁，奈仁，內仁） | **Prinsepia uniflora** | *PRINSEPIA | Semen Prinsepiae |
| 1376 Sui-pu (Ku-sui-pu) | 碎補（骨碎補） | **Drynaria fortunei** | *DRYNARIA | Rhizoma Drynariae |
| 1377 Sung-ch'ên (Sung-ch'ên-p'i) | 宋陳（宋陳皮） | **Citrus reticulata** | MANDARIN ORANGE (salted peel) | Pericarpium Citri Praeparationis |

| Transliteration | Chinese | Botanical Name | English | Pharmaceutical |
|---|---|---|---|---|
| 1378 Sung-chieh | 松節 | **Pinus tabulaeformis** **P. massoniana** | PINE (knots) | *Sungchieh |
| —a Sung-chiu | 松球 | The above species | " (cones) | Fructus Pini |
| Sung-hsiang | 松香 | The above species | " (resin) | Resina Pini |
| Sung-hua-fêng | 松花粉 | **Pinus massoniana** | " (pollen) | Pollen Pini |
| Sung-kên | 松根 | **P. massoniana** | " (root) | Radix Pini |
| Sung-tzǔ | 松子 | See below | " (seeds) | Semen Pini |
| —b Hai-sung-tzǔ | 海松子 | **P. koraiensis** | | |
| —c Pai-sung-tzǔ | 白松子 | **P. armandii** | | |
| 1379 Sung-chün | 松蕈 | **Armillaria matsutake** | *PINE MUSHROOM | Fructificatio Armillariae |
| 1380 Sung-hao | 松蒿 | **Phtheirospermum japonicum** | *JAPANESE LOUSE-SEED | Herba Phtheirospermi |
| 1381 Sung-lan | 松藍 | **Isatis tinctoria** **I. indigotica** | WOAD | Herba Isatidis |
| 1382 Sung-lo | 松蘿 | **Usnea longissima** **U. diffracta** | OLD MAN'S BEARD | Herba Usneae |
| 1382A Suo-yang | 鎖陽 | **Cynomorium songaricum** | APHRODITE CYNOMORIUM | Herba Cynomorii |
| 1383 Ta-ch'a-kên | 大茶根 | **Mussaenda erosa** | WILD MUSSAENDA | Radix Mussaendae |
| 1384 Ta-ch'a-yao (Tuan-ch'ang-ts'ao) | 大茶藥(斷腸草) | **Gelsemium elegans** | YELLOW JESSAMINE | Herba et Radix Gelsemii |
| 1385 Ta-ch'ao-ts'ai | 大巢菜 | **Vicia sativa** | VETCH | Herba Viciae |
| 1386 Ta-chi (Hung-ya-ta-chi) | 大戟(紅芽大戟) | **Knoxia corymbosa** | *KNOXIA | Radix Knoxiae |
| —a Ching-ta-chi | 京大戟 | **Euphorbia pekinensis** | PEKING SPURGE | Radix Euphorbiae Pekinensis |
| 1387 Ta-chi | 大薊 | **Cirsium japonicum** | JAPANESE THISTLE | Herba Cirsii Japonici |

112

| | Transliteration | Chinese | Botanical Name | English | Pharmaceutical |
|---|---|---|---|---|---|
| 1388 | Ta-chiao-p'i | 大蕉皮 | **Musa paradisiaca** | BANANA (skin) | Pericarpium Musae |
| 1389 | Ta-chien | 大箭 | **Alisma canaliculatum** | *CHANNELLED WATER PLANTAIN | Herba Alismatis |
| 1390 | Ta-chin-hua | 大槿花 | **Hibiscus syriacs** | ROSE-OF-SHARON | Flos Hibisci Syriaci |
| 1391 | Ta-chin-pu-huan (Tzŭ-pei-chin-niu) | 大金不換(紫背金牛) | **Polygala chinensis** | *CHINESE MILKWORT | Herba Polygalae Chinensis |
| 1392 | Ta-ch'ing (Ta-ch'ing-yeh) | 大青(大青葉) | **Isatis tinctoria I. indigotica** | WOAD | Herba Isatidis |
| 1393 | Ta-ch'ing-kên (Lu-pien-ch'ing) | 大青根(路邊青) | **Clerodendrum cyrtophyllum** | *GREEN-WHITE CLERODENDRON | Herba et Radix Clerodendri Cyrtophylli |
| 1394 | Ta-ch'ing-ts'ao | 大青草 | **Hygrophila salicifolia** | *HYGROPHILA | Herba Hygrophilae |
| 1395 | Ta-ch'ing-yen (Jung-yen) | 大青鹽(戎鹽) | — | Salt rock (halite) | Halitum |
| 1396 | Ta-chiu-chieh-ling | 大九節鈴 | **Ampelocissus artemisiaefolia** | *AMPELOCISSUS | Radix Ampelocissi |
| 1397 | Ta-chiu-ku-niu | 大九股牛 | **Dobinea delavayi** | *DOBINEA | Radix Dobineae |
| 1398 | Ta-êrh-lang-chien | 大二郎箭 | **Lippia nodiflora** | *LIPPIA | Herba Lippae |
| 1399 | Ta-fei-yang-ts'ao | 大飛揚草 | **Euphorbia hirta** | *HOARY SPURGE | Herba Euphorbiae Hirtae |
| 1400 | Ta-fêng-tzŭ (Ta-fêng-tzŭ-yu) | 大楓子(大楓子油) | **Hydnocarpus anthelmintica H. kurzii** | CHAULMOOGRA | Semen Hydnocarpi |
| 1401 | Ta-fu-p'i (Pin-lang-i) | 大腹皮(檳榔衣) | **Areca catechu** | BETEL (husk) | Pericarpium Arecae |
| 1402 | Ta-fu-p'ing (Chu-mu-lien) | 大浮萍(猪乸蓮) | **Pistia stratiotes** | WATER LETTUCE | Herba Pistiae |

| | Transliteration | Chinese | Botanical Name | English | Pharmaceutical |
|---|---|---|---|---|---|
| 1403 | Ta-hai (Ta-hai-tzǔ, P'ang-ta-hai, P'êng-ta-hai) | 大海(大海子,胖大海, 澎大海) | **Scaphium affine** (Sterculia scaphigera) See 1042 | PANGTAHAI, BUNGTALAI (Siamese) | Semen Scaphii |
| 1404 | Ta-hsüeh-t'êng | 大血藤 | **Sargentodoxa cuneata** | *SARGENTODOXA | Caulis Sargentodoxae |
| 1405 | Ta-hu-ma (Ya-ma) | 大胡麻(亞麻) | **Linum usitatissimum** | FLAX | Semen Lini |
| 1406 | Ta-huang (Chiang-chün) | 大黃(將軍) | **Rheum** spp. | RHUBARB | Rhizoma Rhei |
| −a | Hsi-ning-ta-huang | 西寧大黃 | **R. palmatum** | | |
| −b | Liang-chou-ta-huang | 梁州大黃 | **R. tanguticum** | | |
| −c | Ma-t'i-ta-huang | 馬蹄大黃 | **R. officinale** | | |
| | K'uai-huang | 塊黃 | ,, ,, | ,, (inferior product) | Rhizoma Rhei |
| 1407 | Ta-hung-p'ao | 大紅袍 | **Myrsine africana** | *MYRSINE | Radix et Ramus Myrsinis |
| 1408 | Ta-huo-ts'ao-kên | 大火草根 | **Anemone tomentosa** | *HAIRY ANEMONE | Radix Anemones Tomentosae |
| 1409 | Ta-i-chih-chien | 大一枝箭 | **Lycoris aurea** | *YELLOW LYCORIS | Bulbus Lycoris Aureae |
| 1410 | Ta-i-mien-lo | 大一面鑼 | **Didissandra sesquifolia** | *DIDISSANDRA | Herba Didissandrae |
| 1411 | Ta-li-tzǔ (Niu-p'ang-tzǔ) | 大力子(牛蒡子) | **Arctium lappa** | BURDOCK | Fructus Bardanae |
| 1412 | Ta-lo-san | 大羅傘 | **Ardisia crenata** | HILO HOLLY | Radix et Folium Ardisiae Crenatae |

114

| Transliteration | Chinese | Botanical Name | English | Pharmaceutical |
|---|---|---|---|---|
| 1413 Ta-ma (Ta-ma-shu-chih) | 打馬(璉馬樹脂) | **Balanocarpus heimii** | PENAK DAMMAR | Dammar |
| | | **Hopea micrantha** | MALAYA DAMMAR | ,, |
| | | **Shorea hypochra** | TEMAK DAMMAR | ,, |
| | | **Shorea robusta** | INDIAN DAMMAR | ,, |
| | | **Shorea wiesneri** | INDONESIAN DAMMAR | ,, |
| 1414 Ta-ma-jên | 大麻仁 | **Cannabis sativa** | HEMP (seed) | Semen Cannabis |
| 1415 Ta-mai (Ta-mai-jên, Ta-mai-ya) | 大麥(大麥仁,大麥芽) | **Hordeum vulgare** | BARLEY | Semen et Plantula Hordei |
| 1416 Ta-pai-ting-ts'ao | 大白頂草 | **Senecio orgzetorum** | *SENECIO, TAIPAI RAGWORT | Herba Senecionis Orgzetori |
| 1417 Ta-p'ao-t'ung | 大泡桐 | **Schefflera delavayi** | *SCHEFFLERA | Radix Schefflerae Delavayi |
| 1418 Ta-po-ku-tan | 大駁骨丹 | **Adhatoda ventricosa** **Adhatoda vasica** | Gendarussa | Herba Adhatodae Ventricosae |
| 1419 Ta-sha-yeh | 大沙葉 | **Pavetta hongkongensis** | *PAVETTA | Ramus Pavettae |
| 1420 Ta-shê-yao | 大蛇藥 | **Heteropanax fragrans** | *HETEROPANAX | Radix et Cortex Heteropanacis |
| 1421 Ta-shu-tieh-ta | 大樹跌打 | **Endospermum chinense** | *ENDOSPERMUM | Ramus Endospermi |
| 1422 Ta-suan | 大蒜 | **Allium sativum** | GARLIC | Bulbus Alli Sativi |
| 1423 Ta-ti-tsung-kên | 大地棕根 | **Curculigo capitulata** | *CAPUT CURCULIGO | Rhizoma Curculiginis Capitulatae |
| 1424 Ta-ting-ts'ao | 大丁草 | **Leibnitzia anandria** | *LEIBNITZIA | Herba Leibnitziae |
| 1425 Ta-tou-huang-chuan | 大豆黃捲 | **Glycine max** | SOYBEAN (young sprout) | Plantula Glycines |

115

| | Transliteration | Chinese | Botanical Name | English | Pharmaceutical |
|---|---|---|---|---|---|
| 1426 | Ta-t'ou-ch'ên | 大頭陳 | **Adenosma indianum** | *LESSER ADENOSMA | Herba Adenosmatis Indiani |
| 1427 | Ta-t'ou-ku-hsiao | 大透骨消 | **Gaultheria forrestii** | *GAULTHERIA | Radix et Ramus Gaultheriae |
| 1428 | Ta-t'ou-ku-ts'ao | 大透骨草 | **Vaccinium dunalianum** **var. urophyllum** | *SOUTH CHINA BLUEBERRY | Frutex Vaccini Dunaliani |
| 1429 | Ta-tsao (Hung-tsao) | 大棗(紅棗) | **Zizyphus jujuba** | JUJUBE | Fructus Zizyphi Jujubae |
| 1430 | Ta-ts'ao-k'ou (Yen-shan-chiang, Ts'ao-k'ou) | 大草蔻(艷山薑,草蔻) | **Alpinia zerumbet** **(A. speciosa)** | SHELL GINGER | Fructus Alpiniae zerumbet |
| 1431 | Ta-tu-yeh-ts'ao | 大獨葉草 | **Ligularia lapathifolia** | *LIGULARIA | Herba Ligulariae |
| 1432 | Ta-tuai-ching-ts'ao | 大對經草 | **Hypericum przewalskii** | *WEST CHINA ST. JOHNSWORT | Herba Hyperici Przewalskii |
| 1433 | Ta-tz'ǔ-êrh-ts'ai (Ta-ch'i) | 大刺兒菜(大薊) | **Cirsium eriophoroideum** | TIBETAN THISTLE | Herba Cirsii Eriophoroidei |
| 1434 | Ta-wan-hua | 打碗花 | **Calystegia hederacea** | *CALYSTEGIA | Rhizoma et Flos Calystegiae |
| 1435 | Ta-wei-yao | 大尾搖 | **Heliotropium indicum** | *HELIOTROPIUM | Herba Heliotropii |
| 1436 | Ta-yeh-an | 大葉桉 | **Eucalyptus robusta** | SWAMP MAHOGANY | Ramus Eucalypti Robustae |
| 1437 | Ta-yeh-fêng-sha-t'êng | 大葉風沙藤 | **Kadsura heteroclita** | *KADSURA | Ramus Kadsurae Heteroclitae |
| 1438 | Ta-yeh-fêng-wei | 大葉鳳尾 | **Pteris nervosa** | *GREATER PTERIS | Herba Pteridis Nervosae |
| 1439 | Ta-yeh-hsiang-ju | 大葉香薷 | **Orthodon dianthera** | PRICKLY-HEATWORT | Herba Orthodonis |

116

| Transliteration | Chinese | Botanical Name | English | Pharmaceutical |
|---|---|---|---|---|
| 1440 Ta-yeh-hua-chiao | 大葉花椒 | **Zanthoxylum dissitum** | *GREATER BRAMBLE | Fructus Zanthoxyli Dissiti |
| 1441 Ta-yeh-kou-t'êng | 大葉鈎藤 | **Uncaria macrophylla** | *GREATER UNCARIA | Ramus Uncariae Macrophyllae |
| 1442 Ta-yeh-kuan-mên | 大夜關門 | **Bauhinia pernervosa** | *MANY-NERVED BAUHINIA | Folium Bauhiniae Pernervosae |
| 1443 Ta-yeh-ma-wei-lien | 大葉馬尾蓮 | **Thalictrum faberi** | *FABER'S MEADOW-RUE | Radix et Rhizoma Thalictri Faberi |
| 1444 Ta-yeh-nan-kên | 大葉楠根 | **Machilus leptophylla** | *GREATER NAN | Radix Machili Leptophyllae |
| 1445 Ta-yeh-pai-tou-wêng | 大葉白頭翁 | **Anaphalis margaritacea** | *ANAPHALIS | Herba Anaphalis |
| 1446 Ta-yeh-shan-kuei (Shan-jou-kuei) | 大葉山桂(山肉桂) | **Cinnamomum obtusifolia** | *WILD CINNAMON | Cortex Cinnamomi Obtusifoliae |
| 1447 Ta-yeh-shê-p'ao-lê | 大葉蛇泡簕 | **Rubus alceaefolius** | *ROUGH RASPBERRY | Radix et Folium Rubi Alceaefolii |
| 1448 Ta-yeh-tzŭ-chu | 大葉紫珠 | **Callicarpa macrophylla** | *LARGE-LEAVED CALLICARPA | Radix et Folium Callicarpae Macrophyllae |
| 1449 Ta-yün (Ts'ung-jung) | 大芸(蓯蓉) | **Cistanche salsa** | BROOMRAPE | Herba Cistanchis Salsae |
| 1450 Ta-yün-hsiang (Fêng-hsiang, Yün-hsiang) | 大芸香(楓香,芸香) | **Liquidambar formosana** | CHINESE SWEET GUM (resin) | Resina Liquidambaris |
| 1451 T'a-kan | 獺肝 | — | Otter liver | Iecur Lutrae |

117

| | Transliteration | Chinese | Botanical Name | English | Pharmaceutical |
|---|---|---|---|---|---|
| 1452 | Tai-mao | 玳瑁 | — | Tortoise shell | Carapax Eretmochelytis |
| 1453 | Tai-tai-hua (Suan-ch'êng-hua) | 代代花(酸橙花) | **Citrus aurantium** | SOUR ORANGE (flower) | Flos Citri Aurantii |
| 1454 | T'ai-pai-ai | 太白艾 | **Tanacetum variifolium** | TANSY | Herba Tanaceti |
| 1455 | T'ai-pai-chü | 太白菊 | **Aster flaccidus** | *FLACCID ASTER | Herba Asteris Flaccidi |
| 1456 | T'ai-pai-hsiao-tzŭ-wan | 太白小紫苑 | **Cremanthodium hookerii** | *CREMANTHODIUM | Herba Cremanthodii |
| 1457 | T'ai-pai-hua | 太白花 | Cladonia alpestris | *TAIPAI LICHEN | Herba Cladoniae |
| 1458 | T'ai-pai-lu-chio | 太白鹿角 | **Cladonia gracilis** | *SLENDER CLADONIA | Herba Cladoniae Gracilis |
| 1459 | T'ai-pai-pei-mu | 太白貝母 | **Fritillaria taipaiensis** | *TAIPAI FRITILLARY | Bulbus Fritillariae Taipaiensis |
| 1460 | T'ai-pai-san-ch'i | 太白三七 | **Tongoloa dunnii** | *TONGOLOA | Radix Tongoloae |
| 1461 | T'ai-pai-shên | 太白参 | **Pedicularis davidii** | *DAVID'S PEDICULARIS | Rhizoma Pedicularis |
| 1462 | T'ai-p'ing-mei (Lao-hu-niu) | 太平莓(老虎扭) | **Rubus pacificus** | *PACIFIC RASPBERRY | Herba Rubi Pacifici |
| 1463 | T'ai-tzŭ-shên (Hai-êrh-shên) | 太子参(孩兒参) | **Pseudostellaria hetero-phylla** | LESSER GINSENG | Radix Pseudostellariae |
| 1464 | T'ai-yang-chên | 太陽針 | **Plagiopus oederi** | *PLAGIOPUS | Herba Plagiopi |
| 1465 | T'ai-yang-ts'ao | 太陽草 | **Rhodobryum giganteum** | RHODOBRYUM MOSS | Herba Rhodobryni |
| 1466 | Tan-chu | 淡竹 | **Phyllostachys nigra** | *TANCHU | |
| | Tan-chu-kên | 淡竹根 | " " | " (root) | Radix Phyllostachydis |
| | Tan-chu-ko | 淡竹殼 | " " | " (scale) | Squama Phyllostachydis |
| | Tan-chu-sun | 淡竹笋 | " " | " (shoot) | Gemma Phyllostachydis |
| 1467 | Tan-chu-yeh | 淡竹葉 | **Lophatherum gracile** | *LOPHATHERUM | Herba Lophatheri |

| | Transliteration | Chinese | Botanical Name | English | Pharmaceutical |
|---|---|---|---|---|---|
| 1468 | Tan-fan (Shih-tan) | 胆矾(膽礬,石膽) | — | Blue Vitriol (Copper sulphate) | Chalcanthite |
| 1469 | Tan-hsing (Tan-nan-hsing) | 膽星(膽南星) | See T'ien-nan-hsing | ARISAEMA (powder plus ox gall) | Pulvis Arisaemae cum Felle Bovis |
| 1470 | Tan-kên (Tan-kên-hsü, Tan-hsü) | 丹根(丹根鬚,丹鬚) | **Paeonia suffruticosa** | MOUTAN (root) | *Radix Moutan |
| 1471 | Tan-kên-mu (Chên-t'ien-lui) | 單根木(震天雷) | **Ervatamia hainanensis** | *ERVATAMIA | Radix Ervatamii |
| 1472 | Tan-ku (Wu-tsei-ku) | 淡骨(烏賊骨) | — | Cuttle-fish bone | Os Sepiae |
| 1473 | Tan-mu (Hsiung-tan-shu, Wu-t'an) | 胆木(熊膽樹,烏檀) | **Nauclea officinalis** | *NAUCLEA | Ramulus Naucleae |
| 1474 | Tan-p'i (Mu-tan-pi) | 丹皮(牡丹皮) | **Paeonia suffruticosa** | MOUTAN (root-bark) | Cortex Moutan |
| 1475 | Tan-sha (Chu-sha, Ch'ên-sha) | 丹砂(珠砂,辰砂) | — | Cinnabar | Cinnabaris |
| 1476 | Tan-shên | 丹參 | **Salvia miltiorhiza** **S. przewalskii** | *RED-ROOTED SAGE | Radix Salviae Miltiorhizae |
| 1477 | Tan-tou-shih | 淡豆豉 | **Glycine soja +** **Morus alba +** **Artemisia apiacea** | *Tantoushih | Mistura Glycines, Mori, et Artemisiae Fermentata |
| 1478 | Tan-ts'ai | 淡菜 | — | Mussel (dried) | Mytilus |
| 1479 | Tan-ts'ao (Lung-tan-ts'ao) | 膽草(龍膽草) | **Gentiana scabra** | GENTIAN (root) | Radix Gentianae |
| 1480 | Tan-wei-tang-yao | 淡味當藥 | **Swertia diluta** | SWERTIA | Herba Sweriae Dilutae |

| Transliteration | Chinese | Botanical Name | English | Pharmaceutical |
|---|---|---|---|---|
| 1481 T'an-hsiang (Pai-t'an) | 檀香(白檀) | **Santalum album** | SANDALWOOD | Lignum Santali Albi |
| 1482 T'an-hsiang-yu | 檀香油 | **Santalum album** | SANDALWOOD (oil) | Oleum Santali |
| 1483 Tang-kuei | 當歸(黨歸) | **Angelica sinensis** | *CHINESE ANGELICA | Radix Angelicae Sinensis |
| Chin-kuei (Hsi-kuei) | 秦歸(西歸) | ,, ,, | ,, ,, transported via Hsi-an | |
| Ch'uan-kuei | 川歸 | ,, ,, | ,, ,, transported via Ch'ung-ching | |
| Kuei-shên | 歸身 | ,, ,, | ,, ,, taproot | ,, ,, ,, |
| Kuei-wei | 歸尾 | ,, ,, | ,, ,, branch root ends | ,, ,, ,, |
| Tang-kuei-sui | 當歸碎 | ,, ,, | ,, ,, refuse | ,, ,, ,, |
| 1484 Tang-shên | 黨參 | **Codonopsis pilosula C. tangshen** | *TANGSHEN | Radix Codonopsis |
| Ch'uan-tang | 川黨 | ,, ,, | From Szechuan | |
| Fang-tang | 防黨 | ,, ,, | From Fang-hsien, Hupeh | |
| Fêng-p'i-tang | 鳳皮黨 | ,, ,, | Fastened with red cords | |
| Hsi-tang | 西黨 | ,, ,, | From Shensi | |
| Lu-tang | 潞黨 | ,, ,, | From Lu-an, Shansi | |
| 1485 Tang-yao | 當藥 | **Swertia pseudochinensis** | *TANGYAO | Herba Swertiae |
| 1486 T'ang-chiai | 糖芥 | **Erysimum cheiranthoides** | *ERYSIMUM | Herba Erysimi |
| 1487 Tao-cha-lung | 倒扎龍 | **Rubus pungens** | PIERCING RASPBERRY | Radix Rubi Pungentis |
| 1488 Tao-ch'ih-san | 倒赤傘 | **Ainsliaea latifolia** | *AINSLIAEA | Herba Ainsliaeae |
| 1489 Tao-chü-san (Ch'iang-wei-mei) | 倒觸傘(薔薇莓) | **Rubus rosaefolius** | *ROSE-LEAVED RASPBERRY | Radix Rubi Rosaefolii |

120

| Transliteration | Chinese | Botanical Name | English | Pharmaceutical | Tao |
|---|---|---|---|---|---|
| 1490 Tao-kou-tz'ŭ | 倒鈎刺 | **Rubus delavayi** | *Yunnan Raspberry | Ramus Rubi Delavayi | |
| 1491 Tao-k'ou-ts'ao (Tu-niu-hsi) | 倒扣草(土牛膝) | **Achyranthes aspera** | *Achyranthes | Radix Achyranthis Asperae | |
| 1492 Tao-k'ou-yao | 刀口藥 | **Ainsliaea triflora** | *Three-flowered Ainsliaea | Folium Ainsliaeae Triflorae | |
| 1493 Tao-kua-niu | 倒挂牛 | **Caesalpinia sepiaria** | Mysore Thorn | Radix et Cortex Caesalpiniae Sepiariae | |
| 1494 Tao-shêng-kên | 倒生根 | **Rubus coreanus** | *Korean Raspberry | Radix Rubi Coreani | |
| 1495 Tao-shêng-lien | 倒生蓮 | **Asplenium prolongatum** | *Walking Spleenwort | Herba Asplenii | |
| 1496 Tao-shui-lien | 倒水蓮 | **Thalictrum omeiense** | *Omei Meadowrue | Herba Thalictri Omeiensis | |
| 1497 Tao-ti-ling | 倒地鈴 | **Cardiospermum halicacabum** | Ballon Vine | Herba Cardiospermi | |
| 1498 Tao-t'i-hu (Chieh-ku-ts'ao) | 倒提壺(接骨草) | **Cynoglossum amabile** | Hound's Tongue | Cautex Cynoglossum Amabilis | |
| 1499 Tao-tiao-la-chü (Tao-tiao-pi) | 倒吊燭蠟(倒吊筆) | **Wrightia pubescens** | *Wrightia | Radix, Ramus et Folium Wrightiae | |
| 1500 Tao-tou (Tao-tou-tzŭ, Tao-tou-kên) | 刀豆(刀豆子,刀豆根) | **Canavalia gladiata C. ensiformis** | Jack Bean | Semen et Radix Canavaliae | |
| 1500A T'ao-erh-ch'i | 桃兒七 | (see 0691A) | | | |
| 1501 T'ao-shu | 桃樹 | **Prunus persica** | Peach | | |
| T'ao-jên | 桃仁 | ,,  ,, | ,,  (seed) | Semen Persicae | |
| T'ao-shu-p'i | 桃樹皮 | ,,  ,, | ,,  (bark) | Cortex Persicae | |
| T'ao-yeh | 桃葉 | ,,  ,, | ,,  (leaves) | Folium Persicae | |

| Transliteration | Chinese | Botanical Name | English | Pharmaceutical |
|---|---|---|---|---|
| 1502 Têng-chan-hsi-hsin | 燈盞細辛 | **Erigeron breviscapus** | *ERIGERON | Herba Erigerontis |
| 1503 Têng-hsin-ts'ao (Têng-hsin-ts'ao-kên) | 燈心草(燈心草根) | **Juncus effusus** **J. decipiens** | BOG-RUSH | Medulla et Rhizoma Junci |
| 1504 Têng-lung-kuo | 燈籠果 | **Ribes mandschuricum** | GOOSEBERRY | Fructus Ribis Mandschurici |
| 1505 Têng-lung-ts'ao (Suan-chiang) | 燈籠草(酸漿) | **Physalis minima** **P. peruviana** | GROUND-BERRY | Herba Physalidis |
| 1506 Têng-t'ai-shu | 燈枱樹 | **Alstonia scholaris** | *ALSTONIA | Ramus Alstoniae |
| 1507 T'êng-huang (Yüeh-huang) | 藤黃(月黃) | **Garcinia hanburyi** **C. morella** | GAMBOGE (resin) | Gambogia, Gutti |
| 1508 T'êng-li-kên (Mao-li-tzŭ) | 藤梨根(毛梨子) | **Actinidia chinensis** | *CHINESE ACTINIDIA (root) | Radix Actinidiae Chinensis |
| 1509 Ti-chan-ts'ao (Mao-kao-ts'ai) | 地毡草(毛膏菜) | **Drosera spathulata** | SUNDEW | Herba Droserae |
| 1510 Ti-ch'iang-wei (Chui-fêng-hao) | 地薔薇(追風蒿) | **Chamaerhodos erecta** | *CHAMAERHODOS | Herba Chamaerhodoris |
| 1511 Ti-chiao (Pai-li-hsiang, Yeh-pai-li-hsiang) | 地椒(百里香, 野百里香) | **Thymus serpyllum** **T. mongolicus** | THYME | Herba Thymi |
| 1512 Ti-chieh-tzŭ (T'ung-chui-yü-tai-ts'ao) | 地茄子(銅錘玉帶草) | **Pratia begonifolia** | *PRATIA | Fructus Pratiae |
| 1513 Ti-chin (Huang-mao) | 地筋(黃茅) | **Heteropogon contortus** | TANGLEHEAD | Herba Heteropogonis |

| Transliteration | Chinese | Botanical Name | English | Pharmaceutical |
|---|---|---|---|---|
| 1514 Ti-chin (P'a-shan-hu) | 地錦(爬山虎) | **Parthenocissus tricuspidata** | BOSTON IVY | Ramus Parthenocissi |
| 1515 Ti-chin-ts'ao | 地錦草 | **Euphorbia humifusa** | WOLF'S MILK | Herba Euphorbiae Humifusae |
| 1516 Ti-ching-ts'ao | 地精草 | **Stellaria saxatilis** | CHICKWEED | Herba Stellariae Saxatilis |
| 1517 Ti-êrh-ts'ao (T'ien-chi-huang) | 地耳草(田基黃) | **Hypericum japonicum** | *LESSER ST. JOHNSWORT | Herba Hyperici Japonici |
| 1518 Ti-fêng-p'i | 地楓皮 | **Illicium difengpi** | *DIFENGPI | Cortex Illici Difengpi |
| 1519 Ti-fu (Ti-fu-tzŭ, Ti-fu-miao) | 地膚(地膚子,地膚苗) | **Kochia scoparia** | KOCHIA | Herba et Semen Kochiae |
| 1520 Ti-hsien-t'ao | 地仙桃 | **Lithospermum zollingeri** | *LITHOSPERMUM | Fructus Lithospermi |
| 1521 Ti-hsüeh-hsiang (Ta-fêng-sha-t'êng) | 地血香(大風沙藤) | **Kadsura heteroclita** | KADSURA | Ramus et Flos Kadsurae Heteroclitae |
| 1522 Ti-hua-shêng | 地花生 | **Polygala crotalarioides** | *SZECHUAN POLYGALA | Radix Polygalae Crotalarioidis |
| 1523 Ti-huang | 地黃 | **Rehmannia glutinosa** | CHINESE FOXGLOVE | Radix Rehmanniae |
| Shêng-ti | 生地 | ,,    ,, | ,, (raw root) | Radix Rehmanniae |
| Shu-ti | 熟地 | ,,    ,, | ,, (cooked root) | Radix Rehmanniae Conquitae |
| Ti-huang-hua | 地黃花 | ,,    ,, | ,, (flower) | Flos Rehmanniae |
| Ti-huang-yeh | 地黃葉 | ,,    ,, | ,, (leaf) | Folium Rehmanniae |
| 1524 Ti-huang-kua | 地黃瓜 | **Viola grypoceras** | *SWAMP VIOLET | Herba Violae |

| | Transliteration | Chinese | Botanical Name | English | Pharmaceutical |
|---|---|---|---|---|---|
| 1525 | Ti-huang-lien | 地黃蓮 | **Munronia henryi** | *MUNRONIA | Frutex Munroniae |
| −a | Ai-t'ou-t'ou | 矮沱沱 | **M. sinica** | Chinese Munronia | |
| −b | Hai-nan-ti-huang-lien | 海南地黃蓮 | **M. hainanensis** | Hainan Munronia | |
| −c | Hsiao-fu-jung | 小芙蓉 | **M. heterotricha** | Lesser Munronia | |
| −d | Hu-nan-ti-huang-lien | 湖南地黃蓮 | **M. hunanensis** | Hunan Munronia | |
| −e | Yun-nan-ti-huang-lien | 雲南地黃蓮 | **M. delavayi** | Yunnan Munronia | |
| 1526 | Ti-hung-tzŭ-kên | 地紅子根 | **Cotoneaster horizontalis** | *COTONEASTER | Radix Cotoneastri |
| 1527 | Ti-kao-yao | 地膏藥 | **Gnaphalium adnatum** | *ADNATE CUDWEED | Herba Gnaphalii Adnati |
| 1528 | Ti-ku-lu (Hsien-jên-ku, Lao-lo-po-t'ou) | 地枯蔞(地骷髏,仙人骨,老蘿蔔頭) | **Raphanus sativus** | CHINESE RADISH (after fruiting) | Radix Raphani |
| 1529 | Ti-ku-niu (Chiao-ch'ing-ling, Chin-sha-niu) | 地牯牛(蛟蜻蛉,金沙牛) | — | Damselfly nymph | Myrmeleon |
| 1529A | Ti-ku-p'i | 地骨皮 | (see 0134) | | |
| 1530 | Ti-kua (Ti-kua-tzŭ) | 地瓜(地瓜子) | **Pachyrhizus erosus** | YAM-BEAN | Radix et Semen Pachyrhizi |
| 1531 | Ti-kua-êrh-miao (Ti-sun) | 地瓜兒苗(地笋) | **Lycopus lucidus** | *SHINING WATER HOREHOUND | Herba Lycopi |
| 1532 | Ti-kuei-ts'ao-kên (Ti-kuei-ts'ao) | 地貴草根(地貴草) | **Ophiorrhiza succirubra** | *OPHIORRHIZA | Herba Ophiorrhizae |
| 1533 | Ti-lung | 地龍 | — | Earthworms | Lumbricus |
| 1534 | Ti-ma-huang (Su-mei-ts'ao) | 地麻黃(粟米草) | **Mollugo pentaphylla** | *MOLLUGO | Herba Molluginis |

124

| | Transliteration | Chinese | Botanical Name | English | Pharmaceutical |
|---|---|---|---|---|---|
| 1535 | Ti-mei-tzŭ | 地莓子 | **Rubus xanthocarpus** | *ORANGE RASPBERRY | Radix Rubi Xanthocarpi |
| 1536 | Ti-nien (Ti-jên, P'u-ti-jên) | 地菍(地稔,鋪地稔) | **Melastoma dodecandrum** | *LESSER MELASTOMA | Herba Melastomatis Dodecandri |
| 1537 | Ti-pa-chio | 地八角 | **Astragalus bhotanensis** | *HIMALAYAN MILK VETCH | Herba Astragali Bhotanensis |
| 1538 | Ti-pai-chih | 地柏枝 | **Selaginella moellendorfii** | GROOVED SPIKEMOSS | Herba Selaginellae Moellendorfii |
| 1539 | Ti-pai-ts'ao | 地白草 | **Viola diffusa** | *SPREADING VIOLET | Herba Violae Diffusae |
| 1540 | Ti-pai-yeh | 地柏葉 | **Asplenium incisum** | *INCISED SPLEENWORT | Herba Asplenii Incisi |
| 1541 | Ti-p'i-hsiao | 地皮消 | **Ruellia drymophila** | *RUELLIA | Herba Ruelliae |
| 1542 | Ti-pu-jung (Ti-fu-jung, Shan-wu-kuei) | 地不容(地芙蓉,山烏龜) | **Stephania delavayi S. brachyandra** | *CENTRAL CHINA STEPHANIA | Radix Stephaniae Delavayi et Brachyandrae |
| 1543 | Ti-sê-sê (Hsiao-p'o-p'o-na) | 地澀澀(小婆婆納) | **Veronica serpyllifolia** | THYME-LEAVED SPEEDWELL | Herba Veronicae Serpyllifoliae |
| 1544 | Ti-sha (Mei-yang-shên) | 地沙(米洋參) | **Burmannia coelestis** | *BURMANNIA | Herba Burmanniae |
| 1545 | Ti-shih-liu (Ti-kua-t'êng) | 地石榴(地瓜藤) | **Ficus tikoua** | *TIKOUA FIG | Ramus Fici Tikoua |
| 1546 | Ti-so-lo (Ti-ch'ien) | 地梭羅(地錢) | **Marchantia polymorpha** | LIVERWORT | Herba Marchantiae |
| 1547 | Ti-su-mu | 地蘇木 | **Abacopteris penangiana** | *ABACOPTERIS | Herba Abacopteridis |
| 1548 | Ti-sun (Ti-kua-êrh-miao) | 地笋(地瓜兒苗) | **Lycopus lucidus** | SHINING WATER HOREHOUND | Rhizoma Lycopi |
| 1549 | Ti-tan (Yüan-ch'ing, Ch'ing-mao) | 地膽(芫青,蚖青,青蚖) | — | *Blue-black Beetle | Cantharis |
| 1550 | Ti-tan-t'ou | 地膽頭 | **Elephantopus scaber** | *ELEPHANTOPUS | Herba Elephantopi |

125

| Transliteration | Chinese | Botanical Name | English | Pharmaceutical |
|---|---|---|---|---|
| 1551 Ti-ting | 地釘 | See the following | | |
| −a Lung-tan-ti-ting (South China) | 龍膽地丁(華南) | **Gentiana loureiroi** | *SOUTHERN GENTIAN | Herba Gentianae Loureiroi |
| −b T'ien-ti-ting (North China) | 甜地丁(華北) | **Gueldenstaedtia multiflora** **G. pauciflora** | *GUELDENSTAEDTIA | Herba Gueldenstaedtiae |
| −c Tzǔ-hua-ti-ting (Throughout the country) | 紫花地丁(全國各地) | **Viola chinensis** **V. inconspicua** **V. patrinii** **V. yedoensis** | VIOLET | Radix et Herba Violae |
| 1552 Ti-wu (Wu-kung-san-ch'i) | 地烏(蜈蚣三七) | **Anemone flaccida** | *TIWU, FLACCID ANEMONE | Rhizoma Anemones Flaccidae |
| 1553 Ti-yang-ch'üeh (Pai-mai-kên) | 地羊鵲(百脉根) | **Lotus corniculatus** | LOTUS | Herba Loti |
| 1554 Ti-yang-mei | 地楊梅 | **Luzula capitata** | LUZULA | Herba Luzulae |
| 1555 Ti-yü (Hung-ti-yü) | 地榆(紅地榆) | **Sanguisorba officinalis** | BURNET-BLOODWORT | Radix Sanguisorbae |
| 1556 Ti-yung-chin-lien (Ti-yung-lien) | 地涌金蓮(地涌蓮) | **Ensete lasiocarpum (Musella lasiocarpa)** | *ENSETE | Flos Ensetes |
| 1557 Tiao-chu (Liao-tiao-chu, Hsü-chang-ch'ing) | 刁竹(了刁竹,寮刁竹,徐長卿) | **Cynanchum paniculatum (Pycnostelma paniculatum)** | *LIAOTIAOCHU | Radix Cynanchi Paniculati |
| 1558 Tiao-kan (Tiao-yü-kan) | 釣竿(釣魚竿) | **Veronicastrum axillare** | *VERONICASTRUM | Herba Veronicastri |
| 1559 Tiao-lan | 吊蘭 | **Chlorophytum capense** | CHLOROPHYTUM, SPIDER PLANT | Herba Chlorophyti Capensis |

126

| | Transliteration | Chinese | Botanical Name | English | Pharmaceutical |
|---|---|---|---|---|---|
| 1560 | T'iao-ch'i (Mien-ch'i) | 條芪(綿芪) | **Astragalus membranaceus** | *HUANGCHI | Radix Astragali Membranacei |
| 1561 | T'iao-ts'ao (Kan-ts'ao) | 條草(甘草) | **Glycyrrhiza uralensis** | LIQUORICE | Radix Glycyrrhizae |
| 1562 | T'ieh | 鐵 | — | Iron ore | |
| −a | Chih-t'ieh-k'uang | 赤鐵礦 | — | Hematite | Hematitum |
| −b | Ho-t'ieh-k'uang | 褐鐵礦 | — | Limonite | Limonitum |
| −c | T'ieh-fêng (T'ieh-lo) | 鐵粉(鐵落) | — | Black ferric oxide | $Fe_3O_4$ |
| −d | T'ieh-hsiu | 鐵銹 | — | Iron rust | |
| −e | Tz'ŭ-t'ieh-k'uang | 磁鐵礦 | — | Magnetite | Magnetitum |
| 1563 | T'ieh-chio-fêng-wei-ts'ao (Chu-tsung-ch'i) | 鐵角鳳尾草(猪鬃七) | **Asplenium trichomanes** | *CLIFF SPLEENWORT | Herba Asplenii Trichomanis |
| 1564 | T'ieh-chüeh-chi | 鐵腳鷄 | **Abacopteris multilineata** | *WOODLAND ABACOPTERIS | Herba Abacopteridis Multilineatae |
| 1565 | T'ieh-chüeh-wei-ling-hsien (Huang-yao-tzŭ) | 鐵腳威靈仙(黃藥子) | **Clematis paniculata** | *CLEMATIS | Folium Clematidis Paniculatae |
| 1566 | T'ieh-hai-t'ang (Shih-tzŭ-lê) | 鐵海棠(獅子芀) | **Euphorbia milii** | CROWN-OF-THORN | Radix, Latex, et Flos Euphorbiae Milii |
| 1567 | T'ieh-hsien-chüeh | 鐵綫蕨 | **Adiantum flabellulatum** | FAN-LEAVED MAIDEN-HAIR | Herba Adianti |
| | | | **A. capillus-veneris** | VENUS-HAIR FERN | |

127

| | Transliteration | Chinese | Botanical Name | English | Pharmaceutical |
|---|---|---|---|---|---|
| 1568 | T'ieh-hsien-lien (Wei-ling-hsien) | 鐵綫蓮(威靈仙) | **Clematis florida** | *FLOWERING CLEMATIS | Radix et Herba Clematidis Floridae |
| 1569 | T'ieh-hsien-ts'ai | 鐵莧荣 | **Acalypha australis** | *ANNUAL COPPERLEAF | Herba Acalyphae |
| 1570 | T'ieh-hsien-ts'ao (Pan-kên-ts'ao) | 鐵綫草(絆根草) | **Cynodon dactylon** | BERMUDA GRASS | Herba Cynodontis |
| 1571 | T'ieh-ku-san | 鐵箍散 | **Cynoglossum zeylanicum** | *CEYLON CYNOGLOSSUM | Cortex et Folium Cynoglossi |
| 1572 | T'ieh-k'uai-tzŭ (Hei-mao-ch'i) | 鐵筷子(黑毛七) | **Helleborus thibetanus** | *HELLEBORUS | Radix Hellebori |
| 1573 | T'ieh-k'uai-tzŭ (La-mei-hua) | 鐵筷子(蠟梅花) | **Chimonanthus praecox** | *LAMEI (flower) | Radix et Ramus Chimonanthi |
| 1574 | T'ieh-li-pa-kuo | 鐵籬笆果 | **Paliurus ramosissimus** | *PALIURUS | Fructus Paliuri |
| 1575 | T'ieh-ma-pien | 鐵馬鞭 | **Lespedeza pilosa** | *LESPEDEZA | Herba Lespedezae |
| 1576 | T'ieh-ma-tou | 鐵馬豆 | **Shuteria pampaniniana** | *SHUTERIA | Herba Shuteriae |
| 1577 | T'ieh-pang-ch'ui | 鐵棒錘 | **Aconitum szecheyianum A. flavum** | *YELLOW MONKSHOOD | Radix et Ramus Aconiti Szechenyiani vel Flavi |
| 1578 | T'ieh-pao-chin (Wu-lung-kên) | 鐵包金(烏龍根) | **Berchemia lineata** | *LESSER BERCHEMIA, SUPPLE-JACK | Radix Berchemiae Lineatae |
| 1579 | T'ieh-pien-ts'ao | 鐵鞭草 | **Lespedeza floribunda** | *IRON WHIP | Herba et Radix Lespedezae Floribundae |
| 1580 | T'ieh-sao-chu | 鐵掃竹 | **Indigofera bungeana** | *IRON BROOM, BROOM-INDIGO | Herba et Radix Indigoferae Bungeanae |
| 1581 | T'ieh-sê-chien (Hu-ti-hsiao) | 鐵色箭(忽地笑) | **Lycoris aurea** | *YELLOW LYCORIS | Bulbus Lycoris Aureae |

| | Transliteration | Chinese | Botanical Name | English | Pharmaceutical | T'ieh-s |
|---|---|---|---|---|---|---|
| 1582 | T'ieh-shan-tzŭ | 鐵扇子 | **Adiantum myriosorum** | *IRON-FAN FERN, BOUNTIFUL MAIDEN-HAIR | Herba Adianti Myriosori | |
| 1583 | T'ieh-shu | 鐵樹 | **Cordyline fruticosa** | CORDYLINE | Folium et Flos Cordylines | |
| 1584 | T'ieh-shu-kuo (Su-t'ieh) | 鐵樹果(蘇鐵) | **Cycas revoluta** | CYCAS, SAGOPALM | Semen Cycadis | |
| 1585 | T'ieh-ssŭ-ch'i | 鐵絲七 | **Adiantum pedatum** | *PEDATE ADIANTUM, PALMATE MAIDEN-HAIR | Herba Adianti Pedati | |
| 1586 | T'ieh-t'êng-kên | 鐵藤根 | **Craspedolobium schochii** | *CRASPEDOLOBIUM | Radix Craspedolobii | |
| 1587 | T'ieh-ts'ao-hsieh | 鐵草鞋 | **Hoya pandurata** **H. pottsii** | HOYA | Folium Hoyae Panduratae et pottsii | |
| 1588 | Tien-ch'ieh-kên | 顚茄根 | **Atropa belladonna** | BELLADONNA | Radix Belladonnae | |
| 1589 | Tien-ti-mei | 點地梅 | **Androsace aizoon** **A. umbellata** | *ANDROSACE | Herba Androsaces | |
| 1590 | Tien-t'ou-chü | 點頭菊 | **Cremanthodium plantagineum** | *CREMANTHODIUM | Herba Cremanthodii Plantaginei | |
| 1591 | T'ien-ch'a | 甜茶 | **Hydrangea strigosa** **H. umbellata** | HYDRANGEA (young leaves) | Folium Hydrangeae | |
| 1592 | T'ien-ch'êng | 甜橙 | **Citrus sinensis** | ORANGE | Fructus Citri Sinensis | |
| 1593 | T'ien-chi-huang | 田基黃 | **Hypericum japonicum** | LESSER ST. JOHNSWORT | Herba Hyperici Japonici | |
| 1594 | T'ien-ch'i (San-ch'i) | 田七(三七) | **Panax notoginseng** | *SANCHI | Radix Sanchi | |
| 1595 | T'ien-chiang-ko | 天漿殼 | **Metaplexis japonica** | *METAPLEXIS (husk) | Pericarpium Metaplexis | |

129

| | Transliteration | Chinese | Botanical Name | English | Pharmaceutical |
|---|---|---|---|---|---|
| 1596 | T'ien-chiao-mai-kên | 天蕎麥根 | **Fagopyrum cymosum** | *WILD BUCKWHEAT (root) | Caudex Fagopyri Cymosi |
| 1597 | T'ien-ch'ieh-tzŭ | 天茄子 | **Solanum indicum** | *INDIAN NIGHTSHADE | Fructus Solani Indici |
| 1598 | T'ien-ch'ing-ti-pai (Yeh-hsia-pai) | 天青地白(葉下白) | **Gnaphalium japonicum** | *JAPANESE CUDWEED | Herba Gnaphalii Japonici |
| 1599 | T'ien-chiu (Lü-êrh-chiu) | 天韮(鹿耳韮) | **Allium funckiaefolium** | *DEER-EAR LEEK | Herba Allii Funckiaefolii |
| 1600 | T'ien-chu-huang (Chu-huang) | 天竹黃(竹黃) | see 0244 | Tabasheer | Concretio Silicea Bambusae |
| 1601 | T'ien-chu-tzŭ | 天竹子 | **Nandina domestica** | NANDINA | Fructus Nandinae |
| 1602 | T'ien-chüeh-pan (T'ao-yeh-san-hu) | 天腳板(桃葉珊瑚) | **Aucuba chinensis** | CHINESE AUCUBA | Folium et Fructus Aucubae Chinensis |
| 1603 | T'ien-chun-wu-yin-i | 田脣烏蠅翼 | **Smithia sensitiva** | *SMITHIA | Herba Smithiae |
| 1604 | T'ien-hsiang-lu | 天香爐 | **Osbeckia chinensis** | CHINESE OSBECKIA | Herba Osbeckiae |
| 1605 | T'ien-hsien-t'êng | 天仙藤 | **Aristolochia debilis** | BIRTHWORT | Caulis Aristolochiae |
| 1606 | T'ien-hsien-tzŭ (Lang-tang-tzŭ) | 天仙子(莨菪子) | **Hyoscyamus niger** | HENBANE | Semen Hyoscyami |
| 1607 —a | T'ien-hsing-jên (Pa-tan-hsing-jên) | 甜杏仁 (巴旦杏仁) | **Prunus armeniaca white, detoxified 'Pa-tan'** | SWEET APRICOT (seed) | Semen Pruni Armeniacae |
| 1608 | T'ien-hsüang-hua | 田旋花 | **Convolvulus arvensis** | FIELD MORNING-GLORY | Herba Convolvuli |
| 1609 | T'ien-hsiung (Ch'uan-wu-t'ou) | 天雄(川烏頭) | **Aconitum chinense A. carmichaelii** | CHINESE ACONITE SZECHUAN ACONITE | Radix Aconiti Chinensis |
| 1610 | T'ien-hu-sui | 天胡荽 | **Hydrocotyle sibthorpioides** | PENNYWORT | Herba Hydrocotylis |

130

| Transliteration | Chinese | Botanical Name | English | Pharmaceutical |
|---|---|---|---|---|
| 1611 T'ien-hua-fêng | 天花粉 | **Trichosanthes kirilowii** | TRICHOSANTHES (root) | Radix Trichosanthis |
| 1612 T'ien-ko-ts'ai (T'ang-ko-ts'ai, Kan-ts'ai, Kan-yu-ts'ai) | 田葛菜(塘葛菜, 蔊菜, 旱油菜) | **Rorippa indica (Nasturtium montanum)** | *NASTURTIUM | Herba Rorippae Indicae |
| 1613 T'ien-kua | 甜瓜 | **Cucumis melo** | SWEET MELON | Fructus Cucumis |
| T'ien-kua-chin | 甜瓜莖 | ,,    ,, | ,,    ,,    (stem) | Ramus    ,, |
| T'ien-kua-hua | 甜瓜花 | ,,    ,, | ,,    ,,    (flower) | Flos    ,, |
| T'ien-kua-p'i | 甜瓜皮 | ,,    ,, | ,,    ,,    (peels) | Cortex    ,, |
| T'ien-kua-kên | 甜瓜根 | ,,    ,, | ,,    ,,    (root) | Radix    ,, |
| T'ien-kua-tzŭ | 甜瓜子 | ,,    ,, | ,,    ,,    (seed) | Semen    ,, |
| T'ien-kua-t'i (K'u-ting-hsiang) | 甜瓜蒂(苦丁香) | ,,    ,, | ,,    ,,    (pedicel) | Pedicelli    ,, |
| T'ien-kua-yeh | 甜瓜葉 | ,,    ,, | ,,    ,,    (leaf) | Folium    ,, |
| 1614 T'ien-k'uei | 天葵 | **Semiaquilegia adoxoides** | *SEMIAQUILEGIA | Herba Semiaquilegiae |
| T'ien-k'uei-tzŭ | 天葵子 | ,,    ,, | ,,    (seed) | Semen Semiaquilegiae |
| 1615 T'ien-lo | 田螺 | — | Fresh water snail | Cipangopaludina |
| 1616 T'ien-lo-shui | 天蘿水 | **Luffa cylindrica L. acutangula** | *LUFFA (fresh sap) | Succus Luffae |
| 1617 T'ien-ma (Ch'ih-chien) | 天麻(赤箭) | **Gastrodia elata** | GASTRODIA | Tuber, Semen Gastrodiae |
| 1618 T'ien-mên-tung (T'ien-tung) | 天門冬(天冬) | **Asparagus lucidus A. cochinchinensis** | *CHINESE ASPARAGUS | Tuber Asparagi |
| 1619 T'ien-ming-ching | 天名精 | **Carpesium abrotanoides** | *CARPESIUM | Herba Carpesii |
| 1620 T'ien-mu-mu-chiang-tzŭ (Pa-chiao-yang) | 天目木姜子(芭蕉楊) | **Litsea auriculata** | *AURICULAR LITSEA | Radix, Folium et Fructus Litseae Auriculatae |

| Transliteration | Chinese | Botanical Name | English | Pharmaceutical |
|---|---|---|---|---|
| 1621 T'ien-mu-mu-lan | 天目木蘭 | **Magnolia amoena** | *TIENMU MAGNOLIA | Flos Magnoliae Amoenae |
| 1622 T'ien-nan-hsing | 天南星 | **Arisaema** spp. | JACK-IN-THE-PULPIT | Tuber Arisaematis |
| −a Ch'uan-nan-hsing | 川南星 | **A. lobatum** | SZECHUAN ARISAEMA | ,, ,, |
| −b Han-nan-hsing | 韓南星 | **A. peninsulae** | KOREAN ARISAEMA | ,, ,, |
| −c Kou-chao-nan-hsing | 狗爪南星 | **A. heterophyllum** | *DOG-FEET ARISAEMA | ,, ,, |
| −d Kuei-chü-jo | 鬼蒟蒻 | **A. japonicum** | JAPANESE ARISAEMA | ,, ,, |
| −e Shê-mu-yü | 蛇墨芋 | **A. consanguineum** | *RADIATE ARISAEMA | ,, ,, |
| −f Tien-nan-hsing | 滇南星 | **A. verrucosum** | *YUNNAN ARISAEMA | ,, ,, |
| −g Tung-pei-t'ien-nan-hsing | 東北天南星 | **A. amurense** | AMUR ARISAEMA | ,, ,, |
| 1623 T'ien-p'ao-tzǔ (Huang-ku-niang) | 天泡子(黃姑娘) | **Physalis minima** | *LESSER GROUND-CHERRY | Herba et Fructus Physalis Minimae |
| 1624 T'ien-p'ung-ts'ao (Ch'üeh-shê-ts'ao) | 天蓬草(雀舌草) | **Stellaria alsine** | *LESSER CHICKWEED | Herba Stellariae Alsines |
| 1625 T'ien-shan-hua-ch'iu | 天山花楸 | **Sorbus tianschanica** | *TIENSHAN MOUNTAIN-ASH | Ramus, Cortex et Fructus Sorbi |
| 1626 T'ien-shêng-ts'ao (Ta-lan-hua-shên, Lu-ssǔ-lan) | 天生草(大蘭花參,鷺鷥蘭) | **Diuranthera minor** | *DIURANTHERA | Radix Diurantherae |
| 1627 T'ien-shih-liu (Shih-liu) | 甜石榴(石榴) | **Punica granatum** | POMEGRANATE | Fructus Granati |
| 1628 T'ien-shih-li | 天師栗 | **Aesculus chinensis** | HORSE CHESTNUT | Fructus Aesculi |
| 1629 T'ien-shui-i-ts'ao | 天水蟻草 | **Gnaphalium hypoleucum** | *ASIATIC CUDWEED | Herba Gnaphalii Hypoleuci |

| Transliteration | Chinese | Botanical Name | English | Pharmaceutical |
|---|---|---|---|---|
| 1630 T'ien-ts'ai (T'ien-ts'ai-yeh) | 恭菜(甜菜,甜菜葉) | **Beta vulgaris** | BEET | Radix et Semen Betae |
| 1631 T'ien-tsao-chio | 田皂角 | **Aeschynomene indica** | SENSITIVE JOINT VETCH | Herba Aeschynomenis |
| 1632 T'ien-ts'ao (Yeh-kan-ts'ao) | 甜草(野甘草) | **Hedyotis cantonensis** | *CANTON HEDYOTIS | Herba Hedyotidis Cantonensis |
| 1633 T'ien-tsung | 田葱 | **Philydrum lanuginosum** | *PHILYDRUM | Herba Philydri |
| 1634 T'ien-tung | 天冬 | See T'ien-mên-tung | — | |
| 1635 T'ien-wang-ch'i | 天王七 | **Triosteum pinnatifidum** | *TRIOSTEUM | Radix Triostei |
| T'ien-wang-ch'i-yeh | 天王七葉 | „ „ | „ (leaves) | Folium Triostei |
| Tien-wang-ch'i-kuo | 天王七果 | „ „ | „ (fruit) | Fructus Triostei |
| 1636 T'ien-wên-ts'ao (Chin-niu-k'ou) | 天文草(金扭扣) | **Spilanthes acmella** | *SPILANTHES | Herba Spilanthis |
| 1637 T'ien-yüan-chih (Shên-sha-ts'ao) | 甜遠志(神砂草) | **Polygala sibirica** | *CHINESE SENEGA CHINESE MILKWORT | Radix Polygalae Sibiricae |
| 1638 Ting-ching-ts'ao (Ting-ching) | 定經草(定經) | **Lindernia anagallis** | FALSE PIMPERNEL | Herba Linderniae Anagallis |
| 1639 Ting-hsiang (Hsiung-ting-hsiang) | 丁香(雄丁香) | **Syzygium aromaticum (Eugenia caryophyllata)** | CLOVE | Flos Caryophylli |
| 1640 Ting-hsiang-yu | 丁香油 | „ „ | Clove oil | Oleum Caryophylli |
| 1641 Ting-hsin-san | 定心散 | **Angiopteris officinale** | MULE-FOOT FERN | Rhizoma Angiopteridis |
| 1642 Ting-kuei-ts'ao (Jên-tzŭ-ts'ao) | 丁癸草(人字草) | **Zornia diphylla** | *ZORNIA | Herba Zorniae |
| 1643 Ting-kung-t'êng (Pao-kung-t'êng) | 丁公藤(包公藤) | **Erycibe obtusifolia** | *ERYCIBE | Radix et Ramus Erycibes |

133

| | Transliteration | Chinese | Botanical Name | English | Pharmaceutical |
|---|---|---|---|---|---|
| 1644 | Ting-lang-p'i (Liang-tzŭ-mu) | 丁榔皮(椋子木) | **Cornus macrophylla** | *LARGE-LEAVED CORNEL | Cortex Corni Macrophyllae |
| 1645 | Ting-mu-hsiang (Pai-hsi-hsin) | 定木香(白細辛) | **Beesia calthaefolia** | *BEESIA | Rhizoma Beesiae |
| 1646 | Ting-tzŭ-ts'ao | 丁字草 | See Ting-k'uei-ts'ao | — | — |
| 1647 | T'ing-li-tzŭ (Ting-li-tzŭ) | 葶藶子(丁力子) | **Draba nemorosa** **Lepidium apetalum** | WOODS WHITLOW-GRASS | Semen Drabae |
| 1648 | Tiu-liao-pang (Chui-fêng-kun) | 丟了棒(追風棍) | **Claoxylon polot** | *CLAOXYLON | Radix et Folium Claoxylonis |
| 1649 | T'o-sêng | 佗僧 | See Mi-t'o-sêng | — | — |
| 1650 | Tou-chio-ch'ai | 豆角柴 | **Campylotropis delavayi** | *CAMPYLOTROPIS | Radix Campylotropis |
| 1651 | Tou-fu (Tou-chiang, Tou-fu-cha, Tou-yu) | 豆腐(豆漿,豆腐渣,豆油) | **Glycine max** | SOYBEAN (products) | Effectus Glycines |
| 1652 | Tou-fu-cha-kuo | 豆腐渣果 | **Helicia erratica** | *HELICIA | Radix et Folium Heliciae |
| 1653 | Tou-huang | 豆黃 | **Glycine soja** | BLACK SOYBEAN (cooked and mold yellow) | *Touhuang |
| 1654 | Tou-jên (Pa-tou-jên) | 豆仁(巴豆仁) | **Croton tiglium** | CROTON (seed) | Semen Tiglii |
| 1655 | Tou-kên (Shan-tou-kên) | 豆根(山豆根) | **Sophora tonkinensis** | *BUSHY SOPHORA (root) | Radix Sophorae Subprostratae |
| 1656 | Tou-k'ou (Jou-tou-k'ou) | 豆蔻(肉豆蔻) | **Myristica fragrans** | NUTMEG | Semen Myristicae |

134

| Transliteration | Chinese | Botanical Name | English | Pharmaceutical |
|---|---|---|---|---|
| 1657 Tou-k'ou-hua (Tou-k'ou-k'o) | 豆蔻花(豆蔻殼) | **Amomum krervanh** | KRERVANH | Flos et Pericarpium Amomi Krervanh |
| 1658 Tou-ling | 兜鈴 | See Ma-tou-ling | — | — |
| 1659 Tou-pan-lu (Yen-chin-ts'ao) | 豆瓣綠(岩筋草) | **Peperomia reflexa** | *REFLEX PEPEROMIA | Herba Peperomiae Reflexae |
| 1660 Tou-p'i | 豆皮 | See Lu-tou-p'i | — | — |
| 1661 Tou-shih (Hêh-tou-shih) | 豆豉(黑豆豉) | **Glycine soja** | BLACK SOYBEAN (medicated) | Semen Sojae Praeparationis |
| 1662 Tou-shih-chiang (Shan-tsung-shu) | 豆豉姜(山蒼樹) | **Litsea cubeba** | FRAGRANT LISTSEA | Radix et Ramus Litseae Cubebae |
| 1663 Tou-shih-ts'ao | 豆豉草 | **Iris sanguinea** | *SANGUINE IRIS | Rhizoma Iridis Sanguineae |
| 1664 T'ou-ku-hsiao (Huo-hsüeh-tan) | 透骨消(活血丹) | **Glechoma hederacea** | GROUND IVY | Herba Glechomatis |
| 1665 T'ou-ku-ts'ao | 透骨草 | **Speranskia tuberculata** | *SPERANSKIA | Herba Speranskiae |
| 1666 Ts'ai-kua | 菜瓜 | **Cucumis melo** var. **conomon** | *ORIENTAL PICKLING MELON | *Fructus et Semen Conomonis |
| 1667 Ts'ai-tou-shu (Ta-lang-san) | 菜豆樹(大朗傘) | **Radermachera sinica** | *RADERMACHERA | Radix, Folium et Fructus Radermacherae |
| 1668 Ts'ai-t'ou-shên | 菜頭腎 | **Championella sarcorrhiza** | *CHAMPIONELLA | Herba Championellae |
| 1669 Ts'ai-tzǔ-ch'i | 菜子七 | **Cardamine leucantha** | *WHITE BITTER CRESS | Radix Cardamines |

| | Transliteration | Chinese | Botanical Name | English | Pharmaceutical |
|---|---|---|---|---|---|
| 1670 | Ts'an | 蠶 | — | Silkworm | Bombyx Mori |
| | Ts'an-chien (Ts'an-i) | 蠶繭(蠶衣) | — | Silk cocoon | Bombyx Bombycis |
| | Ts'an-sha | 蠶砂 | — | Silkworm excreta | Excrementum Bombycis |
| | Ts'an-shui (Ts'an-t'ui) | 蠶蛻(蠶退) | — | Silkworm slough | Periostachum Bombycis |
| | Ts'an-yung | 蠶蛹 | — | Silkworm pupa | Pupa Bombycis |
| 1671 | Ts'an-chien-ts'ao | 蠶繭草 | **Polygonum japonicum** | JAPANESE SMARTWEED | Herba Polygoni Japonici |
| 1672 | Ts'an-tou | 蠶豆 | **Vicia faba** | BROAD BEAN | |
| | Ts'an-tou-chin | 蠶豆莖 | ,, ,, | ,, ,, (stem) | Caudex Fabae |
| | Ts'an-tou-hua | 蠶豆花 | ,, ,, | ,, ,, (flower) | Flos Fabae |
| | Ts'an-tou-chia-k'o | 蠶豆莢殼 | ,, ,, | ,, ,, (shell) | Pericarpium Fabae |
| | Ts'an-tou-k'o | 蠶豆殼 | ,, ,, | ,, ,, (testa) | Testa Fabae |
| | Ts'an-tou-yeh | 蠶豆葉 | ,, ,, | ,, ,, (leaf) | Folium Fabae |
| 1673 | Tsang-chieh | 藏茄 | **Anisodus tanguticus (Scopolia tangutica)** | *TSANGCHIEH | Radix et Semen Scopoliae |
| 1674 | Tsang-ch'ing-kuo | 藏青果 | **Terminalia chebula** | MYROBALAN | Fructus Terminaliae |
| 1675 | Tsang-hui-hsiang | 藏茴香 | **Carum carvi** | CARAWAY | Fructus Cari |
| 1676 | Tsang-hung-hua | 藏紅花 | **Crocus sativus** | SAFFRON | Stylus Croci |
| 1677 | Ts'ang-êrh (Ts'ang-êrh-tzŭ, Ts'ang-êrh-kên) | 蒼耳(蒼耳子,蒼耳根) | **Xanthium sibiricum X. strumarium** | COCKLEBUR | Herba, Fructus et Radix Xanthii |
| 1678 | Ts'ang-êrh-ch'ung | 蒼耳虫 | — | Cocklebur Borer | Vermiculus Xanthii |
| 1679 | Ts'ang-pai-ch'êng-kou-fêng | 蒼白秤鈎風 | **Diploclisia glaucescens** | *DIPLOCLISIA | Caudex Diploclisiae |

| Transliteration | Chinese | Botanical Name | English | Pharmaceutical |
|---|---|---|---|---|
| 1680 Ts'ang-shu | 蒼朮 | **Atractylodes** spp. | *TSANGSHU | Radix Atractylodis |
| −a  Nan-ts'ang-shu (Mao-shu, Ching-mao-shu) | 南蒼朮(茅朮, 京茅朮) | **A. lancea** | *SOUTHERN TSANGSHU | Radix Atractylodis Lanceae |
| −b  Pai-ts'ang-shu (Chin-ts'ang-shu) | 北蒼朮(津蒼朮) | **A. chinensis** | *NORTHERN TSANGSHU | Radix Atractylodis Chinensis |
| −c  Tung-ts'ang-shu | 東蒼朮 | **A. japonica** | *EASTERN TSANGSHU | Radix Atractylodis Japonicae |
| 1681 Ts'ang-t'iao-yü-pieh (Shih-chüeh) | 蒼條魚鱉(石蕨) | **Saxiglossum angustissimum** | *SAXIGLOSSUM | Herba Saxiglossi |
| 1682 Ts'ang-yin-ts'ao | 蒼蠅草 | **Indigofera hancockii** | HANCOCK'S INDIGO | Radix Indifogerae Hancockii |
| 1683 Tsao-chio (Ta-tsao) | 皂角(大皂) | **Gleditsia sinensis** | CHINESE HONEY-LOCUST (fruit) | Fructus Gleditsiae |
| 1684 Tsao-chio-tz'ǔ (Tsao-chien, Tsao-tz'ǔ-p'ien, Tz'ǔ-p'ien) | 皂角莿(皂尖, 皂莿片, 莿片) | **Gleditsia sinensis** | CHINESE HONEY-LOCUST (thorn) | Spina Gleditsiae |
| 1685 Tsao-hsiu (Ch'ung-lou, Ch'i-yeh-i-chih-hua) | 蚤休(重樓, 七葉一枝花) | **Paris polyphylla** **P. chinensis** **P. delavayi** **P. quadrifolia** | PARIS | Rhizoma Paris |
| 1686 Tsao-jên (Tsao-chio-tzǔ) | 皂仁(皂角子) | **Gleditsia sinensis** | CHINESE HONEY-LOCUST (seed) | Semen Gleditsiae |

| | Transliteration | Chinese | Botanical Name | English | Pharmaceutical |
|---|---|---|---|---|---|
| 1687 | Tsao-jên (Tsao-hêh) | 棗仁(棗核) | **Zizyphus jujuba** | JUJUBE (seed) | Semen Zizyphi Jujubae |
| | Tsao-jou | 棗肉 | ,, ,, | ,, (fruit) | Fructus Zizyphi Jujubae |
| | Tsao-p'i | 棗皮 | ,, ,, | ,, (peel) | Pericarpium ,, ,, |
| | Tsao-kên | 棗根 | ,, ,, | ,, (root) | Radix ,, ,, |
| | Tsao-yeh | 棗葉 | ,, ,, | ,, (leaf) | Folium ,, ,, |
| 1688 | Tsao-pin-lang | 棗檳榔 | **Areca catechu** | BETEL (immature fruit) | Fructus Arecae |
| 1689 | Ts'ao-chih-chu (Hua-chih-chu) | 草蛛蜘(花蛛蜘) | — | *Grass spider | Agelena |
| 1960 | Ts'ao-chin-shan | 草金杉 | **Pentanema indicum** | *PENTANEMA | Herba Pentanematis |
| 1691 | Ts'ao-chüeh-ming (Chüeh-ming) | 草決明(決明) | **Cassia tora** | FOETID CASSIA | Semen Cassiae Torae |
| 1692 | Ts'ao-ho-ch'ê (Tzŭ-shên, Ch'üan-shên) | 草河車(紫參,拳參) | **Polygonum bistorta P. lapidosum** | ALPINE KNOTWEED | Rhizoma Polygoni Bistortae |
| 1693 | Ts'ao-hsiang-fu | 草香附 | **Juncus amplifolius** | *AMPLE-LEAVED RUSH | Rhizoma Junci Amplifolii |
| 1694 | Ts'ao-hsiao | 草硝 | — | Potash from grass ashes | *Tsaohsiao |
| 1695 | Ts'ao-hsiu-chiu | 草繡球 | **Cardiandra moellendorffii** | *CARDIANDRA | Rhizoma Cardiandrae |
| 1696 | Ts'ao-hsüeh-chieh (I-k'ou-hsüeh) | 草血竭(一口血) | **Polygonum paleaceum** | *BLOOD KNOTWEED | Rhizoma Polygoni Paleacei |
| 1697 | Ts'ao-jên (Ts'ao-k'ou-jên) | 草仁(草蔻仁) | **Alpinia katsumadai** | KATSUMADA'S GALANGAL (seed) | Semen Alpiniae Katsumadai |

| | Transliteration | Chinese | Botanical Name | English | Pharmaceutical |
|---|---|---|---|---|---|
| 1698 | Ts'ao-jung (Tzŭ-ts'ao-jung) | 草蓉(紫草蓉) | **Lithospermum erythrorhizon** | ASIATIC GROOMWELL (refuse) | Radix Lithospermi |
| 1699 | Ts'ao-k'ou (Ts'ao-tou-k'ou) | 草蔻(草豆蔻) | **Alpinia katsumadai** **Amomum globosum** | KATSUMADA'S GALANGAL ROUND CARDAMON | Semen Alpiniae Katsu-madai vel Amomi Globosi |
| 1700 | Ts'ao-kuo Ts'ao-kuo-jên | 草果 草果仁 | **Amomum tsao-ko** „ „ | *TSAOKO CARDAMON „ „ (seed) | Fructus Amomi Tsaoko Semen Amomi Tsaoko |
| 1701 | Ts'ao-kuo-yao | 草果藥 | **Hedychium spicatum** | *HEDYCHIUM | Fructus Hedychii |
| 1702 | Ts'ao-lien | 草蓮 | **Coptis chinensis** | GOLDEN THREAD (inferior kind) | Rhizoma Coptidis |
| 1703 | Ts'ao-ling-chih (Yeh-t'u-shih) | 草靈脂(野兔屎) | — | Wild rabbit dung | Excrementum Cuniculi |
| 1704 | Ts'ao-lung (Shui-ying-ts'ao) | 草龍(水映草) | **Jussiaea linifolia** | *LESSER PRIMROSE WILLOW | Herba Jussiaeae Linifoliae |
| 1705 | Ts'ao-ma-yu (Pei-ma-yu) | 草麻油(蓖麻油) | **Ricinus communis** | CASTOR-OIL-PLANT | Oleum Ricini |
| 1706 | Ts'ao-mu-hsi | 草木犀(樨) | **Melilotus suaveolens** | SWEET CLOVER | Herba Meliloti |
| 1707 | Ts'ao-mu-hui | 草木灰 | — | Plant ash | Cinis Plantae |
| 1708 | Ts'ao-pai-chih | 草柏枝 | **Phtheirospermum tenuisectum** | *YUNNAN LOUSESEED | Radix Phtheirospermi |
| 1709 | Ts'ao-pei-mu (Li-chiang-shan-tz'ŭ-ku) | 草貝母(麗江山慈菇) | **Iphigenia indica** | *IPHIGENIA | Bulbus Iphigeniae |
| 1710 | Ts'ao-pên-san-chio-fêng (Hsiao-hei-yao) | 草本三角楓(小黑藥) | **Sanicula astrantifolia** | SNAKE-ROOT | Herba Saniculae |

| | Transliteration | Chinese | Botanical Name | English | Pharmaceutical |
|---|---|---|---|---|---|
| 1711 | Ts'ao-shih-ts'an (Shih-ch'i-shê, Shih-shêng-chin) | 草石蠶(石奇蛇,石伸筋) | **Humata tyermannii** | *HUMATA | Rhizoma et Herba Humatae |
| 1712 | Ts'ao-shih-ts'an (Kan-lu-tzŭ, Pao-t'a-ts'ai) | 草石蠶(甘露子,寶塔荣) | **Stachys sieboldii** | CHINESE ARTICHOKE | Tuber Stachydis |
| 1713 | Ts'ao-tou-k'ou (Ts'ao-k'ou) | 草豆蔻(草蔻) | **Alpinia katsumadai** | KATSUMADA'S GALANGAL | Semen Alpiniae Katsumadai |
| 1714 | Ts'ao-tsung-jung | 草苁蓉 | **Boschniakia rossica** | *BOSCHNIAKIA | Herba Boschniakiae |
| 1715 | Ts'ao-wei-ling (Hei-wei-ling) | 草威靈(黑威靈) | **Inula nervosa** | *NERVED ELECAMPANE | Radix Inulae Nervosae |
| 1716 | Ts'ao-wu-t'ou | 草烏頭 | Aconitum chinense | MONKSHOOD | Radix Aconiti |
| —a | Hao-yeh-wu-t'ou | 蒿葉烏頭 | **A. artemisaefolium** | *MUGWORT　　　　　" | |
| —b | Pai-wu-t'ou | 北烏頭 | **A. kusnezoffii** | *NORTHERN　　　　　" | |
| —c | Sung-pan-wu-t'ou | 松潘烏頭 | **A. sungpanense** | *SUNGPAN　　　　　" | |
| —d | Ta-ts'ao-wu | 大草烏 | **A. transsectum** | *GREATER　　　　　" | |
| —e | T'ai-pai-wu-t'ou | 太白烏頭 | **A. taipeicum** | *TAIPEI　　　　　" | |
| —f | T'êng-wu-t'ou | 藤烏頭 | **A. hemsleyanum** | *CLIMBING　　　　　" | |
| —g | Tzŭ-ts'ao-wu | 紫草烏 | **A. delavayi** | *YUNNAN　　　　　" | |
| 1717 | Ts'ao-yüan-lao-kuan-ts'ao (Hung-kên-ts'ao) | 草原老鸛草(紅根草) | **Geranium pratense** | *MEADOW CRANESBILL | Herba Geranii Pratensis |
| 1718 | Tsê-ch'i (I-pa-san, Miao-êrh-yen-ching-ts'ao) | 澤漆(一把傘,貓兒眼睛草) | **Euphorbia helioscopia** | *SUN SPURGE | Herba Euphorbiae Helioscopiae |

| Transliteration | Chinese | Botanical Name | English | Pharmaceutical |
|---|---|---|---|---|
| 1719 Tsê-hsieh (Ch'uan-hsieh) | 澤瀉(川瀉) | **Alisma plantago-aquatica** | WATER PLANTAIN | Rhizoma Alismatis |
| Tsê-hsieh-yeh | 澤瀉葉 | ,, ,, | ,, ,, (leaf) | Folium Alismatis |
| Tsê-hsieh-shih | 澤瀉實 | ,, ,, | ,, ,, (fruit) | Fructus Allismatis |
| 1720 Tsê-lan (P'ei-lan) | 澤蘭(佩蘭) | **Eupatorium japonicum E. fortunei** | EUPATORIUM | Herba Eupatorii |
| 1721 Tsê-lan (Ts'ao-tsê-lan, Ti-kua-êrh-miao) | 澤蘭(草澤蘭, 地瓜兒苗) | **Lycopus lucidus** | SHINING WATER HOREHOUND | Herba Lycopi |
| 1722 Ts'ê-pai (Ts'ê-pai-yeh) | 側柏(側柏葉) | **Thuja orientalis (Biota orientalis)** | ARBOR-VITAE | Ramus Thujae |
| 1723 Tso-chiang-ts'ao | 酢漿草 | **Oxalis corniculata** | WOOD-SORREL | Herba Oxalidis |
| 1724 Tsou-ma-chien (Tsou-ma-fêng) | 走馬箭(走馬風) | **Sambucus chinensis** | ELDER | Radix et Ramus Sambuci |
| 1725 Tsou-ma-t'ai | 走馬胎 | **Ardisia gigantifolia** | LARGE-LEAVED ARDISIA | Radix et Folium Ardisiae Gigantifoliae |
| 1726 Tsui-ma-ts'ao | 醉馬草 | **Oxytropis glabra** | *OXYTROPIS | Herba Oxytropis |
| 1727 Tsui-yü-ts'ao | 醉魚草 | **Buddleia lindleyana** | *BUDDLEIA | Ramus Buddleiae |
| Tsui-yü-ts'ao-hua | 醉魚草花 | ,, ,, | ,, (flower) | Flos Buddleiae |
| 1728 Ts'ui-yün-ts'ao | 翠雲草 | **Selaginella uncinata** | HOOKED SPIKEMOSS | Herba Selaginellae Uncinatae |

141

| Transliteration | Chinese | Botanical Name | English | Pharmaceutical |
|---|---|---|---|---|
| 1729 Tsung-lü (Tsung-shu) | 棕櫚(棕樹) | **Trachycarpus fortunei (T. wagnerianus)** | *TRACHYCARPUS | |
| Tsung-shu-hsing | 棕樹心 | ,, ,, | ,, (heart wood) | Xylema Trachycarpi |
| Tsung-shu-kên | 棕樹根 | ,, ,, | ,, (root) | Radix Trachycarpi |
| Tsung-lü-hua | 棕櫚花 | ,, ,, | ,, (flower) | Flos Trachycarpi |
| Tsung-lü-p'i | 棕櫚皮 | ,, ,, | ,, (stipule fiber) | Fibra Stipulae Trachycarpi |
| Tsung-lü-tzǔ | 棕櫚子 | ,, ,, | ,, (fruit) | Fructus Trachycarpi |
| Tsung-lü-yeh | 棕櫚葉 | ,, ,, | ,, (leaf) | Folium Trachycarpi |
| 1730 Ts'ung-jung (Ta-yün, Jou-ts'ung-jung) | 蓯蓉(大芸, 肉蓯蓉) | **Cistanche salsa** | BROOMRAPE | Herba Cistanches |
| 1731 Ts'ung-pai | 葱白 | **Allium fistulosum** | SPRING ONION | Herba Allii Fistulosi |
| 1732 Tu-chiao (Ch'uan-hua-chiu) | 獨椒(川花楸) | **Sorbus unguiculata** | *UNGUICULATE MOUNTAIN ASH | Radix Sorbi Unguiculatae |
| 1733 Tu-ch'in-kên (Tsou-ma-ch'in) | 毒芹根(走馬芹) | **Cicuta virosa** | COW-BANE | Radix Cicutae |
| 1734 Tu-ching-shan | 杜莖山 | **Maesa japonica** | *JAPANESE MAESA | Radix et Folium Maesae Japonicae |
| 1735 Tu-chio-ch'iang-lang (Tu-chio-hsien) | 獨角蜣螂(獨角仙) | — | Rhinoceros Beetle | Xylotropes |
| 1736 Tu-chio-lien (Li-t'ou-chien, Pai-fu-tzǔ) | 獨角蓮(犁頭尖, 白附子) | **Typhonium giganteum** | *GIANT TYPHONIUM | Rhizoma Typhonii Gigantei |

| | Transliteration | Chinese | Botanical Name | English | Pharmaceutical |
|---|---|---|---|---|---|
| 1737 | Tu-chio-yü (Wu-ts'ai-yü) | 獨角芋(五彩芋) | **Caladium bicolor** | CALADIUM | Rhizoma Caladii |
| 1738 | Tu-chuan (Tzǔ-kuei) | 杜鵑(子規) | — | Indian Cuckoo | Caro Cuculi |
| 1739 | Tu-chuan-hua | 杜鵑花 | **Rhododendron simsii** | RED AZALEA | Flos et Fructus Rhododendri Simsii |
| 1740 | Tu-chüeh-ch'i | 獨蕨箕 | **Botrychium lanuginosum** | MOONWORT | Rhizoma Botrychii |
| 1741 | Tu-chüeh-kan (Lu-ts'ao, Kan-ts'ao, Tu-chüeh-chin) | 獨腳柑(鹿草,干草,獨腳金) | **Striga asiatica** | *STRIGA | Herba Strigae |
| 1742 | Tu-chüeh-wu-chiu (Tu-chüeh-wu-chiu-yeh) | 獨腳烏桕(獨腳烏桕葉) | **Cissus modeccoides** | *CISSUS | Radix, Ramus, et Folium Cissi |
| 1743 | Tu-chung (Mian) | 杜仲(楙) | **Eucommia ulmoides** | EUCOMMIA | Cortex Eucommiae |
| 1744 | Tu-chung-t'êng | 杜仲藤 | **Parabarium micranthum** | *PARABARIUM | Ramus Parabarii |
| 1745 | Tu-fên | 凸粉 | — | Prepared chalk | Creta |
| 1746 | Tu-hêng (Nan-hsi-hsin, Ma-hsin) | 杜衡(杜蘅,南細辛,馬辛) | **Asarum forbesii** | *FORBES' WILD GINGER | Herba Asari Forbesii |
| 1747 | Tu-hsing-chien-li | 獨行千里 | **Capparis membranacea** | HONGKONG CAPER | Radix, Ramus et Folium Capparis Membranaceae |

| | Transliteration | Chinese | Botanical Name | English | Pharmaceutical |
|---|---|---|---|---|---|
| 1748 | Tu-huo (Tu-yao-ts'ao) | 獨活(獨搖草) | See the following | *TUHUO | |
| −a | Chiu-yen-tu-huo (T'u-tang-kuei) | 九眼獨活(土當歸) | **Aralia cordata** | *NINE-EYED TUHUO | Radix Araliae Cordatae |
| −b | Juan-mao-tu-huo | 軟毛獨活 | **Heracleum lanatum** | *SOFT-HAIR TUHUO | Radix Heraclei Lanati |
| −c | Mao-tu-huo | 毛獨活 | **Angelica pubescens** | HAIRY TUHUO | Radix Angelicae Pubescentis |
| −d | Niu-wei-tu-huo | 牛尾獨活 | **Heracleum hemsleyanum** | *OX-TAIL TUHUO | Radix Heraclei |
| −e | Tzŭ-ching-tu-huo | 紫莖獨活 | **Angelica porphyrocaulis** | *PURPLE TUHUO | Radix Angelicae Porphyrocaulis |
| 1749 | Tu-i-wei | 獨一味 | **Phlomis rotata** | ROTATING JERUSALEUM SAGE | Radix et Herba Phlomis |
| 1750 | Tu-sung-shih (Tu-sung-tzŭ) | 杜松實(杜松子) | **Juniperus rigida** | *STIFF JUNIPER | Fructus Juniperi Rigidae |
| 1751 | Tu-yeh-i-chih-ch'iang | 獨葉一枝槍 | **Amitostigma gracile** | *AMITOSTIGMA | Herba Amitostigmatis |
| 1752 | Tu-yeh-i-chih-hua | 獨葉一枝花 | **Hemipilia flabellata** | *HEMPILIA | Herba Hemipiliae |
| 1753 | Tu-yeh-pai-chi | 獨葉白芨 | **Pleione yunnanensis** | *PLEIONE | Herba Pleiones |
| 1754 | Tu-yü-t'êng (Pai-yao-kên) | 毒魚藤(白藥根) | **Millettia lasiopetala** | *WOOLLY MILLETTIA | Radix et Ramus Millettiae Lasiopetalae |
| 1755 | T'u-a-wei (Ch'ou-wu-t'ung) | 土阿魏(臭梧桐) | **Clerodendrum trichotomum** | HAIRY CLERODENDRON | Succus Clerodendri Exsiccatus |
| 1756 | T'u-ch'ang-shan (Hsiu-ch'iu) | 土常山(綉球) | **Hydrangea strigosa** **H. umbellata** **H. paniculata** | HYDRANGEA | Radix Hydrangeae |

144

| Transliteration | Chinese | Botanical Name | English | Pharmaceutical |
|---|---|---|---|---|
| 1757 T'u-ch'ên-hsiang | 土沉香 | **Aquilaria sinensis** | CHINESE AGARU | Lignum Aquilariae Sinensis |
| 1758 T'u-ch'iang-huo (Shan-ch'iang-huo, Chiang-hua) | 土羌活(山羌活,薑花) | **Hedychium coronarium** | GINGER LILY | Rhizoma Hedychii |
| 1759 T'u-chien-ch'i | 土箭芪 | **Wikstroemia dolichantha** | *LONG-FLOWERED WIKSTROEMIA | Radix Wikstroemiae Dolichanthae |
| 1760 T'u-chien-nien-chien (Wu-ya-kuo, Wu-fan-tzǔ) | 土千年健(烏鴉果,烏飯子) | **Vaccinium fragile** | BILBERRY | Radix, Ramus, et Fructus Vaccinii Fragilis |
| 1761 T'u-ching-chieh | 土荊芥 | **Chenopodium ambrosioides** | WORMSEED | Herba Chenopodii Ambrosioidis |
| 1762 T'u-ching-p'i (Chin-ch'ien-sung-p'i) | 土荊皮(金錢松皮) | **Pseudolarix amabilis** | GOLDEN LARCH | Cortex Pseudolaricis |
| 1763 T'u-chung-wên (Hsiang-ya-shên) | 土中聞(象牙參) | **Roscoea intermedia** | *ROSCOEA | Radix Roscoeae |
| 1764 T'u-fêng (T'u-fêng-tzǔ) | 土蜂(土蜂子) | — | Wasp and larva | Discolia |
| 1765 T'u-fu (T'u-fu-tzǔ) | 土附(土附子) | — | Fish & egg of goby | Odontobutis |
| 1766 T'u-fu-ling | 土茯苓 | **Smilax glabra** | GLABROUS GREENBRIER | Rhizoma Smilacis Glabrae |
| 1767 T'u-hsiang-fei | 土香榧 | **Cephalotaxus sinensis C. fortunei** | *CEPHALOTAXUS | Fructus Cephalotaxi |

145

| Transliteration | Chinese | Botanical Name | English | Pharmaceutical |
|---|---|---|---|---|
| 1768 T'u-hsiang-ju (Wu-hsiang-ts'ao, Shan-po-ho) | 土香薷(五香草，山薄荷) | **Origanum vulgare** | WILD MARJORAN | Herba Origani |
| 1769 T'u-huang-lien (San-kuo-chin) | 土黃蓮(三顆針) | **Berberis julianae** B. gagnepainii | BARBERRY | Radix et Ramus Berberidis |
| 1770 T'u-i-chih-hao | 土一枝蒿 | **Achillea wilsoniana** | *WILSON'S YARROW | Herba Achilleae Wilsonianae |
| 1771 T'u-jên-shên (Fei-lai-shên) | 土人參(飛來參) | **Talinum paniculatum** | *TALINUM | Radix et Herba Talini |
| 1772 T'u-kên | 吐根 | **Cephaelis ipecacuanha** | IPECAC | Radix Ipecacuanhae |
| 1773 T'u-kua | 土瓜 | **Ipomoea hungaiensis** | *YUNNAN MORNING-GLORY | Radix Ipomoeae Hungaiensis |
| 1774 T'u-kua-lang-tu (Hsiao-lang-tu) | 土瓜狼毒(小狼毒) | **Euphorbia prolifera** | *LESSER WOLFSBANE | Radix Euphorbiae Proliferae |
| 1775 T'u-kuei (Ch'i-pan-ts'ai) | 菟葵(棋盤菜) | **Malva parviflora** | COMMON MALLOW | Herba Malvae Parviflorae |
| 1776 T'u-liang-chiang (Ts'ao-kuo-yao) | 土良薑(草果藥) | **Hedychium spicatum** | HEDYCHIUM | Rhizoma Hedychii Spicati |
| 1777 T'u-lien-ch'iao | 土連翹 | **Hypericum bellum** | *PRETTY ST. JOHNSWORT | Fructus Hyperici Belli |
| 1778 T'u-luan-êrh (T'u-tan) | 土圞兒(土蛋) | **Apios fortunei** | *FORTUNE'S GROUNDNUT | Radix Apioris |
| 1779 T'u-mu-hsiang (Ch'ing-mu-hsiang, Ch'i-mu-hsiang) | 土木香(青木香，祁木香) | **Inula helenium** I. racemosa | ELECAMPANE NORTHERN ELECAMPANE | Radix Inulae Helenii et Racemosae |
| 1779A T'u-mu-kua | 土木瓜 | **Cydonia oblonga** | OBLONG QUINCE | Fructus Cydoniae Oblongae |

146

| Transliteration | Chinese | Botanical Name | English | Pharmaceutical |
|---|---|---|---|---|
| 1780 T'u-mu-tsei (Chieh-chieh-ts'ao) | 土木賊(節節草) | **Equisetum debile** | *WEAK SCOURING RUSH | Herba Equiseti Debilis |
| 1781 T'u-niu-hsi (Niu-hsi, Shan-niu-hsi) | 土牛膝(牛膝,山牛膝) | **Achyranthes aspera A. longifolia** | ACHYRANTHES | Radix Achyranthis |
| 1782 T'u-pa-chio | 土八角 | **Illicium** spp. | STAR ANISE | Fructus Illicii |
| −a Hung-hui-hsiang | 紅茴香 | **I. henryi** | Hupeh ,, ,, | ,, ,, Henryi |
| −b Yün-nan-hui-hsiang | 雲南茴香 | **I. yunnanensis** | Yunnan ,, ,, | ,, ,, Yunnanensis |
| 1783 T'u-pai-chi | 土白芨 | **Platanthera chlorantha** | *PLATANTHERA | Tuber Plantantherae |
| 1784 T'u-pai-lien (Lao-shu-kua) | 土白蘞(老鼠瓜) | **Solena amplexicaulis** | *SOLENA | Radix Solenae |
| 1785 T'u-pan-hsia (Tawahanpa, Tibetan) | 土半夏(藏土半夏) | **Arisaema intermedium** | *TIBETAN ARISAEMA | Tuber Arisaematis Intermedii |
| −a T'u-pan-hsia (Lao-shu-wei, Kwangtung) | 華南土半夏(老鼠尾) | **Typhonium divaricatum** | *LESSER TYPHONIUM | Tuber Typhonii Divaricati |
| 1786 T'u-pei-mu (T'u-pei, Chia-pei-mu) | 土貝母(土貝,假貝母) | **Bolbostemma paniculatum** | *BOLBOSTEMMA | Tuber Bolbostemmatis |
| 1787 T'u-pieh-ch'ung (T'u-pieh) | 土鱉虫(土鱉) | — | Wingless cockroach | Eupolyphaga |
| 1788 T'u-san-ch'i | 土三七 | See the following | *TUSANCHI | |
| −a Hua-nan-t'u-san-ch'i (Hung-pei-san-ch'i) | 華南土三七(紅背三七) | **Gynura segetum** | *CANTON TUSANCHI (VELVET PLANT) | Herba Gynurae Segeti |

147

| Transliteration | Chinese | Botanical Name | English | Pharmaceutical |
|---|---|---|---|---|
| −b Ts'ang-t'u-san-ch'i (Chien-li-kuang) | 藏土三七(千里光) | **Senecio chrysanthemoides** | *TIBETAN TUSANCHI (RAGWORT) | Radix et Herba Senecionis |
| 1789 T'u-ssŭ (T'u-ssŭ-tzŭ) | 菟蘇(菟蘇子) | **Cuscuta japonica C. chinensis** | DODDER | Herba et Semen Cuscutae |
| 1790 T'u-ta-huang | 土大黃 | **Rumex dentatus R. madaio** | DOCK | Radix Rumicis |
| 1791 T'u-tang-kuei (Chiu-yen-tu-huo) | 土當歸(九眼獨活) | **Aralia cordata** | MINE-EYED TUHUO | Radix Araliae Cordatae |
| −a Tung-pê-t'u-tang-kuei (Ta-t'u-huo) | 東北土當歸(大獨活) | **Angelica gigas** | *NORTHEAST ANGELICA | Radix Angelicae Gigatis |
| 1792 T'u-tang-shên | 土黨參 | **Campanumoea javanica** | *CAMPANUMOEA | Radix Campanumoeae |
| 1793 T'u-ting-kuei (Yin-ssŭ-ts'ao) | 土丁桂(銀絲草) | **Evolvulus alsinoides** | *EVOLVULUS | Herba Evolvuli |
| 1794 T'u-ts'an (Chin-kuei-tzŭ) | 土蠶(金龜子) | — | June-Beetle grub | Holotrichia |
| 1795 T'u-yen-wo | 土燕窩 | — | Birdnest | Nidus Collocaliae |
| 1796 T'u-yin-hua-yeh | 土銀花葉 | **Lonicera confusa** | HONEYSUCKLE | Ramus Lonicerae Confusae |
| 1797 T'u-yüan-chih | 土遠志 | **Lysimachia insignis** | LYSIMACHIA | Cordex Lysimachiae |
| 1798 Tung-ch'ing-p'i | 冬青皮 | **Ilex chinensis** | *TUNGCHING (bark) | Cortex Ilicis Chinensis |
| Tung-ch'ing-tzŭ | 冬青子 | " " | " (seed) | Semen " " |
| Tung-ch'ing-yeh | 冬青葉 | " " | " (leaf) | Folium " " |
| 1799 Tung-chung-hsia-ts'ao (Chung-ts'ao) | 冬虫夏草(虫草) | **Cordyceps sinensis** | CHUNGTSAO, WINTER-worm SUMMER-herb | Sclerotium Cordycipitis Sinensis |

| | Transliteration | Chinese | Botanical Name | English | Pharmaceutical |
|---|---|---|---|---|---|
| 1800 | Tung-fêng-chü (Chiu-ping-lê) | 東風橘(酒餅笏) | **Atalantia buxifolia** | *ATALANTIA | Radix et Folium Atalantiae |
| 1801 | Tung-fêng-ts'ai | 東風菜 | **Aster scaber** | *ROUGH ASTER | Herba Aster Scabri |
| 1802 | Tung-kua | 冬瓜 | **Benincasa hispida** | WAX GOURD | |
| | Tung-kua-jang | 冬瓜瓤 | ,,        ,, | ,,      ,, (pulp) | Placenta Benincasae |
| | Tung-kua-p'i | 冬瓜皮 | ,,        ,, | ,,      ,, (peel) | Cortex Fructus Benincasae |
| | Tung-kua-yeh | 冬瓜葉 | ,,        ,, | ,,      ,, (leaf) | Folium Benincasae |
| | Tung-kua-tzǔ | 冬瓜子 | ,,        ,, | ,,      ,, (seed) | Semen Benincasae |
| | Tung-kua-t'êng | 冬瓜藤 | ,,        ,, | ,,      ,, (vine) | Ramus Benincasae |
| 1803 | Tung-kuei | 冬葵 | **Malva verticillata** | MUSK MALLOW | |
| | Tung-kuei-kên | 冬葵根 | ,,        ,, | ,,      ,, (root) | Radix Malvae |
| | Tung-kuei-tzǔ | 冬葵子 | ,,        ,, | ,,      ,, (seed) | Semen Malvae |
| | Tung-kuei-yeh | 冬葵葉 | ,,        ,, | ,,      ,, (leaf) | Folium Malvae |
| 1804 | Tung-li-ma (Shui-ma) | 冬里麻(水麻) | **Debregeasia edulis** | *DEBREGEASIA | Radix et Ramus Debregeasiae |
| 1804A | Tung-ling-ts'ao | 冬凌草 | **Robdosia rubescens** **(Plectranthus rubescens)** | CENTRAL CHINA BALM | Herba Rabdosiae rubescentis |
| 1805 | Tung-mien-ma (Kuan-chung) | 東綿麻(貫眾) | **Dryopteris crassirhizoma** | DRYOPTERIS | Rhizoma Dryopteridis |
| 1806 | Tung-sang-yeh | 冬桑葉 | **Morus alba** | MULBERRY (old leaf) | Folium Mori Vetustum |
| 1807 | Tung-yeh | 冬葉(柊葉, 苓葉) | **Phrynium capitatum** | *PHRYNIUM | Herba Phrynii |
| 1808 | T'ung-chêng-hu (Ting-hsin-ts'ao) | 通城虎(定心草) | **Aristolochia fordiana** **A. tagala** | *FORD'S BIRTHWORT | Radix et Ramus Aristolochiae Fordianae et Tagalae |
| 1809 | T'ung-chi (Sha-wan-tzǔ) | 潼蒺(沙苑子) | **Astragalus complanatus** | *FLAT MILK VETCH | Semen Astragali |

149

| | Transliteration | Chinese | Botanical Name | English | Pharmaceutical | T'ung-c |
|---|---|---|---|---|---|---|
| 1810 | T'ung-chien-ma-huang | 銅錢麻黃 | **Shuteria sinensis** | *SHUTERIA | Radix Shuteriae | |
| 1811 | T'ung-ching-ts'ao | 通經草 | **Aleuritopteris argentea** | *ALEURITOPTERIS | Herba Aleuritopteridis | |
| 1812 | T'ung-ch'ui-ts'ao (Ta-suan-wei-ts'ao) | 銅錘草(大酸味草) | **Oxalis corymbosa** | LAVENDER SORREL | Herba Oxalidis Corymbosae | |
| 1813 | T'ung-ch'ui-yü-tai-ts'ao (Hsiao-t'ung-ch'ui) | 銅錘玉帶草(小銅錘) | **Pratia begonifolia** | *PRATIA | Herba Pratiae | |
| 1814 | T'ung-ku-ch'i (Hsüeh-wu) | 銅骨七(血烏) | **Anemone davidii** | *DAVID'S ANEMONE | Rhizoma et Folium Anemones Davidii | |
| 1815 | T'ung-ku-hsiao | 通骨消 | **Thunbergia grandiflora** | *THUNBERGIA | Radix Thunbergiae | |
| 1816 | T'ung-kuang-san | 通光散 | **Marsdenia tenacissima** | *MARSDENIA | Radix et Folium Marsdeniae Tenacissimae | |
| 1817 | T'ung-lo-san | 銅羅傘 | **Indigofera decora** | *COMELY INDIGO | Herba Indigoferae Decorae | |
| 1818 | T'ung-lu (T'ung-ch'ing) | 銅綠(銅青) | — | Copper rust | *Tunglu | |
| 1819 | T'ung-mu (T'ung-p'i, T'ung-yeh, T'ung-kên) | 桐木(桐皮,桐葉,桐根) | **Paulownia fortunei P. tomentosa** or related species | *TUNG (FOXGLOVE TREE), PAULOWNIA | Radix, Folium, Lignum et Cortex Paulowniae | |
| 1820 | T'ung-pang-ch'ui | 銅棒錘 | **Corydalis linarioides** | *YELLOW CORYDALIS | Radix Corydalis | |
| 1821 | T'ung-t'ien-ts'ao (Pi-chi-kêng) | 通天草(荸薺梗) | **Eleocharis tuberosa (Heleocharis dulcis)** | WATER-CHESTNUT | Herba Eleocharitis | |
| 1822 | T'ung-ts'ao | 通草 | **Tetrapanax papyrifer** | RICE PAPER | Medulla Tetrapanacis | |
| –ᵃ | Hsiao-t'ung-ts'ao | 小通草 | **Stachyurus himalaicus** | STACHYURUS (pith) | Medulla Stachyuri | |

150

| | Transliteration | Chinese | Botanical Name | English | Pharmaceutical |
|---|---|---|---|---|---|
| −b | Fang-t'ung-ts'ao | 方通草 | **Tetrapanax papyrifer** | RICE PAPER (sheet) | *Fangtung |
| | Ssŭ-t'ung-ts'ao | 絲通草 | ,,      ,, | ,,    ,, (shred) | *Ssutung |
| | T'ung-ts'ao-hua | 通草花 | ,,      ,, | ,,    ,, (flower) | Flos Tetrapanacis |
| | T'ung-hua-kên | 通花根 | ,,      ,, | ,,    ,, (root) | Radix    ,, |
| | T'ung-hua-fên | 通花粉 | ,,      ,, | ,,    ,, (pollen) | Pollen    ,, |
| 1823 | T'ung-tzŭ-hua | 桐子花 | **Aleurites fordii** | TUNG-OIL TREE (flower) | Flos Aleurititis |
| 1824 | T'ung-yu (T'ung-tzŭ-yu) | 桐油(桐子油) | **Aleurites fordii** **A. montana** | TUNG-OIL | Oleum    ,, |
| 1825 | Tzŭ-chi-kuan-chung | 紫其貫眾 | **Osmunda japonica** | FLOWERING FERN | Rhizoma Osmundae Japonicae |
| 1826 | Tzŭ-chih | 紫芝 | **Ganoderma japonicum** | GANODERMA | Ganoderma |
| 1827 | Tzŭ-chin (Tuan-chang-ts'ao) | 紫菫(斷腸草) | **Corydalis edulis** | CORYDALIS | Herba et Radix Corydalis |
| 1828 | Tzŭ-chin-hua | 紫菫花 | **Corydalis edulis** | CORYALIS (flower) | Flos Corydalis |
| 1829 | Tzŭ-chin-lien (Pan-tao-chêng) | 紫金蓮(搬倒甑) | **Ceratostigma willmottianum, C. plumbaginoides** | *CERATOSTIGMA | Radix Ceratostigmatis |
| 1830 | Tzŭ-chin-lung | 紫金龍 | **Dactylicapnos scandens** | *DACTYLICAPNOS | Radix Dactylicapnoris |
| 1831 | Tzŭ-chin-niu (Ai-cha-tzŭ, Tzŭ-chin-niu kên) | 紫金牛(矮茶子,紫金牛根) | **Ardisia japonica** | *JAPANESE ARDISIA | Radix, Ramus et Folium Ardisiae Japonicae |
| 1832 | Tzŭ-chin-p'i | 紫金皮 | **Tripterygium hypoglaucum** | *TRIPTERYGIUM | Radix et Ramus Tripterygii |
| 1833 | Tzŭ-chin-piao (Fêng-shih-ts'ao) | 紫金標(風濕草) | **Ceratostigma minus** | *LESSER CERATOSTIGMA | Radix Ceratostigmatis Mini |

| Transliteration | Chinese | Botanical Name | English | Pharmaceutical |
|---|---|---|---|---|
| 1834 Tzŭ-chin-sha | 紫金砂 | **Pternopetalum vulgare** | *PTERNOPETALUM | Radix Pternopetali |
| 1835 Tzŭ-ching | 紫荆 | **Cercis chinensis** | CHINESE REDBUD | |
| Tzŭ-ching-hua | 紫荆花 | ,,        ,, | ,,        ,, (flower) | Flos Cercis |
| Tzŭ-ching-kên | 紫荆根 | ,,        ,, | ,,        ,, (root) | Radix ,, |
| Tzŭ-ching-kuo | 紫荆果 | ,,        ,, | ,,        ,, (fruit) | Fructus ,, |
| Tzŭ-ching-mu | 紫荆木 | ,,        ,, | ,,        ,, (wood) | Lignum ,, |
| Tzŭ-ching p'i | 紫荆皮 | ,,        ,, | ,,        ,, (bark) | Cortex ,, |
| 1836 Tzŭ-ching-ya | 紫荆丫 | **Abelia engleriana** | ABELIA | Flos et Fructus Abeliae |
| 1837 Tzŭ-ch'ing-t'êng kên (Shan-huang-ch'i) | 紫青藤根(山黃芪) | **Berchemia kulingensis** | *KULING SUPPLE JACK | Radix Berchemiae |
| 1838 Tzŭ-chu (Chih-hsüeh-ts'ao) | 紫珠(止血草) | **Callicarpa pedunculata** | *PURPLE PEARL | Folium Callicarpae Pedunculatae |
| 1839 Tzŭ-chu-kên (Wu-chu, Hei-chu) | 紫竹根(烏竹, 黑竹) | **Phyllostachys nigra** | *PURPLE BAMBOO (rhizome) | Rhizoma Phyllostachydi |
| 1840 Tzŭ-ho-ch'ê (Jên-pao, Ho-ch'ê) | 紫河車(人胞, 河車) | — | Human placenta | Placenta Hominis |
| 1841 Tzŭ-hsüeh-hua (Tzŭ-hua-tan) | 紫雪花(紫花丹) | **Plumbago indica** | PURPLE LEADWORT | Herba Plumbaginis |
| 1842 Tzŭ-hua-chiai | 紫花芥 | **Malcolmia africana** | *MALCOLMIA | Semen Malcolmiae |
| 1843 Tzŭ-hua-ch'ien-hu (T'u-ch'ien-hu) | 紫花前胡(土前胡) | **Peucedanum decursivum** | *PEUCEDANUM, MASTERWORT | Radix Peucedani Decursivi |
| 1844 Tzŭ-hua-yü-têng-ts'ao (Tuan-chang-ts'ao) | 紫花魚燈草(斷腸草) | **Corydalis incisa** | PURPLE CORYDALIS | Herba Corydalis Incisae |

| Transliteration | Chinese | Botanical Name | English | Pharmaceutical |
|---|---|---|---|---|
| 1845 Tzǔ-jan-t'ung | 自然銅 | — | Pyrite, COPPER ORE | Pyritum |
| 1846 Tzǔ-k'uei-hua (Ch'ih-k'uei-hua, Shu-k'uei) | 紫葵花(赤葵花,蜀葵) | **Althaea rosea** | HOLLYHOCK | Flos Althaeae Roseae |
| 1847 Tzǔ-lu-ts'ao | 紫綠草 | **Pilea fasciata** | RICHWEED | Herba Pileae |
| 1848 Tzǔ-mo-li | 紫茉莉 | **Mirabilis jalapa** | FOUR O'CLOCK | Herba Mirabilis |
| Tzǔ-mo-li-kên | 紫茉莉根 | ,,　　,, | ,,　　,, | Radix　　,, |
| Tzǔ-mo-li-tzǔ | 紫茉莉子 | ,,　　,, | ,,　　,, | Semen　,, |
| 1849 Tzǔ-nan (Tzǔ-nan-kên) | 紫楠(紫楠根) | **Phoebe sheareri** | *PURPLE NAN | Radix, Cortex, et Folium Phoebes |
| 1850 Tzǔ-pei (Tzǔ-pei-ch'ih, Pei-ch'ih) | 紫貝(紫貝齒,貝齒) | — | Cowry shells | Concha Erosariae, Cypraeae, et Mauritae |
| 1851 Tzǔ-pi-t'ien-kuei (San-hsüeh-tzǔ) | 紫背天葵(散血子) | **Begonia fimbristipulata** | TEA BEGONIA | Herba Begoniae Fimbristipulatae |
| 1852 Tzǔ-pi-t'ien-kuei-ts'ao (Tzǔ-pi-ch'ien-li-kuang) | 紫背天葵草(紫背千里光) | **Senecio nudicaulis** | *PURPLE-LEAVED SENECIO (Ragwort) | Herba et Radix Senecionis Nudicaulis |
| 1853 Tzǔ-p'ing | 紫萍 | **Spirodela polyrrhiza** | *SPIRODELA | Herba Spirodelae |
| 1854 Tzǔ-shan (Tung-pei-hung-tou-shan) | 紫杉(東北紅豆杉) | **Taxus cuspidata** | *ASIATIC YEW | Ramus Taxi Cuspidatae |
| 1855 Tzǔ-shao-hua | 紫梢花 | — | Fresh water sponge | Spongilla |
| 1856 Tzǔ-shên | 紫參 | **Polygonum bistorta** | ALPINE KNOTWEED | Caudex Polygoni Bistortae |
| 1857 Tzǔ-shih-ying | 紫石英 | — | Fluorite | Fluoritum |
| 1858 Tzǔ-su (Tzǔ-su-pao, Tzǔ-su-kêng) | 紫蘇(紫蘇苞,紫蘇梗) | **Perilla frutescens** var. **crispa** | PURPLE PERILLA | Herba, Ramus, et Calyx Perillae Crispae |

| | Transliteration | Chinese | Botanical Name | English | Pharmaceutical |
|---|---|---|---|---|---|
| 1859 | Tzŭ-t'an | 紫檀 | **Pterocarpus indicus** | BURMESE ROSEWOOD | Lignum Centrale Pterocarpi |
| 1860 | Tzŭ-t'an-shu | 紫彈樹 | **Celtis biondii** | HACKBERRY | Ramus, Folium et Cortex Celtis |
| 1861 | Tzŭ-t'êng | 紫藤 | **Wisteria sinensis** | WISTERIA | Ramus et Folium Wisteriae |
| | Tzŭ-t'êng-kên | 紫藤根 | ,,        ,, | ,,   (root) | Radix Wisteriae |
| | Tzŭ-t'êng-tzŭ | 紫藤子 | ,,        ,, | ,,   (seed) | Semen  ,, |
| 1862 | Tzŭ-ts'ao | 紫草 | See the following | — | — |
| —a | Juan-tzŭ-ts'ao | 軟紫草 | **Arnebia euchroma A. guttata** | *ARNEBIA | Radix Arnebiae |
| —b | Tien-tzŭ-ts'ao | 滇紫草 | **Onosma paniculatum O. hookeri** | *ONOSMA | Radix Onosmatis |
| —c | Ying-tzŭ-ts'ao | 硬紫草 | **Lithospermum erythrorhizon** | GROOMWELL | Radix Lithospermi |
| 1863 | Tzŭ-ts'ao-jung (Tzŭ-chiao) | 紫草茸(紫膠) | — | Insect secretion on *Dalbergia, Ficus,* etc. | Lacca |
| 1864 | Tzŭ-ts'ao-wu | 紫草烏 | **Aconitum delavayi** | YUNNAN MONKSHOOD | Radix Aconiti Delavayi |
| 1865 | Tzŭ-tu-chuan | 紫杜鵑 | **Rhododendron mariae** | PURPLE RHODODENDRON | Ramus et Radix Rhododendri Mariae |
| 1866 | Tzŭ-t'ung-k'uang | 紫銅礦 | — | Bornite copper ore | Bornitum |
| 1867 | Tzŭ-t'ung-ts'ao-kên | 紫筒草根 | **Arnebia saxatilis** | *ROCK ARNEBIA | Radix Arnebiae |
| 1868 | Tzŭ-wei-hua | 紫薇花 | **Lagerstroemia indica** | CRAPE MYRTLE | Flos, Folium et Radix Lagerstroemiae |

154

| | Transliteration | Chinese | Botanical Name | English | Pharmaceutical |
|---|---|---|---|---|---|
| 1869 | Tzŭ-wei-kên | 紫葳根 | **Campsis grandiflora** | TRUMPET-FLOWER | Radix Campsis |
| 1870 | Tzŭ-ya-chih-ts'ao | 紫鴨跖草 | **Tradescantia virginiana** | SPIDERWORT | Herba Tradescantiae |
| 1871 | Tzŭ-yen-ts'ao | 紫燕草 | **Lobelia hybrida** | *HYBRID LOBELIA | Herba Lobeliae Hybridae |
| 1872 | Tzŭ-yu-chan | 紫玉簪 | **Hosta ventricosa** | BLUE PLANTAIN-LILY | Herba et Radix Hostae |
| 1873 | Tzŭ-yu-mu | 紫油木 | **Pistacia weinmannifolia** | *YUNNAN PISTACIA | Folium et Cortex Pistaciae Weinmanni-foliae |
| 1874 | Tzŭ-yüan | 紫苑 | **Aster tataricus** | PURPLE ASTER | Radix Asteris |
| 1875 | Tzŭ-yün-ying-tzŭ | 紫雲英子 | **Astragalus sinicus** | CHINESE MILK-VETCH | Semen Astragali Sinici |
| 1876 | Tz'ŭ-chi-li | 刺蒺藜 | **Tribulus terrestris** | CALTROP | Fructus Tribuli |
| 1877 | Tz'ŭ-chiu-shu | 刺楸樹 | **Kalopanax septemlobus** | *KALOPANAX | Cortex et Radix Kalopanacis |
| 1878 | Tz'ŭ-chu-sun (Lê-chu) | 刺竹笋(筋竹) | **Babusa sinospinosa** | SPINY BAMBOO | Gemma Bambusae Sinospinosae |
| 1879 | Tz'ŭ-hsien-ts'ai | 刺莧荣 | **Amaranthus spinosus** | SPINY AMARANTH | Radix Amaranthi Spinosi |
| 1880 | Tz'ŭ-hu-yeh | 刺虎葉 | **Damnacanthus indicus** | *DAMNACANTHUS | Ramus Damnacanthi |
| 1881 | Tz'ŭ-huai-hua | 刺槐花 | **Robinia pseudoacacia** | BLACK LOCUST | Flos Robiniae |
| 1882 | Tz'ŭ-huang | 雌黃 | — | Orpiment, or Auripigment | Orpimentum, or Auripigmentum |
| 1883 | Tz'ŭ-huang-lien | 刺黃蓮 | **Berberis soulieana** | *TIBETAN BARBERRY | Radix et Cortex Berberidis |
| 1884 | Tz'ŭ-huang-pai | 刺黃柏 | **Mahonia gracilipes** <br> **M. ganpinensis** <br> **M. fortunei** <br> **Berberis anhweiensis** | *SLENDER MAHONIA <br> *GANPIN MAHONIA <br> *FORTUNE'S MAHONIA <br> *ANHWEI BARBERRY | Radix Mahoniae <br><br><br> Cortex Berberidis |

| Transliteration | Chinese | Botanical Name | English | Pharmaceutical | |
|---|---|---|---|---|---|
| 1885 Tz'ŭ-jên-shên | 刺人参 | **Oplopanax elatus** | *OPLOPANAX | Radix Oplopanacis | |
| 1886 Tz'ŭ-kai-ts'ao | 刺蓋草 | **Cirsium belingschanicum** | *PLUMED THISTLE | Radix Cirsii Belingschanici | |
| 1887 Tz'ŭ-kua-mi-ts'ao (Tz'ŭ-so-lo) | 刺瓜米草(刺梭羅) | **Smilax nana** | *SMALL CATBRIER | Caudex Smilacis Nanae | |
| 1888 Tz'ŭ-kuo-su-mu (Mang-kuo-ting) | 刺果蘇木(杧果釘) | **Caesalpinia crista** | *TUFTED SAPPAN | Folium Caesalpiniae Cristae | |
| 1889 Tz'ŭ-kuo-wei-mao (K'ou-tzŭ-hua) | 刺果衞矛(扣子花) | **Euonymus wilsonii** | *WILSON'S EUONYMUS | Radix Euonymi Wilsonii | |
| 1890 Tz'ŭ-lao-ya | 刺老鴉 | **Aralia elata** | HERCLES'-CLUB | Cortex Araliae Elatae | |
| 1891 Tz'ŭ-li | 刺藜 | **Chenopodium aristatum** | *AWNED GOOSEFOOT | Herba Chenopodii Aristati | |
| 1892 Tz'ŭ-li (Tibetan) | 刺李 | **Ribes alpestre** | *THORNY PLUM | Fructus Ribis | |
| 1893 Tz'ŭ-li-hua | 刺梨花 | **Rosa roxburghii** | *SPINY PEAR | Flos Rosae Roxburghii | |
| Tz'ŭ-li-kên | 刺梨根 | ,, ,, | ,, ,, (root) | Radix ,, ,, | |
| Tz'ŭ-li-yeh | 刺梨葉 | ,, ,, | ,, ,, (leaf) | Folium ,, ,, | |
| Tz'ŭ-li-kuo | 刺梨果 | ,, ,, | ,, ,, (fruit) | Fructus ,, ,, | |
| 1894 Tz'ŭ-li-tzŭ | 刺栗子 | **Rosa graciliflora** | *SPINY CHESTNUT | Fructus Rosae Graciliflorae | |
| 1895 Tz'ŭ-ling (Tz'ŭ-ling-kên) | 刺菱(刺菱根) | **Trapa incisa** var. **quadricaudata** | WATER CALTROP | Fructus et Radix Trapae Incisae | |
| 1896 Tz'ŭ-lung-pao (Ts'ung-mu) | 刺龍包(楤木) | **Aralia decaisneana** | ANGELICA TREE | Radix Araliae Decaisneanae | |
| 1897 Tz'ŭ-mei-hua (Tz'ŭ-mei-kuo) | 刺玫花(刺莓果) | **Rosa davurica** | *SIBERIAN ROSE | Flos et Fructus Rosae Davuricae | |

156

| | Transliteration | Chinese | Botanical Name | English | Pharmaceutical | Tz'u-m |
|---|---|---|---|---|---|---|
| 1898 | Tz'ŭ-mi (Ts'ao-mi, Tz'ŭ-t'ang) | 刺密(草蜜, 刺糖) | **Alhagi pseudalhagi** | ALHAGI-HONEY | Mel Alhagi | |
| 1899 | Tz'ŭ-mo-ling-ts'ao (Tz'ŭ-shên) | 刺蘑苓草(刺参) | **Morina coulteriana M. betonicoides** | *MORINA | Herba Morinae | |
| 1900 | Tz'ŭ-nan-shê-t'êng (Pa-shan-hu) | 刺南蛇藤(爬山虎) | **Celastrus flagellaris** | *SPINY CELASTRUS | Ramus et Fructus Celastri Flagellaris | |
| 1901 | Tz'ŭ-pei-hsieh | 刺萆薢 | **Smilax ferox** | CAT BRIER | Caudex Smilacis Ferici | |
| 1902 | Tz'ŭ-p'ien | 刺片 | **Gleditsia sinensis** | SWEET LOCUST | Spina Gleditsiae | |
| 1903 | Tz'ŭ-po | 刺泡 | **Rubus hirsutus** | *PRICKLY RASPBERRY | Radix et Folium Rubi Hirsuti | |
| 1904 | Tz'ŭ-san-chia (Wu-chia-p'i) | 刺三加(五加皮) | **Eleutherococcus trifoliatus** | ACANTHOPANAX | Radix Eleutherococci Trifoliati | |
| 1905 | Tz'ŭ-sha-p'êng (Fêng-kun-ts'ao) | 刺沙蓬(風滾草) | **Salsola ruthenica S. collina** | SALSOLA | Herba Salsolae | |
| 1906 | Tz'ŭ-shên | 刺参 | **Morina delavayi** | *YUNNAN MORINA | Radix Morinae Delavayi | |
| 1907 | Tz'ŭ-shih | 磁石 | — | Magnetite | Magnetitum | |
| 1908 | Tz'ŭ-shih-liu (Shan-shih-liu) | 刺石榴(山石榴) | **Rosa omeiensis** | OMEI ROSE | Fructus et Radix Rosae Omeiensis | |
| 1909 | Tz'ŭ-t'ien-ch'ieh (K'u-t'ien-ch'ieh) | 刺天茄(苦天茄) | **Solanum khasianum** | *HIMALAYAN NIGHTSHADE | Fructus et Folium Solani Khasiani | |
| 1910 | Tz'ŭ-t'ung-hua (Tz'u-t'ung-yeh) | 刺桐花(刺桐葉) | **Erythrina variegata** var. **orientalis** | SPINY ERYTHRINA | Flos et Folium Erythrinae Variegatae | |
| 1911 | Tz'ŭ-wei-p'i | 刺猬皮 | | Hedgehog skin | Corium Erinacei | |
| 1911A | Tz'ŭ-wu-chia | 刺五加 | **Eleutherococcus senticosus** | ELEUTHERO, (Sibirian Ginseng) | Coudex et Ramus Eleutherococci senticosi | |
| 1912 | Wa-lêng-tzŭ | 瓦楞子 | — | Cockle shells | Concha Arcae | |
| 1913 | Wa-sung | 瓦松 | **Orostachys fimbriatus O. erudescens** | *CHINESE HENS-AND-CHICKENS | Herba Orastachydis | |

| | Transliteration | Chinese | Botanical Name | English | Pharmaceutical |
|---|---|---|---|---|---|
| 1914 | Wa-wei | 瓦韋 | **Lepisorus thunbergianus** | *LEPISORUS | Herba Lepisori |
| 1915 | Wai-yüan | 外苑 | See Sha-yüan | — | — |
| 1916 | Wan-chang-shên | 萬丈深 | **Crepis lignea** | *CREPIS | Radix et Folium Crepidis |
| 1917 | Wan-nien-ch'ing | 萬年青 | **Rohdea japonica** | ROHDEA | |
| | Wan-nien-ch'ing-kên | 萬年青根 | ,,　　,, | ,,　(rhizome) | Rhizoma Rohdeae |
| | Wan-nien-ch'ing-hua | 萬年青花 | ,,　　,, | ,,　(flower) | Flos　,, |
| | Wan-nien-ch'ing-yeh | 萬年青葉 | ,,　　,, | ,,　(leaf) | Folium　,, |
| 1918 | Wan-nien-sung | 萬年松 | **Lycopodium pulcherrimum (Phegmariurus pulcherrimus)** | *BEAUTIFUL CLUB MOSS | Herba Lycopodii |
| 1919 | Wan-nien-sung (Chuan-pai) | 萬年松(卷柏) | **Selaginella involvens** | *SELAGINELLA | Herba Selaginellae Involventis |
| 1920 | Wan-shou-chü | 萬壽菊 | **Tagetes erecta** | AFRICAN MARIGOLD | Herba et Flos Tagetis |
| 1921 | Wang-chiang-nan (Yang-chiao-tou) | 望江南(羊角豆) | **Cassia occidentalis** | COFFEE SENNA | Semen Cassiae Occidentalis |
| 1922 | Wang-kua | 王瓜 | **Trichosanthes cucumeroides** | CUCUMBER GOURD | Fructus et Semen Trichosanthis Cucumeroidis |
| | Wang-kua-kên | 王瓜根 | **Trichosanthes cucumeroides** | CUCUMBER GOURD (root) | Radix Trichosanthis Cucumeroidis |
| 1923 | Wang-pu-liu-hsing (Liu-hsin) | 王不留行(留心) | **Vaccaria segetalis** | *VACCARIA, COW COCKLE | Semen Vaccariae |

| | Transliteration | Chinese | Botanical Name | English | Pharmaceutical | Wang |
|---|---|---|---|---|---|---|
| 1924 | Wang-sun | 王孫 | **Paris tetraphylla** | *FOUR-LEAVED PARIS | Rhizoma Paris Tetraphyllae | |
| 1925 | Wang-yao-sha | 望月砂 | — | Rabbit dung | Excrementum Lepi | |
| 1926 | Wei-jui | 萎蕤 | **Polygonatum odoratum** | SOLOMON'S SEAL | Rhizoma Polygoni Odorati | |
| 1927 | Wei-ling-hsien (Ling-hsien) | 威靈仙(靈仙) | **Clematis chinensis** | CHINESE CLEMATIS | Radix Clematidis | |
| 1928 | Wei-ling-ts'ai | 委陵菜 | **Potentilla chinensis** | *CHINESE SILVER-WEED | Radix Potentillae Chinensis | |
| 1929 | Wên-ching | 問荊 | **Equisetum arvense** | COMMON HORSETAIL | Herba Equiseti Arvensis | |
| 1930 | Wên-chu | 文竹 | **Asparagus plumosus** | ASPARAGUS FERN | Herba Asparagi Plumosi | |
| 1931 | Wên-ko (Ko-k'o) | 文蛤(蛤殼) | — | Clam shell | Concha Meretricis | |
| 1932 | Wên-kuan-kuo | 文冠果 | **Xanthoceras sorbifolia** | *XANTHOCERAS | Lignum et Ramus Xanthoceratis | |
| 1932A | Wên-p'u, (Mu-kua) | 榲桲(木瓜) | **Cydonia oblonga** | OBLONG QUINCE | Fructus Cydoniae Oblongae | |
| 1933 | Wên-shu-lan-kuo | 文殊蘭果 | **Crinum asiaticum** | ST. JOHNS LILY | Fructus Crini Asiatici | |
| 1934 | Wên-yao-yü | 文鰩魚 | — | Flying Fish | Cypsilurus | |
| 1935 | Wu-chao-chin-lung | 五爪金龍 | **Tetrastigma hypoglaucum** | TETRASTIGMA | Radix et Herba Tetrastigmatis | |
| 1936 | Wu-chao-fêng | 五爪楓 | **Rubus blinii** | *BLIN'S RASPBERRY | Herba Rubi Blinii | |
| 1937 | Wu-chao-lung (Wu-chao-chin lung) | 五爪龍 (五爪金龍) | **Ipomoea cairica** | CAIRO MORNING-GLORY | Radix et Ramus Ipomoea Cairicae | |
| | Wu-chao-lung-hua | 五爪龍花 | „ „ | „ „ (flower) | Flos Ipomoeae Cairicae | |

| | Transliteration | Chinese | Botanical Name | English | Pharmaceutical |
|---|---|---|---|---|---|
| 1938 | Wu-ch'i-ch'ao-yang-ts'ao (Chui-fêng-ch'i) | 五氣朝陽草(追風七) | **Geum aleppicum** | AVENS | Radix et Herba Gei |
| 1939 | Wu-chia-p'i (Nan-wu-chia-p'i) | 五加皮(南五加皮) | **Eleuteroccus gracilistylis (Acanthopanax)** | *WUCHIAPI, Acanthopanax | Cortex Eleutherococci |
| —a | Ch'iao-mu-wu-chia | 橋木五加 | **E. evodiaefolius** | ,, | ,, ,, |
| —b | Hung-mao-wu-chia | 紅毛五加 | **E. giraldii** | ,, | ,, ,, |
| —c | Lun-san-wu-chia | 輪傘五加 | **E. verticillatus** | ,, | ,, ,, |
| —d | Shu-wu-chia | 蜀五加 | **E. setchuenensis** | ,, | ,, ,, |
| —e | T'êng-wu-chia | 藤五加 | **E. leucorrhizus** | ,, | ,, ,, |
| —f | Ts'ao-yeh-wu-chia | 糙葉五加 | **E. henryi** | ,, | ,, ,, |
| —g | Tz'ŭ-wu-chia | 刺五加 | **E. senticosus** | ,, | ,, ,, |
| —h | Wu-chia | 五加 | **E. gracilistylus** | ,, | ,, ,, |
| —i | Wu-kêng-wu-chia | 無梗五加 | **E. sessiliflorus** | ,, | ,, ,, |
| —j | T'o-chia-p'i Ku-le-ch'iang Pai-le-kên | 土加皮 苦簕薳 白簕根 | **Eleutherococcus trifoliatus** | ,, | ,, ,, |
| 1940 | Wu-chih-mao-t'ao | 五指毛桃 | **Ficus simplicissima** | *FIVE-FINGER FIG | Radix Fici Simplicissimae |
| 1941 | Wu-chih-shan-shên | 五指山參 | **Abelmoschus moschatus (A. sagittifolius)** | *HAINAN-OKRA (root) | Radix Abelmoschi |
| 1942 | Wu-chin-ts'ao | 烏金草 | **Swertia heterantha** | *ALPINE SWERTIA | Herb Swertiae Heteranthae |
| 1943 | Wu-chio-fêng-kên | 五角楓根 | **Acer sinense** | *CHINESE MAPLE | Radix Aceris Sinensis |
| 1944 | Wu-chio-yeh-p'u-t'ao (Yeh-p'u-t'ao) | 五角葉葡萄(野葡萄) | **Vitis quinquangularis** | CHINESE WILD GRAPE | Cortex Radicis Vitis Quinquangularis |

160

| | Transliteration | Chinese | Botanical Name | English | Pharmaceutical |
|---|---|---|---|---|---|
| 1945 | Wu-chiu | 烏桕 | **Sapium sebiferum** | CHINESE VEGETABLE TALLOW | |
| | Wu-chiu-kên-p'i | 烏桕根皮 | ,,　　　,, | ,,　,,　,, (root-bark) | Cortex Radicis Sapii |
| | Wu-chiu-tzŭ | 烏桕子 | ,,　　　,, | ,,　,,　,, (seed) | Semen Sapii |
| | Wu-chiu-yeh | 烏桕葉 | ,,　　　,, | ,,　,,　,, (leaf) | Folium ,, |
| 1946 | Wu-chu-yeh (T'ieh-ku-san) | 五除葉(鐵骨散) | **Evodia trichotoma** | *SOUTHERN EVODIA | Frutex Evodiae Trichotomae |
| 1947 | Wu-chu-yü | 吳茱萸 | **Tetradium rutaecarpum** (Evodia rutaecarpa) | EVODIA | Fructus Evodiae |
| | Wu-chu-yü-kên | 吳茱萸根 | ,,　　　,, | ,, (root) | Radix ,, |
| | Wu-chu-yü-yeh | 吳茱萸葉 | ,,　　　,, | ,, (leaf) | Folium ,, |
| 1948 | Wu-chuan-ch'i | 五轉七 | **Triosteum fargesii** | *TRIOSTEUM | Frutex Triostei |
| 1949 | Wu-fan-tzŭ | 烏飯子 | **Vaccinium fragile** | LESSER BILBERRY | Fructus Vaccinii Fragilis |
| 1950 | Wu-fêng-chao-yang-ts'ao | 五鳳朝陽草 | **Pedicularis rex** | *PEDICULARIS | Herba Pedicularis |
| 1951 | Wu-hsiang-hsüeh-t'êng (Ta-huo-hsüeh) | 五香血藤(大活血) | **Kadsura longipedunculata** | LONG-STALKED KADSURA | Ramus Kadsurae et Ramus Schisandrae |
| | | | **Schisandra sphenanthera** | *SPHERE-SCHISANDRA | |
| 1952 | Wu-hsiang-ts'ao | 五香草 | **Mosla soochouensis** | *SOOCHOU MOSLA | Herba Moslae Soochouensis |
| 1953 | Wu-hsien-lin-mu | 五腺槤木 | **Prunus brachypoda** var. **eglandulosa** | *SHORT-STALKED WILD CHERRY | Radix, Folium et Fructus Pruni Brachypodae |

| Transliteration | Chinese | Botanical Name | English | Pharmaceutical |
|---|---|---|---|---|
| [1954] Wu-hsin-hao | 五星蒿 | **Echinopsilon divaricatum** | *ECHINOPSILON | Herba Echinopsilonis |
| [1955] Wu-hua-kuo | 無花果 | **Ficus carica** | FIG (fruit) | Fructus Fici |
| Wu-hua-kuo-kên | 無花果根 | ,, ,, | ,, (root) | Radix ,, |
| [1956] Wu-huan-tzǔ | 無患子 | **Sapindus mukorossi** | SOAPBERRY | Semen Sapindi |
| Wu-huan-shu-p'i | 無患樹皮 | ,, ,, | ,, (bark) | Cortex ,, |
| Wu-huan-shu-chiang | 無患樹薑 | ,, ,, | ,, (root) | Radix ,, |
| Wu-huan-tzǔ-p'i | 無患子皮 | ,, ,, | ,, (pericarp) | Pericarpium ,, |
| Wu-huan-tzǔ-yeh | 無患子葉 | ,, ,, | ,, (leaf) | Folium ,, |
| Wu-huan-tzǔ-chung-jên | 無患子種仁 | ,, ,, | ,, (cotyledons) | Cotyledones ,, |
| [1957] Wu-i (K'u-i) | 武夷(蕪荑, 苦夷) | **Ulmus macrocarpa** | STINKING ELM (medicine cake) | Pasta Ulmi |
| [1958] Wu-kên-t'êng (Wu-yeh-t'êng, Lo-wang-t'êng) | 無根藤(無葉藤, 羅網藤) | **Cassytha filiformis** | CASSYTHA | Liana Cassythae |
| [1959] Wu-ku-chi (Wu-chi) | 烏骨鷄(烏鷄) | — | Black-bone Fowl | Pullus cum Osse Nigro |
| [1960] Wu-ku-chung (Ch'ü, Shui-hsien-tzǔ) | 五谷虫(蛆, 水仙子) | — | Maggots | Larva Chrysomyiae |
| [1961] Wu-ku-t'êng | 烏骨藤 | **Fissistigma glaucescens** | *FISSISTIGMA | Radix Fissistigmatis |
| [1962] Wu-kung | 蜈蚣 | — | Centipedes | Scolopendra |
| [1963] Wu-kung-ch'i | 蜈蚣七 | **Cypripedium macranthum** | MOCCASIN-FLOWER | Caudex et Flos Cypripedii |

| | Transliteration | Chinese | Botanical Name | English | Pharmaceutical |
|---|---|---|---|---|---|
| 1964 | Wu-kung-ch'i-kên | 蜈蚣旗根 | **Woodsia polystichoides** | WOODSIA | Rhizoma Woodsiae |
| 1965 | Wu-kung-lan | 蜈蚣蘭 | **Sarcanthus scolopen-driifolius** | *CENTIPEDE ORCHID | Herba Sarcanthi Scolopendriifolii |
| 1966 | Wu-kung-p'ing | 蜈蚣萍 | **Salvinia natans** | SALVINIA | Herba Salviniae |
| 1967 | Wu-kung-t'êng | 蜈蚣藤 | **Zanthoxylum multijugum** | *CENTIPEDE BRAMBLE | Ramus Zanthoxyli Multijugi |
| 1968 | Wu-kung-ts'ao | 蜈蚣草 | **Pteris vittata** | *CENTIPEDE FERN | Rhizoma Pteridis Vittatae |
| 1969 | Wu-lan (Wu-kan-lan) | 烏欖(烏橄欖) | **Canarium pimela** | BLACK CHINESE OLIVE | Fructus Canarii Pimelae |
| | Wu-lan-kên | 烏欖根 | ,, ,, | ,, ,, ,, (root) | Radix Canarii Pimelae |
| | Wu-lan-jên | 烏欖仁 | ,, ,, | ,, ,, ,, (seed) | Semen ,, ,, |
| | Wu-lan-yeh | 烏欖葉 | ,, ,, | ,, ,, ,, (leaf) | Folium ,, ,, |
| 1970 | Wu-lien-mei (Lung-kê, Hu-kê) | 烏蘞莓(龍葛, 虎葛) | **Cayratia japonica** | *CAYRATIA | Radix et Ramus Cayratiae |
| 1971 | Wu-ling-chih | 五靈脂 | — | Cave bat dung | Excrementum Pteropi |
| 1972 | Wu-liu-kên | 烏柳根 | **Salix microstachya** | *DESERT WILOW | Radix Salicis Microstachyae |
| 1973 | Wu-lou-tzǔ (Hai-tsao, Po-ssǔ-tsao) | 無漏子(海棗, 波斯棗) | **Phoenix dactylifera** | DATE | Fructus Phoenicis |
| 1974 | Wu-lung-kên | 五龍根 | **Ficus simplicissima** | *ROUGH FIG | Radix Fici Simplicissimae |
| 1975 | Wu-lung-pai-wei (Wu-pao) | 烏龍擺尾(烏泡) | **Rubus tephrodes** | *ASH RASPBERRY | Radix et Folium Rubi Tephrodis |

| | Transliteration | Chinese | Botanical Name | English | Pharmaceutical |
|---|---|---|---|---|---|
| 1976 | Wu-mai-lu-jung-hao-hua (Mao-yeh-t'u-êrh-fêng) | 五脈綠絨蒿花(毛葉兔耳風) | **Meconopsis quintuplinervia** | *MECONOPSIS | Flos Meconopsis |
| 1977 | Wu-mei (Mei-shih) | 烏梅(梅實) | **Prunus mume** | *WUMEI | Fructus Pruni Mume |
| 1978 | Wu-ming-i | 無名異 | — | Pyrolusite | Pyrolusitum |
| 1979 | Wu-ming-tzǔ | 無名子 | **Pistacia vera** | PISTACHIO | Fructus Pistaciae |
| 1980 | Wu-mu-hsieh | 烏木屑 | **Diospyros ebenum** | MACASSAR EBONY (sawdust) | Scobis Diospyroris Ebeni |
| 1981 | Wu-nu-lung-tan | 烏奴龍膽 | **Gentiana urnula** | *URN GENTIAN | Herba Gentianae Urnulae |
| 1982 | Wu-pan-chi-shêng | 五瓣寄生 | **Loranthus pentapetalus** | *GREATER LORANTHUS | Ramus Loranthi Pentapetali |
| 1983 | Wu-pei-tzǔ (Wên-chia, Pei-tzǔ) | 五倍子(文甲,倍子) | **Rhus chinensis** **R. potaninii** | CHINESE SUMAC (gallnut) | Galla Rhi Chinensis et Potaninii |
| 1984 | Wu-pei-tzǔ-miao | 五倍子苗 | **Rhus chinensis** | CHINESE SUMAC (young shoot) | Ramulus Immaturus Rhi Chinensis |
| 1985 | Wu-pei-tzǔ-nei-ch'ung | 五倍子內虫 | — | Gall insect | Melaphis |
| 1986 | Wu-piao-lien | 烏薸連 | **Viola vaginata** | *VAGINANT VIOLET | Herba Violae Vaginatae |
| 1987 | Wu-sao-fêng (Ch'ing-shê-t'êng) | 烏騷風(青蛇藤) | **Periploca calophylla** | *PRETTY-LEAVED PERIPLOCA | Ramus Periplocae Calophyllae |
| 1988 | Wu-sê-mei (Ma-ying-tan) | 五色梅(馬櫻丹) | **Lantana camara** | LANTANA | Ramus Lantanae Camarae |
| | Wu-sê-mei-hua | 五色梅花 | ,, ,, | ,, (flower) | Flos Lantanae Camarae |
| | Wu-sĕ-mei-kên | 五色梅根 | ,, ,, | ,, (root) | Radix ,, ,, |

164

| Transliteration | Chinese | Botanical Name | English | Pharmaceutical |
|---|---|---|---|---|
| 1989 Wu-shê (Hei-hua-shê, Wu-fêng-shê) | 烏蛇(黑花蛇,烏風蛇) | — | Black-Striped Snake | Zaocys |
| 1990 Wu-shih-tzŭ | 無食子 | See Mu-shih-tzŭ | — | — |
| 1991 Wu-shui-kê | 霧水葛 | **Pouzolzia zeylanica** | *POUZOLZIA | Herba Pouzolziae |
| 1992 Wu-tou-kên | 烏豆根 | **Sophora mairei** | *MAIRE'S SOPHORA | Radix Sophorae Mairei |
| 1993 Wu-t'ou | 烏頭 | See Ch'uan-wu and Ts'ao-wu-t'ou | — | — |
| 1994 Wu-tsei (Wu-tsei-jou, Wu-tsei-fu-chung-mê, Wu-tsei-ku) | 烏賊(烏賊肉,烏賊腹中墨,烏賊骨) | — | Cuttle-fish (meat, ink-sac, or internal bone) | Sepia, or Sepiella |
| 1995 Wu-t'ung | 梧桐 | **Firmiana simplex** | CHINESE PARASOL TREE | See the following |
| Wu-t'ung-kên | 梧桐根 | ,,      ,, | ,, ,, ,, (root) | Radix Firmianae |
| Wu-t'ung-hua | 梧桐花 | ,,      ,, | ,, ,, ,, (flower) | Flos      ,, |
| Wu-t'ung-pai-p'i | 梧桐白皮 | ,,      ,, | ,, ,, ,, (bark) | Cortex      ,, |
| Wu-t'ung-tzŭ | 梧桐子 | ,,      ,, | ,, ,, ,, (seed) | Semen      ,, |
| Wu-t'ung-yeh | 梧桐葉 | ,,      ,, | ,, ,, ,, (leaf) | Folium      ,, |
| 1996 Wu-tz'ŭ-kên | 無莿根 | **Ampelopsis cantoniensis** | *CANTON AMPELOPSIS | Radix et Ramus Ampelopsis Cantoniensis |
| 1997 Wu-wei-ts'ao | 五味草 | **Corydalis stenantha** | *STRAIGHT-FLOWERED CORYDALIS | Herba Corydalis Stenanthae |
| 1998 Wu-wei-tzŭ (Pei-wei-tzŭ) | 五味子(北味子) | **Schisandra chinensis** | SCHISANDRA | Fructus Szhisandrae Chinensis |

165

| | Transliteration | Chinese | Botanical Name | English | Pharmaceutical |
|---|---|---|---|---|---|
| 1999 | Wu-ya (Lao-ya) | 烏鴉(老鴉) | — | Crow | Corvus |
| –a | Wu-ya-tan | 烏鴉膽 | — | Crow's gall bladder | Fel Corvi |
| 2000 | Wu-yao, T'ai-wu | 烏藥, 台烏 | **Lindera aggregata** | *CHINESE ALLSPICE | Radix Linderae aggretae |
| | T'ai-wu-ch'iu | 台烏球 | **L. chunii** | DINGHU ALLSPICE | Radix Linderae chunii |
| | Wu-yao-tzŭ | 烏藥子 | **L. aggregata** | ALLSPICE (seed) | Semen Linderae |
| | Wu-yao-yeh | 烏藥葉 | „ „ | „ „ (leaf) | Folium „ |
| 2001 | Wu-yao-hua | 烏藥花 | **Clerodendrum yunnanense** | *YUNNAN CLERODENDRUM | Flos Clerodendri Yunnanensis |
| 2002 | Wu-yeh-p'ao | 五葉泡 | **Rubus cochinchinensis** | *FIVE-LEAVED BLACKBERRY | Radix et Folium Rubi Cochinchinensis |
| 2003 | Wu-yeh-t'êng | 無爺藤 | See Wu-kên-t'êng | — | |
| 2004 | Wu-yen-kuo-shu-p'i (Suan-tsao-p'i) | 五眼果樹皮(酸棗皮) | **Choerospondias axillaris** | *SOUR DATE | Cortex Choerospondiatis |
| 2005 | Wu-yü | 吳萸 | See Wu-chu-yü | — | — |
| 2006 | Wu-yü-tan | 烏魚蛋 | — | Cuttle-fish egg | Ovum Sepiae |
| 2007 | Wu-yüeh-ai | 五月艾 | **Artemisia vulgaris A. argyi** | COMMON MUGWORT | Herba Artemisiae |
| 2008 | **Ya** | 鴨 | — | Duck | Anas |
| 2009 | Ya-chê-ts'ao | 鴨跖草 | **Commelina communis** | DAY FLOWER | Herba Commelinae |
| 2010 | Ya-chüeh-ai (Ya-chüeh-ts'ai) | 鴨腳艾(鴨腳荣) | **Artemisia lactiflora** | DUCK-FOOT MUGWORT | Herba Artemisiae Lactiflorae |
| 2011 | Ya-chüeh-mu (Ya-chüeh-shu-p'i, Ya-chüeh-shu-kên) | 鴨腳木(鴨腳樹皮, 鴨腳樹根) | **Schefflera octophylla** | SCHEFFLERA | Ramus cum Folia, Cortex et Radix Schefflerae |

166

| Transliteration | Chinese | Botanical Name | English | Pharmaceutical |
|---|---|---|---|---|
| 2012 Ya-chüeh-pan-ts'ao (La-tzŭ-ts'ao) | 鴨腳板草(辣子草) | **Ranunculus sieboldii** | CROWFOOT | Herba Ranuculi Sieboldii |
| 2013 Ya-êrh-ch'in | 鴨兒芹 | **Cryptotaenia japonica** | CRYPTOTAENIA | Herba Cryptotaeniae |
| 2014 Ya-fêng-yeh (Fêng-shu-yeh) | 椏楓葉(楓樹葉) | **Acer trifidum** | MAPLE (twig) | Ramus Aceris trifidi |
| 2015 Ya-hu | 雅斛 | **Dendrobium nobile** | DENDROBIUM | Herba Dendrobii Nobilis |
| 2016 Ya-kan-yao | 鴉疳藥 | **Hedyotis uncinella (Oldenlandia uncinella)** | *MEADOW HEDYOTIS | Herba Hedyotidis Uncinellae |
| 2017 Ya-ma-jên | 亞麻仁 | **Linum usitatissimum** | LINSEED | Semen Lini |
| 2018 Ya-p'ien | 鴉片 | **Papaver somniferum** | OPIUM POPPY | Opium, Morphine |
| 2019 Ya-shê-ts'ao | 鴨舌草 | **Monochoria vaginalis** | DUCK'S TONGUE MONOCHORIA | Herba Monochoriae |
| 2020 Ya-tan (Ya-tan-k'o) | 鴨蛋(鴨蛋殼) | — | Duck egg and shell | Ovum Anatis |
| 2021 Ya-tan-tzŭ | 鴉膽子 | **Brucea javanica** | *BRUCEA | Fructus et Radix Bruceae |
| 2022 Ya-tsao (Ya-tsao-chieh, Chu-ya-tsao) | 牙皂(牙皂莢,猪牙皂) | **Gleditsia sinensis** | SWEET LOCUST | Fructus Gleditsiae |
| 2023 Ya-tsao-shu-p'i (Ya-tsao-shu-kên) | 鴨皂樹皮(鴨皂樹根) | **Acacia farnesiana** | ACACIA | Cortex et Radix Acaciae Farnesianae |
| 2024 Ya-tsui-huang (T'ao-ching-ts'ao) | 鴨嘴癀(調經草) | **Lindernia ruellioides** | *DUCK-BILL PIMPERNEL | Herba Linderniae Ruellioidis |
| 2025 Ya-ts'ung | 鴉葱 | **Scorzonera austriaca** | *SCORZONERA | Caudex Scorzonerae |
| 2026 Ya-yung-ts'ao | 牙痈草 | **Cynoglossum lanceolatum** | *CYNOLOSSUM | Herba Cynoglossi |

| Transliteration | Chinese | Botanical Name | English | Pharmaceutical |
|---|---|---|---|---|
| 2027 Yai-chiao (T'u-hua-chiao) | 崖椒(土花椒) | **Zanthoxylum schinifolium** | *CLIFF PRICKLY ASH | Fructus Zanthoxyli Schinifolii |
| 2028 Yai-sung | 崖松 | **Sedum elatinoides** | STONECROP | Herba Sedi Elatinoidis |
| 2029 Yai-ts'ung-kên | 崖棕根 | **Carex siderostica** | *PALM SEDGE | Rhizoma Caricis |
| 2030 Yang | 羊 | — | Goat or sheep | Capra vel Ovis |
| 2031 Yang-chi-chü-kên (Nao-yang-hua-kên) | 羊躑躅根(鬧羊花根) | **Rhododendron molle** | YELLOW AZALEA (root) | Radix Rhododendri Mollis |
| 2032 Yang-ch'i-shih (Ch'i-shih) | 陽起石(起石) | — | Actinolite | Actinolitum |
| 2033 Yang-ch'i-ts'ao | 洋蓍草 | **Achillea millefolium** | YARROW | Herba Achilleae |
| 2034 Yang-chin hua (Man-t'o-lo-hua) | 洋金花(曼陀羅花) | **Datura** spp. | DATURA | Flos Daturae |
| −a Nan-yang-chin-hua (Pai-man-t'o-lo) | 南洋金花(白曼陀羅) | **D. metel** | WHITE-FLOWERED DATURA | ,, ,, metel |
| −b Pei-yang-chin hua (Mao-man-t'o-lo) | 北洋金花(毛曼陀羅) | **D. innoxia** | HAIRY DATURA | ,, ,, innoxiae |
| 2035 Yang-ch'ing | 秧青 | **Dalbergia yunnanense** | *YUNNAN DALBERGIA | Radix Dalbergiae Yunnanensis |
| 2036 Yang-chio-au | 羊角拗 | **Strophanthus divaricatus** | *STROPHANTHUS | Radix, Ramus et Semen Strophanthi |
| 2037 Yang-chio-shên | 羊角參 | **Polygonatum verticillatum P. roseum** | SOLOMON'S SEAL | Caudex Polygonati Verticillati et Rosei |
| 2038 Yang-chio-t'êng (Shan-pa-chiao) | 羊角藤(山八角) | **Morinda umbellata** | *MORINDA | Radix Morindae Umbellatae |

| Transliteration | Chinese | Botanical Name | English | Pharmaceutical |
|---|---|---|---|---|
| 2039 Yang-chio-ts'ao | 羊角草 | **Lindernia angustifolia** | *NARROW-LEAVED PIMPERNAL | Herba Linderniae Angustifoliae |
| 2040 Yang-chüeh-hua | 洋雀花 | **Caragana franchetiana** | *CARAGANA | Flos et Radix Caraganae |
| 2041 Yang-ch'ung (Chiu-lung-ch'ung) | 洋虫(九龍虫) | — | *Exotic Worm | Martianus |
| 2042 Yang-êrh-chü (Shan-pai-chih) | 羊耳菊(山白芷) | **Inula cappa** | GOAT-EAR ELECAMPANE | Herba Inulae |
| 2043 Yang-êrh-suan | 羊耳蒜 | **Liparis japonica** | *GOAT-EAR-LIPARIS | Herba Liparis |
| 2044 Yang-hêh-tzŭ (Yang-ts'ao-chieh) | 羊胲子(羊草結) | — | Nodules in goat stomach | Calculi Caprae |
| 2045 Yang-ho | 羊藿 | See Yin-yang-ho | — | — |
| 2046 Yang-ho-hsiang | 洋藿香 | **Pogostemon cablin** | PATCHOULI | Herba Patchouli |
| 2047 Yang-hu-hsü-ts'ao | 羊胡鬚草 | **Carex lanceolata** | *CAREX | Herba Caricis |
| 2048 Yang-mei-shu | 楊梅樹 | **Myrica rubra** | *CHINESE MYRICA | Radix, Cortex, et Semen Myricae Rubrae |
| 2049 Yang-pien (Yang-shên) | 羊鞭(羊腎) | — | Penis of sheep or goat | Penis Ovis vel Caprae |
| 2050 Yang-shan-tz'ŭ | 羊山刺 | **Zanthoxylum dimorphophyllum** | *DIMORPHOUS PRICKLY ASH | Ramus et Fructus Zanthoxyli Dimorphophylli |
| 2051 Yang-shih-mu | 羊屎木 | **Osmanthus matsumuranus** | *GOAT-DUNG TREE | Cortex et Folium Osmanthi Matsumurani |
| 2052 Yang-shih-t'iao-kên (Yang-shih-tzŭ-kên | 羊屎條根(羊食子根) | **Viburnum utile** | ARROW WOOD | Radix Viburni Utilis |

169

| | Transliteration | Chinese | Botanical Name | English | Pharmaceutical |
|---|---|---|---|---|---|
| 2053 | Yang-t'ao | 楊桃 | **Averrhoa carambola** | CARAMBOLA | Radix, Folium, Flos et Fructus Carambolae |
| 2054 | Yang-ti-huang | 洋地黃 | **Digitalis purpurea** | FOX GLOVE | Folium Digitalis |
| 2055 | Yang-t'i (T'u-ta-huang, Ya-chiao-ta-huang) | 羊蹄(土大黃,鴨腳大黃) | **Rumex japonicus** **R. nepalensis** | DOCK | Caudex, Folium et Fructus Rumicis |
| 2056 | Yang-t'i-an-hsiao | 羊蹄暗消 | **Passiflora altebilobata** | *YUNNAN PASSION FLOWER | Radix et Ramus Passiflorae Altebilobatae |
| 2057 | Yang-t'i-ts'ao (I-tien-hung) | 羊蹄草(一點紅) | **Emilia sonchifolia** | *EMILIA | Herba Emiliae |
| 2058 | Yang-ts'ung | 洋葱 | **Allium cepa** | ONION | Bulbus Allii Cepae |
| 2059 | Yang-tu-chun | 羊肚菌 | **Morchella esculenta** | MORELS | Fructificatio Morchellae |
| 2060 | Yang-yü (Ma-ling-shu) | 洋芋(馬鈴薯) | **Solanum tuberosum** | IRISH POTATO | Tuber Solani Tuberosi |
| 2061 | Yao-hua (Yao-hung-hua) | 藥花(藥紅花) | **Carthamus tinctorius** | SAFFLOWER (Inferior quality) | Flos Carthami |
| 2062 | Yao-hui-hsiang | 藥茴香 | **Pleurospermum giraldii** | *MONTANE PARSLEY | Herba Pleurospermi |
| 2063 | Yao-lao (Tsui-ma-ts'ao) | 藥老(醉馬草) | **Achnatherum inebrians** | *ACHNATHERUM | Herba et Radix Achnatheri |
| 2064 | Yao-wang-cha (Mu-pên-wei-ling-ts'ai) | 藥王茶(木本委陵菜) | **Dasiphora fruticosa** | *DASIPHORA | Folium Dasiphorae |
| 2065 | Yao-yung-tao-t'i-hu | 藥用倒提壺 | **Cynoglossum officinale** | *OFFICINAL CYNOGLOSSUM | Radix Cynoglossi Officinalis |

| Transliteration | Chinese | Botanical Name | English | Pharmaceutical |
|---|---|---|---|---|
| 2066 Yeh-cha-tzŭ | 野茶子 | **Eurya obtusifolia** | *EURYA | Fructus Euryae |
| 2067 Yeh-chi-ts'ao (Hsiao-hsien-mao) | 野鷄草(小仙茅) | **Hypoxis aurea** | *HYPOXIS | Herba Hypoxis |
| 2068 Yeh-ch'i-shu | 野漆樹 | **Rhus sylvestris** | CHINESE SUMAC | Radix et Folium Rhi Sylvestris |
| 2069 Yeh-chiao-t'êng (Ho-shou-wu) | 夜交藤(何首烏) | **Polygonum multiflorum** | *CHINESE CORNBIND | Ramus Polygoni Multiflori |
| 2070 Yeh-chien-hu | 野前胡 | **Aquilegia ecalcarata** | *SPURLESS COLUMBINE | Herba Aquilegiae |
| 2071 Yeh-chih-ma | 野芝麻 | **Lamium barbatum** | *BARBATE DEAD NETTLE | Herba et Radix Lamii |
| 2072 Yeh-chiu-hua (Hsiang-shê-ma, P'i-chiu-hua) | 野酒花(香蛇麻, 啤酒花) | **Humulus lupulus** var. **cordifolius** | HOPS | Flos Humuli |
| 2073 Yeh-chu | 野猪 | — | Wild pig | Sus Scrofa |
| Yeh-chu-p'i | 野猪皮 | | ,, ,, (hide) | |
| Yeh-chu-t'i | 野猪蹄 | | ,, ,, (feet) | |
| Yeh-chu-t'ou-ku | 野猪頭骨 | | ,, ,, (head bone) | |
| Yeh-chu-wai-shêng | 野猪外腎 | | ,, ,, (testicles) | |
| 2074 Yeh-chu-lan | 野竹蘭 | **Epipactis helleborine** | *EPIPACTIS | Herba Epipactinis |
| 2075 Yeh-chu-ma | 野苧麻 | **Boehmeria siamensis** | WILD RAMIE | Herba Boehmeriae Siamensis |
| 2076 Yeh-chü | 野菊 | **Chrysanthemum indicum** | WILD CHRYSANTHEMUM | Herba et Radix Chrysanthemi Indici |
| 2077 Yeh-chü-hua | 野菊花 | **Chrysanthemum indicum** **C. boreale** **C. lavandulaefolium** | ,, ,, (flower) | Flos Chrysanthemi |

171

| | Transliteration | Chinese | Botanical Name | English | Pharmaceutical |
|---|---|---|---|---|---|
| 2078 | Yeh-chüeh-ming | 野決明 | **Thermopsis lupinoides** | *THERMOPSIS | Ramus et Semen Thermopsis |
| 2079 | Yeh-fêng-hsien-hua | 野鳳仙花 | **Impatiens textori** | SNAPWEED | Herba Impatientis Textoris |
| 2080 | Yeh-hai-chiao | 野海椒 | **Solanum capsicastrum** | *CHILI NIGHTSHADE | Herba Solani Capsicastri |
| 2081 | Yeh-hai-t'ang | 野海棠 | **Begonia aptera** | BEGONIA | Radix Begoniae |
| 2082 | Yeh-hêh-t'ao-jên | 野核桃仁 | **Juglans cathayensis** | WILD WALNUT | Semen Juglandis Cathayensis |
| 2083 | Yeh-ho-hua | 夜合花 | **Magnolia coco** | DWARF MAGNOLIA | Flos Magnoliae Cocinis |
| 2084 | Yeh-hsi-kua-miao | 野西瓜苗 | **Hibiscus trionum** | *ANNUAL HIBISCUS | Herba Hibisci Trioni |
| 2085 | Yeh-hsi-ts'ao-kên | 野席草根 | **Juncus setchuensis** | *SZECHUAN RUSH | Rhizoma Junci Setchuensis |
| 2086 | Yeh-hsia-hua | 葉下花 | **Ainsliaea pertyoides** | *AINSLIAEA | Herba Ainsliaoae |
| 2087 | Yeh-hsiang-hua | 葉象花 | **Euphorbia heterophylla** | SUMMER POINSETTIA | Herba Euphorbiae Heterophyllae |
| 2088 | Yeh-hsiang-mao | 野香茅 | **Cymbopogon goeringii** | *WILD CAMEL HAY | Herba Cymbopogonis |
| 2089 | Yeh-hsiang-niu (Shang-han-ts'ao) | 夜香牛(傷寒草) | **Vernonia cinera** | ERECT VERNONIA | Herba Vernoniae |
| 2090 | Yeh-hsien-ts'ai | 野莧荣 | **Amaranthus ascendens** | AMARANTH | Herba et Semen Amaranthi Ascendentis |
| 2091 | Yeh-hua-chiao | 野花椒 | **Zanthoxylum tibetanum** | WILD PRICKLY ASH | Fructus Zanthoxyli Tibetani |
| 2092 | Yeh-hua-shêng | 野花生 | **Cassia tora** | FOETID CASSIA | Herba Cassiae Torae |
| 2093 | Yeh-hua-t'êng | 夜花藤 | **Hypserpa nitida** | *HYPSERPA | Liana Hypserpae |
| 2094 | Yeh-huang-kua | 野黃瓜 | **Dichocarpum fargesii** | *DICHOCARPUM | Herba Dichocarpi |

| Transliteration | Chinese | Botanical Name | English | Pharmaceutical |
|---|---|---|---|---|
| 2095 Yeh-huang-p'i | 野黃皮 | **Clausena dentata** | WILD WAMPEE | Folium et Radix Clausenae Dentatae |
| 2096 Yeh-huo-hsiang | 野藿香 | **Microtoena insuavis** | *MICROTOENA | Herba Microtoenae |
| 2097 Yeh-kan-ts'ao | 野甘草 | **Scoparia dulcis** | *SCOPARIA | Herba Scopariae |
| 2098 Yeh-kao-liang | 野高粱 | **Astilbe rivularis** | FALSE GOAT'S BEARD | Radix et Herba Astilbes |
| 2099 Yeh-ku | 野菰 | **Aeginetia indica** | *AEGINETIA | Herba Aeginetiae |
| 2100 Yeh-k'u-li-kên | 野苦梨根 | **Cotoneaster coriaceus** | *COTONEASTER | Radix Cotoneastri |
| 2101 Yeh-kuan-men | 夜關門 | **Lespedeza cunneata** | *CUNEATE-LEAVED LESPEDEZA | Herba Lespedezae Cuneatae |
| 2102 Yeh-la-tzǔ | 野辣子 | **Hypoestes poilanei** | *HYPOESTES | Herba Hypoestidis |
| 2103 Yeh-li-chih | 野荔枝 | **Cornus kousa** var. **angustata** | CHINESE DOGWOOD | Flos et Folium Corni Kousae |
| 2104 Yeh-li-chih-yeh | 野梨枝葉 | **Pyrus calleryana** | WILD PEAR | Folium Pyri Calleryanae |
| 2105 Yeh-liao-tou | 野料豆 | **Glycine soja** | WILD SOYBEAN | Semen Glycines Soja |
| 2106 Yeh-lu-tou (Yeh-huang-tou) | 野綠豆(野黃豆) | **Laportea bulbifera** | *LAPORTEA | Herba Laporteae |
| 2107 Yeh-ma-chui | 野馬追 | **Eupatorium lindleyanum** | *EUPATORIUM | Herba Eupatorii Lindleyani |
| 2108 Yeh-ma-jou | 野馬肉 | — | Wild horse meat | Equus Przewalskii |
| 2109 Yeh-ma-t'i-ts'ao | 野馬蹄草 | **Scirpus juncoides** | BULRUSH | Herba Scirpi Juncoidis |
| 2110 Yeh-mai-tzǔ | 野麥子 | **Avena fatua** | WILD OAT | Semen Avenae Fatuae |
| 2111 Yeh-mien-hua | 野棉花 | **Anemone vitifolia** | *GRAPE-LEAVED ANEMONE | Caudex Anemones Vitifoliae |
| 2112 Yeh-ming-sha (Ming-sha) | 夜明砂(明砂) | — | Bat's dung | Excrementum Vespertilii |

| | Transliteration | Chinese | Botanical Name | English | Pharmaceutical |
|---|---|---|---|---|---|
| 2113 | Yeh-mu-hsü | 野苜蓿 | **Medicago falcata** | *YELLOW CLOVER | Herba Medicaginis Falcatae |
| 2114 | Yeh-mu-kua | 野木瓜 | **Stauntonia hexaphylla** | *STAUNTONIA | Radix et Ramus Stauntoniae Hexaphyllae |
| 2115 | Yeh-mu-tan (Chu-ku-nien) | 野牡丹(猪古惢) | **Melastoma candidum** | *MELASTOMA | Herba Melastomatis Candidi |
| 2116 | Yeh-pa-tzǔ | 野巴子 | **Elsholtzia rugulosa** | *WRINKLED ELSHOLTZIA | Herba Elsholtziae Rugulosae |
| 2117 | Yeh-pai-ho (Kou-ling-ts'ao) | 野百合(狗鈴草) | **Crotalaria sessiliflora** | NARROW-LEAVED RATTLEBOX | Herba Crotalariae Sessiliflorae |
| 2118 | Yeh-pien-tou | 野扁豆 | **Dunbaria villosa** | *DUNBARIA | Herba et Semen Dunbariae |
| 2119 | Yeh-pin-lang (Pai-p'i-k'o) | 野檳榔(白皮柯) | **Lithocarpus dealbatus** | *LITHOCARPUS | Inflorescentia Lithocarpi Dealbati |
| 2120 | Yeh-p'u-t'ao | 野葡萄 | **Vitis wilsonae** **V. romanetii** | *WILD GRAPE | Radix Vitis Wilsonae „ „ Romanetii |
| 2121 | Yeh-p'u-t'ao-t'êng (Ta-fêng-t'êng) | 野葡萄藤(大風藤) | **Vitis quinquangularis** | *FIVE-ANGLED GRAPE | Ramus Vitis Quinquangularis |
| 2122 | Yeh-shan-hua-kuo (Wei-yu) | 野扇花果(胃友) | **Sarcococca ruscifolia** | *SARCOCOCCA | Fructus Sarcococcae |
| 2123 | Yeh-shan-ma-huang | 野山螞蝗 | **Bothriospermum secundum** | *BOTHRIOSPERMUM | Herba Bothriospermi |
| 2124 | Yeh-shang-chu | 葉上珠 | **Helwingia japonica** | *HELWINGIA | Folium et Fructus Helwingiae |

| | Transliteration | Chinese | Botanical Name | English | Pharmaceutical |
|---|---|---|---|---|---|
| 2125 | Yeh-shang-kuo-kên (Tuan-shu-kên) | 葉上果根(椴樹根) | **Tilia tuan** | LINDEN (root) | Radix Tiliae Tuan |
| 2126 | Yeh-shêng-ma | 野昇麻 | **Cimicifuga simplex** | *CIMICIFUGA | Caudex Cimicifugae |
| 2127 | Yeh-su-hsing | 野素馨 | **Jasminum polyanthum** | *WILD JASMINE | Herba et Flos Jasmini Polyanthi |
| 2128 | Yeh-su-ma | 野蘇麻 | **Isodon coetsa** | *ISODON | Herba Isodonis |
| 2129 | Yeh-ta-tou-t'êng | 野大豆藤 | **Glycine soja** | WILD SOYBEAN | Herba et Radix Glycines Soja |
| 2130 | Yeh-tan-shên | 野丹參 | **Salvia cavaleriei** | *CAVALERIE'S SAGE | Radix Salviae Cavaleriei |
| 2131 | Yeh-ti-chu I-yeh-ch'iu | 葉底珠，一葉萩 | **Securinega suffruticosa** | *SECURINEGA | Ramus et Flos Securinegae |
| 2132 | Yeh-tien-chieh | 野顛茄 | **Solanum surattense** | *TOXIC NIGHTSHADE | Herba Solani Surattensis |
| 2133 | Yeh-tien-ch'ing | 野靛青 | **Peristrophe bivalvis** | *PERISTROPHE | Herba Peristrophis |
| 2134 | Yeh-ting-hsiang | 野丁香 | **Syringa persica** | *WILD LILAC | Flos Immaturus Syringae Persicae |
| 2135 | Yeh-ting-hsiang (Chiu-p'ing-hua) | 野丁香(酒瓶花) | **Luculia intermedia** | *LUCULIA | Radix, Flos et Fructus Luculiae |
| 2136 | Yeh-tsung | 野棕 | **Didymospermum caudatum** | *WILD PALM | Radix Didynospermatis |
| 2137 | Yeh-ts'ung | 野葱 | **Allium prattii** | *WILD ONION | Herba Allii Prattii |
| 2138 | Yeh-tu-chung | 野杜仲 | **Euonymus grandiflorus** | *LARGE-FLOWERED EUONYMUS | Cortex Euonymi Grandiflori |
| 2139 | Yeh-tung-ch'ing | 野冬青 | **Syzygium cumini S. brachyantherum** | *SYZYGIUM | Cortex et Fructus Syzygii |

| | Transliteration | Chinese | Botanical Name | English | Pharmaceutical |
|---|---|---|---|---|---|
| 2140 | Yeh-tung-chü | 野東菊 | **Aster oreophilus** | *MOUNTAIN ASTER | Flos Asteris Oreophili |
| 2141 | Yeh-tzŭ-hua (Pao-chin) | 葉子花(寶巾) | **Bougainvillea glabra** | BOUGAINVILLEA | Flos Bougainvilleae |
| 2142 | Yeh-tzŭ-p'i | 椰子皮 | **Cocos nucifera** | COCONUT (root) | Radix Cocoris |
| | Yeh-tzŭ-k'o | 椰子殻 | ,,      ,, | ,,      (husk) | Pericarpium   ,, |
| | Yeh-tzŭ-yu | 椰子油 | ,,      ,, | ,,      (oil) | Oleum       ,, |
| | Yeh-tzŭ-chiang | 椰子漿 | ,,      ,, | ,,      (milk) | Endospermum ,, |
| | Yeh-tzŭ-jang | 椰子瓤 | ,,      ,, | ,,      (copra) | Endospermum ,, |
| 2143 | Yeh-tz'ŭ-ku (Shui-tz'ŭ-ku) | 野慈菇(水慈菇) | **Sagittaria sagittifolia (S. trifolia var. angustifolia)** | ARROWHEAD | Herba Sagittariae |
| 2144 | Yeh-wu-t'ung | 野梧桐 | **Mallotus japonicus** | *MALLOTUS | Cortex Malloti Japonici |
| 2145 | Yeh-ya-ch'ung (Yeh-ya-ch'ung-tzŭ, Yeh-ya-ch'ung-hua, Yeh-ya-ch'ung-kên) | 野鴉椿(野鴉椿子, 野鴉椿花, 野鴉椿根) | **Euscaphis japonica** | *EUSCAPHIS | Radix, Flos et Semen Euscaphis |
| 2146 | Yeh-yang-shên | 野洋参 | **Primula sinodenticulata** | PRIMROSE | Herba Primulae |
| 2147 | Yeh-yang-yen-kên (Shan-k'u-ts'ai) | 野洋烟根(山苦荬) | **Lactuca elata (L. raddeana)** | *WILD LETTUCE | Radix Lactucae Elata |
| 2148 | Yeh-yen | 野烟 | **Lobelia seguinii** | *SEGUIN'S LOBELIA | Radix et Folium Lobeliae Seguinii |
| 2149 | Yeh-yen-yeh | 野烟葉 | **Solanum verbascifolium** | TOBACCO NIGHT-SHADE | Folium Solani Verbascifolii |
| 2150 | Yeh-ying-su | 野罌粟 | **Papaver nudicaule** | WILD POPPY | Herba et Fructus Papaveris Nudicaulis |

| | Transliteration | Chinese | Botanical Name | English | Pharmaceutical |
|---|---|---|---|---|---|
| 2151 | Yeh-ying-t'ao | 野櫻桃 | **Prunus discadenia** | *WILD CHERRY | Fructus et Semen Pruni Discadeniae |
| | Yeh-ying-t'ao-kên | 野櫻桃根 | ,,　　,, | ,,　　,, (root) | Radix Pruni Discadeniae |
| 2152 | Yeh-yu-ma | 野油麻 | **Stachys oblongifolia** | *CHINESE HEDGE NETTLE | Herba et Radix Stachydis Oblongifoliae |
| 2153 | Yeh-yü-yeh | 野芋葉 | **Colocasia antiquorum** | WILD TARO | Folium Colocasiae |
| | Yeh-yü-kên | 野芋根 | ,,　　,, | ,,　　,, (root) | Caudex ,, |
| | Yeh-yü-shih | 野芋實 | ,,　　,, | ,,　　,, (fruit) | Fructus ,, |
| 2154 | Yeh-yüan-sui | 野芫荽 | **Eryngium foetidum** | ERYNGO | Herba Eryngii |
| 2155 | Yen-chiao | 烟膠 | — | Solidified oily mass from tannery smoke | Massa Oleosa Fumi Coriarii |
| 2156 | Yen-ching-shê | 眼鏡蛇 | — | Cobra | Naja Naja |
| −a | Yen-ching-shê-shên-ching-tu | 眼鏡蛇神經毒 | — | Cobra neurotoxin | Cobratoxin |
| 2157 | Yen-chou-chuan-pai | 兗州卷柏 | **Selaginella involvens** | SPIKEMOSS | Herba Selaginellae |
| 2158 | Yen-fu-mu | 鹽麩木 | **Rhus chinensis** | CHINESE SUMAC | See following |
| | Yen-fu-mu-hua | 鹽麩木花 | ,,　　,, | ,,　　,, (flower) | Flos Rhi Chinensis |
| | Yen-fu-tzŭ-kên | 鹽麩子根 | ,,　　,, | ,,　　,, (root) | Radix ,,　　,, |
| | Yen-fu-kên-pai-p'i | 鹽麩根白皮 | ,,　　,, | ,,　　,, (root-bark) | Cortex Radicis Rhi Chinensis |
| | Yen-fu-tzŭ | 鹽麩子 | ,,　　,, | ,,　　,, (fruit) | Fructus Rhi Chinensis |
| | Yen-fu-shu-pai-p'i | 鹽麩樹白皮 | ,,　　,, | ,,　　,, (bark) | Cortex ,,　　,, |
| | Yen-fu-yeh | 鹽麩葉 | ,,　　,, | ,,　　,, (leaf) | Folium ,,　　,, |

| Transliteration | Chinese | Botanical Name | English | Pharmaceutical |
|---|---|---|---|---|
| 2159 Yen-hu-suo (Yen-hu, Yüan-hu) | 延胡索 (延胡，芫胡) | Corydalis yanhusuo C. ambigua C. remota, C. hamosa | CORYDALIS (tuber) | Tuber Corydalis |
| 2160 Yen-k'o-t'u | 燕巢土 | — | SWALLOW nest mud | Lutum Nidi Hirundinis |
| 2161 Yen-kuo-ts'ao | 烟鍋草 | Thalictrum thunbergii | MEADOW-RUE | Caudex Thalictri Thunbergii |
| 2162 Yen-mai-ling | 燕麥靈 | Ainsliaea yunnanensis | *YUNNAN AINSLIAEA | Herba Ainsliaeae Yunnanensis |
| 2163 Yen-mai-ts'ao | 燕麥草 | Avena fatua | WILD OAT | Herba Avenae Fatuae |
| 2163A Yen-pai-ts'ai | 岩白菜 | Bergenia crassifolia B. purpurascens | *BERGENIA | Herba Bergeniae |
| 2164 Yen-shê (Lei-kung-shê) | 鹽蛇(雷公蛇) | — | *Tree lizard | Japalura |
| 2165 Yen-tan-shui (Lu-shui) | 鹽膽水(鹵水) | — | *Residual brine | *Lushui |
| 2166 Yen-t'ang | 鹽湯 | — | *Salty tea | *Yentang |
| 2167 Yen-ts'ao (Yen-yeh) | 烟草(菸葉) | Nicotiana tabacum | TOBACCO | Folium Nicotianae |
| 2168 Yen-tzǔ-ts'ai (Shui-huang-lien) | 眼子菜(水黃連) | Potamogeton franchetii P. cristatus | PONDWEED | Herba Potamogetonis |
| 2169 Yen-wo | 燕窩 | — | Sea Swallow nest | Secretio Collocaliae |
| 2170 Yen-yu (Yen-kau) | 烟油(烟膏) | — | Deposit in tobacco pipe | *Yenyu |
| 2171 Yin-ch'ai-hu (Yin-ch'ai, Yin-hu) | 銀柴胡(銀柴，銀胡) | Stellaria dichotoma var. lanceolata | *STELLARIA | Radix Stellariae Dichotomatis |
| —a Shan-yin-ch'ai-hu | 山銀柴胡 | Arenaria juncea Gypsophila oldhamiana Silene jenisseensis | *WILD YINCHAIHU | Radix Arenasiae Radix Gypsophilae Radix Silenes |

| Transliteration | Chinese | Botanical Name | English | Pharmaceutical |
|---|---|---|---|---|
| 2172 Yin-ch'ên-hao (Mien-yin-ch'ên, Yin-ch'ên) | 茵陳蒿(綿茵陳,茵陳) | **Artemisia capillaris** | *CAPILLARY ARTEMISIA | Herba Artemisiae Capillaris |
| 2173 Yin-ching-shih (Yin-mêng-shih) | 銀精石(銀礞石) | — | Silvery colored Mica schist | *Yinchingshih |
| 2174 Yin-chu (Ling-sha) | 銀硃(靈砂) | — | Vermilion (Artificial cinnabar) | *Yinchu |
| 2175 Yin-êrh (Pai-mu-êrh) | 銀耳(白木耳) | **Tremella fuciformis** | SILVER EAR | Fructificatio Tremellae |
| 2176 Yin-hsiang | 陰香 | **Cinnamomum burmannii** | CINNAMON TREE | |
| Yin-hsiang-kên | 陰香根 | ,, ,, | ,, ,, (root) | Radix Cinnamomi Burmanni |
| Yin-hsiang-p'i | 陰香皮 | ,, ,, | ,, ,, (bark) | Cortex ,, ,, |
| Yin-hsiang-yeh | 陰香葉 | ,, ,, | ,, ,, (leaf) | Folium ,, ,, |
| 2177 Yin-hsien-ts'ao | 銀綫草 | **Chloranthus japonicus** | *CHLORANTHUS | Herba Cloranthi Japonici |
| 2178 Yin-hsing-ts'ao | 陰行草 | **Siphonostegia chinensis** | *SIPHONOSTEGIA | Herba Siphonostegiae |
| 2179 Yin-hua-tzǔ | 銀花子 | **Lonicera japonica** | HONEYSUCKLE | Fructus Lonicerae Japonicae |
| 2180 Yin-kou | 陰蠅 | — | *Hooked-jaw Turtle | Platysternon |
| 2181 Yin-lao-mei | 銀老梅 | **Dasiphora davurica** | *DASIPHORA | Ramus, Folium et Flos Dasiphorae |

179

| | Transliteration | Chinese | Botanical Name | English | Pharmaceutical |
|---|---|---|---|---|---|
| 2182 | Yin-pien-tan | 銀扁擔 | **Aquilegia incurvata** | *INCURVED COLUMBINE | Caudex Aquilegiae Incurvatae |
| 2183 | Yin-po (Tzŭ-jan-yin) | 銀箔(自然銀) | — | Native silver | Argentum |
| 2184 | Yin-pu-huan | 銀不換 | **Cyclea barbata** | *BARBATE CYCLEA | Radix et Ramus Cycleae Barbatae |
| 2185 | Yin-so-shih (Pai-chieh, Hei-p'i-shê) | 銀鎖匙(百解,黑皮蛇) | **Cyclea hypoglauca** | *CYCLEA | Radix et Folium Cycleae Hypoglaucae |
| 2186 | Yin-ti-chüeh (I-tuo-yün) | 陰地蕨(一朵雲) | **Botrychium ternatum** | MOONWORT | Herba Botrychii Ternati |
| 2187 | Yin-yang-huo (Yin-yang-hua) | 淫羊霍(銀羊花) | **Epimedium** spp. | *EPIMEDIUM | Herba Epimedii |
| | | | **E. grandiflorum** | ,, | ,,   ,, |
| –a | Chien-yeh-yin-yang-huo | 箭葉淫羊霍 | **E. sagittatum** | ,, | ,,   ,, |
| –b | Hsing-yeh-yin-yang-huo | 心葉淫羊霍 | **E. brevicornum** | ,, | ,,   ,, |
| –c | Ch'ien-yeh-yin-yang-huo | 尖葉淫羊霍 | **E. acuminatum** | ,, | ,,   ,, |
| 2188 | Yin-yü | 茵芋 | **Skimmia reevesiana** | *SKIMMIA | Ramus et Folium Skimmiae |
| 2189 | Yin-yü | 銀魚 | — | Glassfish | Hemisalanx |
| 2190 | Ying (Huang-niao) | 鶯(黃鳥) | — | Oriole | Oriolus |
| 2191 | Ying-ê (Ying-ê-li) | 櫻額(櫻額梨) | **Prunus padus** | BIRD CHERRY | Fructus Pruni Padi |

| | Transliteration | Chinese | Botanical Name | English | Pharmaceutical |
|---|---|---|---|---|---|
| 2192 | Ying-ku | 鷹骨 | — | Eagle bone | Ossis Accipiteris |
| | Ying-t'ou | 鷹頭 | — | Eagle head | Caput ,, |
| | Ying-tsui-chao | 鷹嘴爪 | — | Eagle beak and claw | Rostrum et Ungula Accipiteris |
| | Ying-yen-ching | 鷹眼睛 | — | Eagle eyes | Pupula Accipiteris |
| 2193 | Ying-pu-po (Ying-pu-fu) | 鷹不泊(鷹不伏) | **Zanthoxylum avicennae** | PRICKLY ASH | Radix Zanthoxyli Avicennae |
| 2194 | Ying-pu-po-yuan | 鷹不泊蓮 | ,, ,, | PRICKLY ASH (tender shoot) | Ramus Immaturus Zanthoxyli Avicennae |
| 2195 | Ying-pu-p'u (Lui-kung-mu) | 鷹不撲(雷公木) | **Aralia armata** | HERCULES'-CLUB | Cortex et Ramus Araliae Armatae |
| 2196 | Ying-su | 罌粟 | **Papaver somniferum** | OPIUM POPPY (seed) | Semen Papaveris Somniferi |
| | Ying-su-k'o | 罌粟殼 | ,, ,, | POPPY CAPSULE | Pericarpium Papaveris Somniferi |
| | Ying-su-nun-miao | 罌粟嫩苗 | ,, ,, | YOUNG POPPY PLANT | Planta Immatura Papaveris Somniferi |
| 2197 | Ying-t'ao | 櫻桃 | **Prunus pseudocerasus** | CHERRY | Fructus Pruni Pseudocerasi |
| | Ying-t'ao-shui | 櫻桃水 | ,, ,, | ,, (juice) | Succus ,, ,, |
| | Ying-t'ao-kên | 櫻桃根 | ,, ,, | ,, (root) | Radix ,, ,, |
| | Ying-t'ao-chih | 櫻桃枝 | ,, ,, | ,, (branch) | Ramus ,, ,, |
| | Ying-t'ao-yeh | 櫻桃葉 | ,, ,, | ,, (leaf) | Folium ,, ,, |
| | Ying-t'ao-hêh | 櫻桃核 | ,, ,, | ,, (seed) | Semen ,, ,, |

| | | | | | |
|---|---|---|---|---|---|
| 2198 Ying-ts'ao-kên | 櫻草根 | **Primula patens** | PRIMROSE | Caudex Primulae Patentis | |
| 2199 Ying-yü (Shan-p'u-t'ao) | 蘡薁(山葡萄) | **Vitis thunbergii** | WILD GRAPE | Radix Vitis Thunbergii | |
| 2200 Yu (Lan-hsiang-ts'ao) | 蕕(藍香草) | **Caryopteris incana** | *CARYOPTERIS | Herba Caryopteridis | |
| 2201 Yu (Wên-tan) | 柚(文旦) | **Citrus grandis** | POMELO | Fructus Citri Grandis | |
| Yu-hêh | 柚核 | ,,     ,, | ,,     (seed) | Semen   ,,     ,, | |
| Yu-hua | 柚花 | ,,     ,, | ,,     (flower) | Flos     ,,     ,, | |
| Yu-p'i | 柚皮 | ,,     ,, | ,,     (peel) | Pericarpium ,,  ,, | |
| Yu-yeh | 柚葉 | ,,     ,, | ,,     (leaf) | Folium     ,,     ,, | |
| 2202 Yu-hu-t'ao | 油胡桃 | **Juglans regia** | WALNUT | Semen Juglandis Regiae | |
| 2203 Yu-kan-tzŭ | 油柑子 | **Phyllanthus emblica** | MYROBALAN | Fructus Phyllanthi Emblicae | |
| Yu-kan-tzŭ-kên | 柚柑子根 | ,,     ,, | ,,     (root) | Radix   ,,     ,, | |
| Yu-kan-tzŭ-yeh | 柚柑子葉 | ,,     ,, | ,,     (left) | Folium   ,,     ,, | |
| Yu-kan-chung-chieh | 柚柑虫節 | ,,     ,, | ,,     (insect gall) | Galla   ,,     ,, | |
| 2204 Yu-shu-chi-shêng (Yu-chi-shêng) | 柚樹寄生(柚寄生) | **Viscum orientale** | ORIENTAL MISTLETOE | Ramus et Folium Visci Orientalis | |
| 2205 Yu-sung-chieh | 油松節 | **Pinus tabulaeformis P. massoniana** | PINE (knotty wood) | Lignum Pini Nodi Tumorisati | |
| 2206 Yu-ts'ai-tzŭ-yu (Ts'ai-tzŭ-yu) | 油菜子油(菜子油) | **Brassica campestris var. oleifera** | RAPESEED (oil) | Oleum Brassicae | |
| 2207 Yu-ts'ao (Niu-ts'ao) | 游草(牛草) | **Leersia hexandra** | SWAMP RICE GRASS | Herba Leersiae | |

| Transliteration | Chinese | Botanical Name | English | Pharmaceutical |
|---|---|---|---|---|
| 2208 Yu-ts'ao (Ch'ien-chin-tzǔ) | 油草(千金子) | **Leptochloa chinensis** | *LEPTOCHLOA (Field grass) | Herba Leptochloae |
| 2209 Yu-t'ung | 油桐 | **Aleurites fordii** | TUNG-OIL TREE | |
| Yu-t'ung-kên | 油桐根 | ,, ,, | ,, ,, (root) | Radix Aleurititis |
| Yu-t'ung-tzǔ | 油桐子 | ,, ,, | ,, ,, (seed) | Semen ,, |
| Yu-t'ung-yeh | 油桐葉 | ,, ,, | ,, ,, (leaf) | Folium ,, |
| Yu-t'ung-mu-p'i | 油桐木皮 | ,, ,, | ,, ,, (bark) | Cortex ,, |
| 2210 Yu-yü (Ch'üan-shui-yü) | 油魚(泉水魚) | — | Spring Fish | Pseudogyrinocheilus |
| 2211 Yü-chien (Kuei-yü-chien) | 羽箭(鬼羽箭) | **Buchnera cruciata** | *BUCHNERA | Herba Buchnerae |
| 2212 Yü-chih-tzǔ | 預知子 | **Akebia quinata** **A. trifoliata** | AKEBIA (seed) | Semen Akebiae |
| 2213 Yü-chin | 郁金(鬱金,玉金) | **Curcuma aromatica** | TURMERIC | Tuber Curcumae Aromaticae |
| —a Wên-yü-chin | 溫郁金 | C. 'Wenyujin' | — | |
| 2214 Yü-chin-hsiang | 鬱金香 | **Tulipa gesneriana** | TULIP | Flos et Folium Tulipae Gesnerianae |
| 2215 Yü-chu | 玉竹 | **Polygonatum odoratum** **P. macropodium** **P. involucratum** **P. inflatum** | SOLOMON'S SEAL | Rhizoma Polygonati |
| 2216 Yü-fu-jung | 玉芙蓉 | **Opuntia dillenii** | CACTUS (dried sap) | Succus Desiccatus Cacti |
| 2217 Yü-hsieh (Pai-yü-hsieh) | 玉屑(白玉屑) | — | Nepherite grains | Nepheritum |

| | Transliteration | Chinese | Chinese | English | Pharmaceutical |
|---|---|---|---|---|---|
| 2218 | Yü-hsing-ts'ao | 魚腥草 | **Houttuynia cordata** | *FISHWORT | Herba Houttuyniae |
| 2219 | Yü-jou (Shan-yü-jou) | 萸肉(山萸肉) | **Cornus officinalis** | ASIATIC CORNEL | Mesocarpium Corni Officinalis |
| 2220 | Yü-kan-tzǔ | 餘甘子 | **Phyllanthus emblica** | MYROBALAN | Fructus Phyllanthi Emblicae |
| 2221 | Yü-kua (Mu-kua) | 玉瓜(木瓜) | **Chaenomeles cathayensis (C. sinensis)** | *SUPERIOR MUKUA | Fructus Chaenomelis |
| 2222 | Yü-lan-hua | 玉蘭花 | **Magnolia denudata** | MAGNOLIA (flower) | Flos Magnoliae |
| 2223 | Yü-li-jên | 郁李仁 | **Prunus japonica P. humilis** | PLUM (seed) | Semen Pruni Japonicae et Humilis |
| 2224 | Yü-li-kên | 郁李根 | **Prunus japonica** | PLUM (root) | Radix Pruni Japonicae |
| 2225 | Yü-liang-shih (Yü-liang-shih, Ju-liang-shih, Yü-liang) | 禹粮石(餘粮石, 乳粮石, 于良) | **—** | Limonite (Clay Ironstone) | Limonitum |
| 2226 | Yü-lung-pien (Chia-ma-pien) | 玉龍鞭(假馬鞭) | **Stachytarpheta jamaicensis** | JAMAICA VERVAIN | Herba Stachytarphetae |
| 2227 | Yü-mei (Yü-shu-shu) | 玉米(玉蜀黍) | **Zea mays** | CORN (MAIZE) | See the following |
| | Yü-mei-hsü | 玉米鬚 | „ „ | „ (silk) | Stylus Zeae |
| | Yü-mei-ch'u | 玉米軸 | „ „ | „ (cob) | Rhachis „ |
| 2228 | Yü-mo | 榆蘑 | **Pleurotus citrinopileatus** | MUSHROOM (on elm stump) | Fructificatio Meuroti |
| 2229 | Yü-pai (Wan-nien-sung) | 玉柏(萬年松) | **Lycopodium obscurum** | *OBSCURE CLUB-MOSS | Herba Lycopodii Obscuri |

| Transliteration | Chinese | Botanical Name | English | Pharmaceutical | Yü-p |
|---|---|---|---|---|---|
| 2230 Yü-pai-fu | 禹白附 | **Typhonium giganteum** | GIANT TYPONIUM | Rhizoma Typhonii Gigantei | |
| 2231 Yü-p'iao (Yü-tu) | 魚鰾(魚肚) | — | Fish swim bladder | Colla Piscis, Ichthyocolla | |
| 2232 Yü-san-hu-kên | 玉珊瑚根 | **Solanum pseudo-capsicum** | JERUSALEM-CHERRY | Radix Solani Pseudocapsici | |
| 2233 Yü-shou-shih | 魚首石 | — | Auricular bones in fish head | *Os Auriculae Piscis | |
| 2234 Yü-shu | 於朮 | See Pai-shu | — | — | |
| 2235 Yü-shu | 榆樹 | **Ulmus pumila** | CHINESE ELM | See the following | |
| Yü-chia-jên | 榆荚仁 | ,,    ,, | ELM (seed) | Semen Ulmi Pumilae | |
| Yü-jên-chiang | 榆仁醬 | ,,    ,, | FERMENTED ELM (seed jam) | Savillum Seminis Ulmi Pumilae | |
| Yü-hua | 榆花 | ,,    ,, | ELM (flower) | Flos    ,,    ,, | |
| Yü-pai-p'i | 榆白皮 | ,,    ,, | ,, (white bark) | Cortex    ,,    ,, | |
| 2236 Yü-shu-shu-kên | 玉蜀黍根 | **Zea mays** | CORN (root) | Radix Zeae | |
| Yü-shu-shu-yeh | 玉蜀黍葉 | ,,    ,, | ,, (leaf) | Folium  ,, | |
| 2237 Yü-tai-kên (Yü-san-hu) | 玉帶根(玉珊瑚) | **Pedilanthus tithymaloides** | *PEDILANTHUS | Herba Pedilanthi | |
| 2238 Yü-t'êng | 魚藤 | **Derris elliptica** | FISH POISON | Radix Derritis | |
| 2239 Yü-ts'an-yeh | 玉簪葉 | **Hosta plantaginea** | PLANTAIN-LILY | Folium Hostae | |
| Yü-ts'an-hua | 玉簪花 | ,,    ,, | ,,    ,, | Flos    ,, | |
| 2240 Yü-yeh-san-ch'i | 羽葉三七 | **Panax bipinnatifidus** | CUT-LEAVED GINSENG | Rhizoma Panacis bipinnatifidi | |

| | Transliteration | Chinese | Botanical Name | English | Pharmaceutical |
|---|---|---|---|---|---|
| 2241 | Yü-yeh-ting-hsiang (Shan-chên-hsiang) | 羽葉丁香(山沉香) | **Syringa pinnatifolia** | PINNATE-LEAVED LILAC | Radix et Ramus Syringae Pinnatifoliae |
| 2242 | Yüan-chih (Yüan-chih-jou, Chih-jou, Chih-t'ung) | 遠志(遠志肉,志肉,志通) | **Polygala sibirica** **P. tenuifolia** | CHINESE SENEGA | Radix Polygalae |
| 2243 | Yüan-ching-shih (Hsüan-ching-shih) | 元精石(玄精石) | — | Selenite | Selenitum |
| 2244 | Yüan-hu (Yüan-hu-p'ien) | 元胡(元胡片) | **Corydalis yanhusuo** | CORYDALIS (tuber and slices) | Tuber Corydalis |
| 2245 | Yüan-hua (Huan-hua) | 芫花(莞花) | **Daphne genkwa** | DAPHNE | Flos Daphnes Genkwae |
| 2246 | Yüan-ming-fên (Hsüan-ming-fên) | 元明粉(玄明粉) | — | Powder of Liquorice, radish root, treated with Sodium sulphate | *Yuanmingfen |
| 2247 | Yüan-pao-ts'ao | 元寶草 | **Hypericum sampsonii** | SOUTH CHINA ST. JOHNSWORT | Herba Hyperici Sampsonii |
| 2248 | Yüan-shên (Hsüan-shên, Hsiao-yüan-shên) | 元參(玄參,小元參) | **Scrophularia ningpoensis** | FIGWORT | Radix Scrophulariae |
| 2249 | Yüan-shu | 元朮 | See Pai-shu | — | — |
| 2250 | Yüan-sui-jên (Yüan-sui-tzŭ) | 芫荽仁(芫荽子) | **Coriandrum sativum** | CORIANDER (seed) | Semen Coriandri |
| 2251 | Yüan-yang | 鴛鴦 | — | Mandarin Duck | Caro Aicis Galericulatae |

186

| Transliteration | Chinese | Botanical Name | English | Pharmaceutical |
|---|---|---|---|---|
| 2252 Yüeh-chi-hua | 月季花 | **Rosa chinensis** | CHINESE TEA ROSE | Flos Rosae Chinensis |
| Yüeh-chi-hua-kên | 月季花根 | ,,    ,, | ,,   ,,   ,,   (root) | Radix   ,,       ,, |
| Yüeh-chi-hua-yeh | 月季花葉 | ,,    ,, | ,,   ,,   ,,   (leaf) | Folium   ,,       ,, |
| 2253 Yüeh-chien-ts'ao | 月見草 | **Oenothera erythrosepala** **O. odorata** | EVENING PRIMROSE | Radix Oenotherae |
| 2254 Yüeh-kuei-tzŭ | 月桂子 | **Laurus nobilis** | LAUREL, SWEET BAY | Fructus Lauri Nobilis |
| 2255 Yüeh-sha (Wan-yüeh-sha, Ming-yüeh-sha) | 月砂(望月砂, 明月砂) | — | Rabbit's dung | Faeces Cuniculi |
| 2256 Yüeh-shih (P'êng-sha) | 月石(硼砂) | — | Borax | Borax |
| 2256A Yün-chih | 雲芝 | **Coriolus versicolor (Polystichus versicolor)** | YUNCHIH | Yunchih |
| 2257 Yün-hsiang (Pai-yün-hsiang, Ta-yün-hsiang) | 芸香(白芸香, 大芸香) | **Liquidambar formosana** | CHINESE SWEET-GUM | Resina Liquidambaris Formosananae |
| 2258 Yün-hsiang (Ch'ou-ts'ao) | 芸香(臭草) | **Ruta graveolens** | COMMON RUE | Herba Rutae graveolensis |
| 2259 Yün-hsiang-ts'ao | 雲香草 | **Cymbopogon distans** | *CHINESE CITRONELLA | Herba Cymbopogonis Distantis |
| 2260 Yün-lien | 雲連 | **Coptis chinensis** | YUNNAN GOLDEN THREAD | Rhizoma Coptidis |
| 2261 Yün-mu (Yün-mu-shih) | 雲母(雲母石) | — | Common mica | Muscovitum |
| 2262 Yün-nan-ch'ien-ts'ao | 雲南茜草 | **Rubia yunnanensis** | YUNNAN MADDER | Herba et Radix Rubiae Yunnanensis |

187

| Transliteration | Chinese | Botanical Name | English | Pharmaceutical |
|---|---|---|---|---|
| 2263 Yün-niu-hsi (T'u-niu-hsi) | 雲牛膝(土牛膝) | **Achyranthes aspera** var. **rubrafusca** | YUNNAN ACHYRANTHES | Radix Achyranthis Asperae |
| 2264 Yün-p'ien | 雲片 | **Poria cocos** | YUNNAN CHINA-ROOT | Sclerotium Poriae |
| 2265 Yün-shih-kên | 雲實根 | **Caesalpinia sepiaria** | MYSORE THORN | Radix Caesalpiniae |
| 2266 Yün-shih-chu-ch'ung | 雲實蛀虫 | — | Long-horn Beetle larva in Caesalpinia seed | Insecta Semen Casealpinine |
| 2267 Yün-t'ai (Yu-ts'ai) | 蕓苔(油菜) | **Brassica campestris** var. **oleifera** | OIL-RAPE (young shoots) | Herba Tenera Brassicae |
| 2268 Yün-t'ai-tzǔ (Yu-ts'ai-tzǔ) | 蕓苔子(油菜子) | **Brassica campestris** var. **oleifera** | OIL-RAPESEED | Semen Brassicae |
| 2269 Yün-wu-ch'i | 雲霧七 | **Delphinium giraldii** | TSINLING LARK-SPUR | Caudex Delphinii Giraldii |
| 2270 Yung-shu | 榕樹 | **Ficus microcarpa** | BANYAN TREE | See the following |
| Yung-shu-kuo | 榕樹果 | ,, ,, | ,, (fruit) | Fructus Banyan |
| Yung-shu-p'i | 榕樹皮 | ,, ,, | ,, (bark) | Caudex ,, |
| Yung-shu-yeh | 榕樹葉 | ,, ,, | ,, (leaf) | Folium ,, |
| Yung-shu-chiao-chi | 榕樹膠汁 | ,, ,, | ,, (latex) | Latex ,, |
| Yung-hsü | 榕鬚 | ,, ,, | ,, (aerial root) | Radix Aerio ,, |

# PART II

## A Systematic Arrangement

Plants, Animals, Minerals, and
Miscellaneous Preparations

# SYSTEMATIC LISTS

# PLANTS

## THALLOPHYTES

### ALGAE (Alg)

*Caloglossa leprieurii* (Mont.) J. Arg. (042)
*Codium fragile* (Sur.) Har. (1332)
*Ecklonia kurome* Okam (702c)
*Eucheuma gelatina* (Esp.) J. Ag. (1248)
*Gelidium amansii* Lamx. (238)
*Gracilaria verrucosa* (Huds.) Papenf. (103A, 811A)
*Laminaria japonica* Aresch. (388, 702)
*Nostoc commune* Vaucher (632)
*N. flagelliforme* Born. et Flah (317)
*Sargassum fusiforme* (Harv.) Setch. (390)
*S. kjellmanianum* Yendo (390)
*S. pallidum* (Turn.) C. Ag. (390)
*S. thunbergii* (Mert.) O. Ktze. (390)
*S. tortile* C. Ag. (390)
*Ulva lactuca* L. (1237)
*Undaria pinnatifida* (Harv.) Sur. (702a)

### FUNGI

#### ASCOMYCETES (A-myc)

*Claviceps purpurea* (Fr.) Tul. (846)
*Cordyceps scotianus* Olliff. (024, 1174)
*C. sinensis* (Berk.) Sacc. (311, 449, 1799)
*C. sobolifera* (Hill.) Berk. et Br. (024)
*Monascus purpureus* Went (126, 566, 1220)
*Morchella esculenta* (L.) Pers. (2059)
*Shiraia bambusicola* P. Henn. (243)

#### BASIDIOMYCETES (B-myc)

*Agaricus bisporus* (Lange) Sing. (887)
*Armillaria matsutake* Ito et Imai (1379)
*Auricularia auricula-judas* (L. ex HK.) Underw. (894A, 2256A)
*Clitocybe gigantea* (Sow. ex Franch.) Quél (722)
*Coriolus versicolor* (L. ex Fr.) Quél. (2256A)

*Ganoderma japonicum* (Fr.) Lloyd (1826)
*G. lucidum* (Leyss. ex Fr.) Karst. (745)
*Lentinus edodes* (Berk.) Sing. (453, 457)
*Pleurotus citrinopileatus* Sing. (2228)
*Polyporus mylittae* Cook et Mass. (724, 808) (*Omphalia lapidescens* Schroeter)
*P. umbellatus* (Pers.) Fr. (247) (Polystictus versicolor (L.) Fr.) = Coriolus versicolor
*Poria cocos* (Schw.) Wolf (370, 373, 2264)
*Tremella fuciformis* Berk (997, 2175)
*Tricholoma mongolicum* Imai (995)
*Umbilicaria esculenta* (Miyoshi) Minks (1239)

#### GASTEROMYCETES (G-myc)

*Calvatia gigantea* (Balsch ex Pers.) Lloyd (835b)

191

*Calvatia lilacina* (Mont. ex Berk.)
Lloyd (835c)
*Geastrum hygrometricum* Pers. (1172)
*Lasiosphaera fenzlii* Reich. (835)
*L. nipponica* (Kawam.) Y. Kobayasi
ex Asahima (835)
*Lycoperdon gemmatum* Batsch. (826)
*L. perlatum* Pers. (835a)

### LICHENS (Lich)

*Cladonia alpestris* (L.) Rabht. (1457)
*C. gracilis* (L.) Willd. (718, 1458)
*Lobaria isidiosa* Wain. (718)
*L. pulmonaria* (L.) Hoffm. var.
*meridionals* Zahlbr. (379)
*L. retigera* Trevis (718)
*Parmelia saxatilis* Ach. (1247)
*Stereocaulon paschale* Hoffm. (1231)
*Usnea diffracta* Vain. (382, 716, 1382)
*U. longissima* Ach. (1382)

## BRYOPHYTES (Bryo)

*Marchantia polymorpha* L. (1546)
*Mnium cuspidata* Hedw. (1323)
*Plagiopus oederi* (Brid.) Limpr.
(1464)

*Rhodobryum giganteum* (Schwaeger)
Par. (1465)

## PTERIDOPHYTES

### PSILOTACEAE (F1)

*Psilotum nudum* (L.) Griseb. (1272)

### LYCOPODIACEAE (F2)

*Lycopodium cernuum* L. (1108, 1219)
*L. clavatum* L. (1219, 1275)
*L. obscurum* L. (2229)
*L. pulcherrimum* Wall. (1918)

### SELAGINELLACEAE (F3)

*Selaginella doederleinii* Hieron. (1271)
*S. involvens* (Sw.) Spring. (1919,
2157)
*S. moellendorfil* Hieron. (1538)
*S. tamariscina* (Beauv.) Spring. (295,
542)
*S. uncinata* (Desv.) Spring. (1728)

### EQUISETACEAE (F5)

*Equisetum arvense* L. (1929)

*Equisetum debile* Roxb (1780)
*E. hiemale* L. (908)

### OPHIOGLOSSACEAE (F6)

*Ophioglossum thermale* Kom. (587)
*O. vulgatum* L. (587)

### BOTRYCHIACEAE (F7)

*Botrychium lanuginosum* Wall. (1740)
*B. ternatum* (Thunb.) Swartz (2186)

### HELMINTHOSTACHYACEAE (F8)

*Helminthostachys zeylanica* (L.)
Hook. (081)

### ANGIOPTERIDACEAE (F9)

*Angiopteris fokiensis* Hieron. (840)
*A. magna* Ching (840)
*A. officinalis* Ching (1641)

### OSMUNDACEAE (F10)

*Osmunda japonica* Thunb. (1825)

### LYGODIACEAE (F12)

*Lygodium japonicum* (Thunb.)
Swartz (380)

DICKSONIACEAE (F18)

*Cibotium barometz* (L.) J. Sm. (182)

LINDSAEACEAE (F20)

*Stenoloma chusana* (L.) Ching (178)

DAVALLIACEAE (F21)

*Nephrolepis cordifolia* (L.)
Presl (1249)

PTERIDACEAE (F24)

*Pteris multifida* Poir. (355)
*P. nervosa* Thunb. (1438)
*P. semipinnata* L. (1035)
*P. vittata* L. (1968)

SINOPTERIDACEAE (F25)

*Aleuritopteris argentea* (Gmel.)
Fée (1811)

ADIANTACEAE (F26)

*Adiantum capillus-veneris* L. (1567)
*A. flabellulatum* L. (1567)
*A. myriosorum* Baker (1582)
*A. pedatum* L. (1585)

ASPLENIACEAE (F30)

*Asplenium incisum* Thunb. (1540)
*A. prolongatum* Hook. (1495)
*A. trichomanes* L. (1563)

THELYPTERIDACEAE (F31)

*Abacopteris multilineata* (Wall.)
Ching (1564)
*A. penangiana* (Hook.) Ching (1547)

BLECHNACEAE (F32)

*Blechnum orientale* L. (403)
*Woodwardia japonica* (L. f.) Sm.
(639)
*W. unigemmata* (Makino) Nakai
(639)

WOODSIACEAE (F34)

*Woodsia polystichoides* Eaton (1964)

DRYOPTERIDACEAE (F37)

*Cyrtomium fortunei* J. Sm. (673)
*Dryopteris crassirhizoma* Nakai
(673, 1805)

DIPTERIDACEAE (F41)

*Humata tyermannii* Moore (1711)

POLYPODIACEAE (F42)

*Drymotaenium miyoshianum*
(Makino) Makino (1352)
*Drynaria fortunei* (Kze.) J. Sm. (657,
885, 1105, 1218, 1376)
*Lepisorus eilophyllus* (Diels) Ching
(1232)
*L. thunbergianus* (Kaulf.) Ching
(1914)
*Polypodium nipponicum* Mett. (1322)
*Pyrrosia davidii* (Gies) Ching (1281)
*P. lingua* (Thunb.) Farw. (1281)
*P. sheareri* (Baker) Ching (1281)
*Saxiglossum angustissimum* (Gies)
Ching (1681)

MARSILEACEAE (F48)

*Marsilea quadrifolia* L. (1095)

SALVINIACEAE (F49)

*Salvinia natans* (L.) All. (1966)

# SPERMATOPHYTES

## CYCADACEAE 1

*Cycas revoluta* Thunb. (354, 1584)

## GINKGOACEAE 4

*Ginkgo biloba* L. (985)

## TAXACEAE 5

*Taxus cuspidata* Sieb. et Zucc. (1854)
*Torreya grandis* Fort. (330, 454)

## CEPHALOTAXACEAE 5b

*Cephalotaxus fortunei* Hook. f.
　(1767)
*C. sinensis* (Rehd. et Wils.)
　Li (1767)

## PINACEAE 6

*Pinus armandii* Franch. (1378c)
*P. koraiensis* Sieb. et Zucc. (1378b)
*P. massoniana* Lamb. (844, 1378a,
　2205)
*P. tabulaeformis* Carr. (1378a, 2205)

*Pseudolarix amabilis* (Nelson) **Rehd.**
　(166, 1762)

## TAXODIACEAE 6a

*Cunninghamia lanceolata* (Lamb.)
　Hook (1129)
*Glyptostrobus pensilis* (Lamb.) K.
　Koch (1333)

## CUPRESSACEAE 6c

*Juniperus formosana* Hayata (1196)
*J. rigida* Sieb. et Zucc. (1750)
*Thuja orientalis* L. (982, 1019, 1085,
　1722) (*Biota orientalis* (L.) Endl.)

## EPHEDRACEAE 7

*Ephedra equisetina* Bunge (828)
*E. sinica* Stapf (828)

## GNETACEAE 7a

*Gnetum parvifolium* (Warb.) C. Y.
　Cheng (476)

## TYPHACEAE 8

*Typha angustata* Bory et Chaub.
　(462)

*Typha angustifolia* L. (462, 1110)
*T. latifolia* L. (462)
*T. orientalis* Presl (1110)

## PANDANACEAE 9

*Pandanus tectorius* Soland. (795,
　799)

## SPARGANIACEAE 10

*Sparganium simplex* Huds. (1127)
*S. stenophyllum* Maxim. (1127)
*S. stoloniferum* Buch.-Ham. ex Royle
　(1127)

## POTAMOGETONACEAE 11

*Potamogeton cristatus* Regel et Maack
　(2168)
*P. franchetii* A. Bennett (2168)
*P. natans* L. (1293)
*P. perfoliatus* L. (1372)

## ALISMATACEAE 15

*Alisma canaliculatum* A. Br. et
　Bouche (1389)
*A. plantago-aquatica* L. (041, 129,
　277, 1719)

*Sagittaria sagittifolia* L. (2143)
  (*S. trifolia* L. var. *angustifolia*
  (Sieb.) Kitag.)

## GRAMINEAE 19

*Achnatherum inebrians* (Hance)
  Keng (2063)
*Apluda mutica* L. (1295)
*Avena fatua* L. (2110, 2163)
*Bambusa sinospinosa* McClure
  (1878)
*B. textilis* McClure (244, 1600)
*Coix lacryma-jobi* L. (589)
*Cymbopogon citratus* (DC.) Stapf
  (458)
*C. distans* (Nees) W. Wats. (2259)
*C. goeringii* (Steud.) A. Camus
  (2088)
*Cynodon dactylon* (L.) Pers. (1570)
*Heteropogon contortus* (L.) Beauv.
  (1513)
*Hordeum vulgare* L. (592, 849, 850,
  1415)
*Imperata cylindrica* (L.) Beauv.
  (860, 992)
*Leersia hexandra* Swartz (2207)
*Leptochloa chinensis* (L.) Nees
  (2208)

*Lophatherum gracile* Brongn. (1467)
*Oryza glutinosa* Lour. (941)
*O. sativa* L. (487, 566, 628, 659)
*Phragmites communis* Trin. (788)
  (*P. australis* (Cav.) Trin.)
*P. karka* (Retz.) Trin. (788)
*Phyllostachys nigra* (Lodd.) Munro
  (244, 245, 246, 779, 1466, 1600,
  1839)
*P. reticulata* (Rupr.) K. Koch (244,
  1600)
*Pleioblastus amarus* (Keng) Keng
  (661)
*Pogonatherum paniceum* (Lam.)
  Hack. (174)
*Saccharum officinarum* L. (1012A,
  1094A)
*Saccharum sinense* Roxb. (609)
*Setaria italica* (L.) Beauv. (471)
*Sorghum bicolor* (L.) Moench. (592,
  624)
  (*S. vulgare* Pers.)
*Triticum aestivum* L. (364, 849)
*Zea mays* L. (2227, 2236)
*Zizania caduciflora* (Turcz. ex Trin.)
  Hand.-Mazz. (112)

## CYPERACEAE 20

*Carex lanceolata* Boott (2047)

*C. siderostica* Hance (2029)
*Cyperus rotundus* L. (455)
*Eleocharis tuberosa* (Roxb.) Roemer et
  Schultes (838, 1068, 1821)
  (*Heleocharis dulcis* (Burm. f.) Trin.)
*Kyllinga brevifolia* Rottb. (1342)
*Scirpus juncoides* Roxb. (2109)
*S. lacustris* L. (1339)
*S. validus* Vahl (1339)
*S. yagara* Ohwi (201, 409)

## PALMAE 21

*Areca catechu* L. (376, 1092, 1093,
  1401, 1688)
*Cocos nucifera* L. (2142)
*Daemonorops draco* (Willd.) Blume
  (507)
*Didymospermum caudatum* (Lour.) H.
  Wendl. et Drude (2136)
*Livistona chinensis* R. Br. (1111)
*Lodoicea maldivica* (Gmelin) Pers.
  (389A)
*Phoenix dactylifera* L. (1973)
*Trachycarpus fortunei* Hook. (056,
  1729)

## ARACEAE 23

*Acorus calamus* L. (038, 958)
*A. gramineus* Soland. (1228)
*Aglaonema modestum* Schott (686)

195

*Alocasia macrorhiga* (L.) Schott (393)
*Amorphophylla rivieri* Durien (260A)
*Arisaema ambiguum* Engler (1083)
*A. amurense* Maxim. (1083, 1469, 1622g)
*A. consanguineum* Schott (913, 1083, 1469, 1622e)
*A. heterophyllum* Blume (913, 1469, 1622c)
*A. intermedium* Blume (1785)
*A. japonicum* Blume (1469, 1622d)
*A. lobatum* Engler (1469, 1622a)
*A. peninsulae* Nakai (1469, 1622b)
*A. verrucosum* Schott (1469, 1622f)
*Caladium bicolor* (Ait) Vent. (1737)
*Colocasia esculenta* (L.) Schott (2153)
 (*C. antiquorum* Schott)
*Homalomena occulata* (Lour.) Schott (144, 927)
*Pinellia pedatisecta* Schott (242)
*P. ternata* (Thunb.) Breit. (242, 1031, 1356)
*Pistia stratiotes* L. (1402)
*Pothos chinensis* (Raf.) Merr. (1251)
*Typhonium divaricatum* (L.) Dcne. (733, 1785a)
*T. giganteum* Engler (972, 1736, 2230).

## LEMNACEAE 24

**Lemna minor** L. (365)
*Spirodela polyrrhiza* (L.) Schleid. (366, 1853)

## ERIOCAULACEAE 30

*Ericaulon buergerianum* Koern. (652)
*E. wallichianum* Mart. (652)

## COMMELINACEAE 33

*Commelina communis* L. (2009)
*Rhoeo discolor* Hance (1039)
*Tradescantia virginiana* L. (1870)

## PONTEDERIACEAE 34

*Eichhornia crassipes* (Mert.) Solms. (1311)
*Monochoria vaginalis* (Burm. f.) Presl ex Kunth (2019)

## PHILYDRACEAE 35

*Philydrum lanuginosum* Banks (1633)

## JUNCACEAE 36

*Juncus amplifolius* A. Camus (1693)

*Juncus decipiens* (Buch.) Nakai (1262, 1503)
*J. effusus* L. (1503)
*J. setchuensis* Buch. (2085)
*Luzula capitata* (Miq.) Miq. (1554)

## STEMONACEAE 37

*Stemona japonica* (Blume) Miq. (1005)
*S. sessilifolia* (Miq.) Miq. (1005)
*S. tuberosa* Lour. (1005)

## LILIACEAE 38

*Allium cepa* L. (2058)
*A. chinense* G. Don (115, 480)
 (*A. bakeri* Regel)
*A. fistulosum* L. (1731)
*A. funckiaefolium* Hand.-Mazz. (1599)
*A. nipponicum* Franch. et Sav. (1188)
*A. prattii* C. H. Wright (2137)
*A. sativum* L. (1422)
*A. tuberosum* Rottler ex Sprengel (234)
*Aloe barbadensis* Miller (785)
 (*A. vera* L.)
*A. ferox* Miller (785)

*Anemarrhena asphodeloides* Bunge (155, 251)

*Asparagus cochinchinensis* (Lour.) Merr. (870, 1618, 1634)

*A. lucidus* Lindl. (870, 1618, 1634)

*A. plumosus* Baker (1930)

*Cardiocrinum cathayanum* (Wils.) Stearn (1326)

*Chlorophytum capense* Kuntze (1559)

*C. laxum* R. Br. (1119)

*Cordyline fruticosa* (L.) A. Cheval (579, 1583)

*Crinum asiaticum* L. (1933)

*Diuranthera minor* (C. H. Wright) Hemsl. (1626)

*Fritillaria cirrhosa* D. Don (288, 1051b)

*F. delavayi* Franch. (1051e)

*F. pallidiflora* Schrenk (1051c)

*F. przewalskii* Maxim. (1051e)

*F. roylei* Hook. (1051b)

*F. taipaiensis* P. Y. Li (1459)

*F. thunbergii* Miq. (044, 460, 1051a) (*F. verticillata* var. *thunbergii* Baker)

*F. unibracteata* Hsiao et Hsia (460)

*F. ussuriensis* Maxim. (1051d)

*F. walujewii* Regel (1051c)

*Hemerocallis citrina* Baroni (551)

*H. fulva* L. (506)

*Hemerocallis lilioasphodelus* L. (551)

*H. minor* Miller (551)

*Hosta plantaginea* (Lam.) Ascherson (2239)

*H. ventricosa* (Salisb.) Stearn (1872)

*Iphigenia indica* Kunth (1709)

*Lilium brownii* F. E. Br. (973)

*L. concolor* Salisb. (973, 1190c)

*L. lancifolium* Thunb. (1190a) (*L. tigrinum* Ker.-Gawl.)

*L. pumilum* DC. (973, 1190b) (*L. tenuifolium* Fischer)

*Liriope gramifolia* (L.) Baker (848)

*Liriope spicata* Lour. (848)

*Ophiopogon japonicus* (L. f.) Ker-Gawl. (848, 1354)

*Paris chinensis* Franch. (1685)

*P. delavayi* Franch. (1685)

*P. polyphylla* Sm. (091, 1685)

*P. quadrifolia* L. (1685)

*P. tetraphylla* A. Gray (1924)

*Polygonatum cirrhifolium* (Wall.) Royle (546)

*P. inflatum* Komarov (2215)

*P. involucratum* Maxim. (2215)

*P. macropodium* Turcz. (2215)

*P. multiflorum* All. (546)

*P. odoratum* (Miller) Druce (1926, 2215)

*P. roseum* (Ledeb.) Kunth (2037)

*Polygonatum sibiricum* Redouté (546)

*P. verticillatum* (L.) All. (2037)

*Rohdea japonica* (Thunb.) Roth (1917)

*Scilla sinensis* (Lour.) Merr. (880)

*Smilax china* L. (179)

*S. ferox* Wall. ex Kunth (1901)

*S. glabra* Roxb. (1766)

*S. nana* Wang (1887)

*Tulipa edulis* (Miq.) Baker (683, 1195)

*T. gesneriana* L. (2214)

*Urginea maritima* Baker (391)

*Veratrum maackii* Regel (731)

*V. nigrum* L. (731)

## AMARYLLIDACEAE 40

*Curculigo capitulata* (Lour.) O. Ktze. (1423)

*C. orchioides* Gaertn. (486)

*Hypoxis aurea* Lour. (2067)

*Lycoris aurea* L'Hérit. (1409, 1581)

*L. radiata* (L'Hérit.) Herb. (1274)

*Narcissus tazetta* L. (1306)

## TACCACEAE 42

*Schizocapsa plantaginea* Hance (1335)

(*Tacca plantaginea* (Hance)
Drenth.)

## DIOSCOREACEAE 43

*Dioscorea bulbifera* L. (559)
*D. cirrhosa* Lour. (1289)
*D. futschauensis* Uline (1048)
*D. hispida* Dennst. (1011)
*D. opposita* Thunb. (132, 539, 1199)
  (*D. batatas* Dcne.)
*D. tokoro* Makino (1048)

## IRIDACEAE 44

*Belamcanda chinensis* (L.) DC. (1211)
*Crocus sativus* L. (319, 442, 1676)
*Iris ensata* Thunb. (831)
  (*I. pallasii* Fischer var.
  *chinensis* Koidz.)
*I. sanguinea* Hornem. (1663)

## MUSACEAE 45

*Musella lasiocarpa* (Franch.) C. Y. Wu
  Ex H. W. Li (1556)
  (*Ensete lasiocarpum* (Franch.) E. E.
  Cheesman)
*Musa basjoo* Sieb. (113)

*M. paradisiaca* L. (1388)

## ZINGIBERACEAE 46

*Alpinia galanga* (L.) Willd. (570,
  574, 650)
*A. katsumadai* Hayata (1697, 1699,
  1713)
*A. officinarum* Hance (625, 734, 1159)
*A. oxyphylla* Miq. (586)
*A. zerumbet* (Pers.) Burtt et Smith
  (1430)
*Amomum globosum* Lour. (1699)
*A. krervanh* Pierre ex Gagnep. (1015,
  1657)
*A. tsao-ko* Crevost et Lemaire (1700)
*A. villosum* Lour. (304, 1147)
*A. xanthioides* Wall. (1147)
*Caulokaempferia yunnanensis*
  (Gagnep.) R. M. Smith (105)
*Costus speciosus* (Koenig) Sm. (029)
*Curcuma aromatica* Salisb. (858, 2213)
*C. longa* L. (103)
*C. kwangsiensis* Lee et Liang (946,
  948)
*C. 'Wênyujin'* (2213A)
*C. zedoaria* (Berg.) Rosc. (925, 946,
  948, 1063, 1286a)
*Elettaria cardamomum* (L.) Maton

(475, 1015)
*Hedychium coronarium* Koenig (1758)
*H. spicatum* Buch.-Ham. ex Sm. (1701,
  1776)
*Kaempferia galanga* L. (1130, 1145,
  1184)
*Roscoea intermedia* Gagnep. (1763)
*Stahlianthus involucratus* (King ex
  Baker) Craib (105)
*Zingiber officinale* Rosc. (100, 104,
  108, 611)
*Z. zerumbet* (L.) Smith (565)

## CANNACEAE 47

*Canna indica* L. (868)

## MARANTACEAE 48

*Phrynium capitatum* Willd. (1807)

## BURMANNIACEAE 49

*Burmannia coelestis* D. Don (1544)

## ORCHIDACEAE 50

*Amitostigma gracile* (Blume) Schltr.
  (1751)

*Bletilla striata* (Thunb.) Reichb. f. (959)

*Bulbophyllum inconspicuum* Maxim. (847)

*B. radiatum* Lindl. (1280)

*Cremastra variabilis* (Blume) Nakai (1195)

*Cypripedium macranthum* Swartz (1963)

*Dendrobium aduncum* Wall. ex Lindl. (898)

*D. chrysanthum* Lindl. (898)

*D. crispulum* Kimura et Migo (1245f)

*D. hancockii* Rolfe (1245c)

*D. hercoglossum* Reichb. f. (1245g)

*D. linawianum* Reichb. f. (187)

*D. loddigesii* Rolfe (1245b)

*D. lohohense* Tang et Wang (541, 1245d)

*D. nobile* Lindl. (161, 485, 898, 1245a, 2015)

*D. officinale* Kimura et Migo (485, 1245e)

*Epipactis helleborine* (L.) Crantz (2074)

*Gastrodia elata* Blume (1617)

*Goodyera procera* (Ker-Gawl.) Hook. (1241)

*Hemipilia flabellata* Bur. et Franch. (1752)

*Liparis japonica* (Miq.) Maxim. (2043)

*Ludisia discolor* (Ker.-Gawl.) A. Rich. (1279)

*Pholidota chinensis* Lindl. (1244)

*Platanthera chlorantha* Custor ex Reichb. (1783)

*Pleione yunnanensis* (Rolfe) Rolfe (1195, 1753)

*Sarcanthus scolopendriifolius* Makino (1965)

*Spiranthes sinensis* (Pers.) Ames (1038)

### SAURURACEAE 52

*Gymnotheca involucrata* P'ei (1294)

*Houttuynia cordata* Thunb. (088, 2218)

*Saururus chinensis* (Lour.) Merr. (1131)

### PIPERACEAE 53

*Peperomia dindygulensis* Miq. (1270)

*P. reflexa* (L. f.) A. Dietr. (1659)

*Piper betle* L. (209, 721)

*Piper cubeba* L. f. (057, 1067)

*P. hainanense* Hemsl. (386)

*P. hancei* Maxim. (1166)

*P. kadsura* (Choisy) Ohwi (352, 382) (*P. futokadsura* Sieb. et Zucc.)

*P. longum* L. (1071)

*P. nigrum* L. (513)

*P. puberulum* (Benth.) Maxim. (920, 1256)

*P. sarmentosum* Roxb. (094)

*P. wallichii* (Miq.) Hand.-Mazz. (920, 1256, 1266)

*P. wallichii* var. *hupehense* (DC.) Hand.-Mazz. (1266)

### CHLORANTHACEAE 54

*Chloranthus japonicus* Sieb. (2177)

*C. serratus* (Thunb.) R. et S. (062)

*Sarcandra glabra* (Thunb.) Kakai (226)

### SALICACEAE 56

*Populus davidiana* Dode (1021)

*P. diversifolia* Schrenk (526)

*P. euphratica* Oliver (526)

*Salix babylonica* L. (753)

*S. microstachya* Turcz. (1972)

*S. purpurea* L. (1343)

199

## MYRICACEAE 57

*Myrica rubra* Sieb. et Zucc. (2048)

## JUGLANDACEAE 60

*Carya cathayensis* Sarg. (1170)
*Juglans cathayensis* Dode (2082)
*J. regia* L. (420, 2202)
*Pterocarya stenoptera* DC. (357)

## BETULACEAE 61

*Betula platyphylla* Suk. (533, 1351)
*Corylus heterophylla* Fischer et Bess.
(051)

## FAGACEAE 62

*Castanea mollissima* Blume (729)
*Lithocarpus dealbatus* Rehd. (2119)
*Quercus acutissima* Carr. (732)
*Q. infectoria* Oliver (904, 1990)
*Q. mongolica* Fischer (732)

## ULMACEAE 63

*Celtis biondii* Skan (1860)
*C. bungeana* Blume (1041)
*Ulmus macrocarpa* Hance (1957)
*U. parvifolia* Jacq. (715)
*U. pumila* L. (464, 2235)

## MORACEAE 64

*Antiaris toxicaria* (Pers.) Lesch. (130)
*Artocarpus hypargyraeus* Hance (694,
984)
(*A. nitidus* Trec.)
*Broussonetia papyrifera* (L.)
L'Héritier (256)
*Cannabis sativa* L. (582, 829, 1414)
*Cudrania cochinchinensis* (Lour.)
Kudo et Masam. (290, 1179)
*Debregeasia edulis* (Sieb. et Zucc.)
Wedd. (1804)
*Ficus carica* L. (1955)
*F. martinii* Lévl. et Vant. (352)
*F. microcarpa* L. (2270)
(*F. retusa* auct. non L.)
*F. pumila* L. (013, 693, 735, 1075)
*F. sarmentosa* Buch.-Ham. ex J. E.
Sm. (1268)
*F. simplicissima* Lour. (1940, 1974)
*F. tikoua* Bur. (1545)
*Humulus lupulus* L. var. *cordifolius*
(Miq.) Maxim. (2072)
*Humulus scandens* (Lour.) Merr. (805)
(*H. japonicus* Sieb. et Zucc.)
*Morus alba* L. (1139, 1141, 1144,
1477, 1806)

## URTICACEAE 65

*Boehmeria nivea* (L.) Gaud. (249)
*B. siamensis* Craib (2075)
*Laportea bulbifera* (Sieb. et Zucc.)
Wedd. (2106)
*Pilea fasciata* Franch. (1847)
*Pouzolzia zeylanica* Benn. (1991)

## PROTEACEAE 66

*Helicia erratica* Hook. f. (1652)

## LORANTHACEAE 67

*Loranthus pentapetalus* Roxb. (1982)
*Scurrula parasiticus* L. (1140D)
*Taxillus chinensis* (DC.) Danser (1140)
*T. sutchuensis* (Lecomte) Danser
(1140)
*Viscum articulatum* Burm. f. (338)
*V. coloratum* (Kom.) Nakai (076, 580,
752, 1140)
*V. orientale* Willd. (2204)

## SANTALACEAE 69

*Santalum album* L. (1481, 1482)

*Thesium chinensis* Turcz. (983)

### ARISTOLOCHIACEAE 74

*Aristolochia contorta* Bunge (842, 1658)

*A. debilis* Sieb. et Zucc. (219, 842, 1605, 1658)

*A. fangchi* Wu ex Chow et Hwang (324c, 681)

*A. fordiana* Hemsl. (1808)

*A. heterophylla* Hemsl. (324a, 394)

*A. mandshuriensis* Kom. (675, 909) (*Hocquartia mandshuriensis* (Kom.) Nakai)

*A. mollissima* Hance (491)

*A. tagala* Champ. et Schlecht (1808)

*A. westlandii* Hemsl. (324c, 681)

*Asarum forbesii* Maxim. (1746)

*A. gracilipes* Yang ex Liang (173)

*A. heterotropoides* F. Schmidt (431)

*A. insigne* Diels (173)

*A. longepedunculatum* O. C. Schmidt (173)

*A. sagittarioides* C. F. Liang (1195)

*A. sieboldii* Miq. (1049)

### POLYGONACEAE 77

*Antenoron neofiliforme* (Nakai) Hara (177)

*Calligonum mongolicum* Turcz. (1148)

*Fagopyrum cymosum* Meissner (1596)

*F. esculentum* Moench (116)

*Oxyria digyna* (L.) Hill (1366)

*Polygonum amplexicaule* D. Don (117)

*P. aviculare* L. (1084)

*P. bistorta* L. (267, 1692, 1856)

*P. chinense* L. (584)

*P. cuspidatum* Sieb. et Zucc. (512, 1032)

*P. divaricatum* L. (1371)

*P. hypdropiper* L. (740, 1319)

*P. japonicum* Meissner (1671)

*P. lapathifolium* L. (1314)

*P. lapidosum* Kitagawa (1692)

*P. multiflorum* Thunb. (040, 419, 1285, 2069)

*P. paleaceum* Wall. (1696)

*P. perfoliatum* L. (622)

*P. tinctorium* Ait. (222a)

*Rheum officinale* Baill. (1406c)

*R. palmatum* L. (1406a)

*Rheum tanguticum* Maxim. (1406b)

*Rumex acetosa* L. (1369)

*R. dentatus* L. (1790)

*R. japonicus* Houtt. (2055)

*R. madaio* Makino (1790)

*R. nepalensis* Spreng. (2055)

### CHENOPODIACEAE 78

*Beta vulgaris* L. (1630)

*Chenopodium album* L. (725)

*C. ambrosioides* L. (1761)

*C. aristatum* L. (1891)

*Echinopsilon divaricatum* Kar. et Kir. (1954)

*Kochia scoparia* (L.) Schrad. (1519)

*Salsola collina* Pall. (250, 1905)

*S. pestifera* A. Nelson (250)

*S. ruthenica* Iljin (1905)

### AMARANTACEAE 79

*Achyranthes aspera* L. (931b, 1491, 1781)

*A. aspera* var. *rubrafusca* (Wight) Hook. (2263)

*A. bidentata* Blume (931)

*A. longifolia* Makino (1781)

*Alternanthera sessilis* R. Br. (445)

*Amaranthus ascendens* Loisel (2090)
*A. spinosus* L. (1879)
*Celosia argentea* L. (215)
*C. cristata* L. (071)
*Cyathula capitata* Moq. (931a)
*C. officinalis* Kuan (276, 286)
*Gomphrena globosa* L. (141)

## NYCTAGINACEAE 80

*Bougainvillea glabra* Choisy (2141)
*Mirabilis jalapa* L. (1848)

## PHYTOLACCACEAE 83

*Phytolacca acinosa* Roxb. (1203)

## AIZOACEAE 84

*Mollugo pentaphylla* L. (1534)

## PORTULACAEAE 85

*Portulaca oleracea* L. (825)
*Talinum paniculatum* (Jacq.)
　Gaertn. (1771)

## CARYOPHYLLACEAE 87

*Arenaria juncea* Bieb. (2171)
*Dianthus chinensis* L. (266)

*Dianthus superbus* L. (266, 1235)
*Gypsophila oldhamiana* Miq. (2171a)
*G. pacifica* Kom. (2171a)
*G. paniculata* L. (2171a)
*Lychnis coronata* Thunb. (127)
*Pseudostellaria heterophylla* (Miq.)
　Pax ex Pax et Hoffm. (1463)
*Silene fortunei* Vis. (2171a)
*S. jenisseensis* Willd. (2171a)
*Stellaria alsine* Grimm. (1624)
*S. dichotoma* L. var. *lanceolata* Bunge
　(2171)
*S. saxatilis* Buch.-Ham. ex D. Don
　(1516)
*Vaccaria segetalis* (Neck.) Garcke
　(754, 1106, 1923)
　(*V. pyramidata* Medic.)

## NYMPHAEACEAE 88

*Euryale ferox* Salisb. (146)
*Nelumbo nucifera* Gaertn. (214, 417,
　744, 949)

## RANUNCLULACEAE 91

*Aconitum artemisaefolium* Bar. et Skv.
　(1716a)
*A. bullatifolium* Levl. var.
　*homotrichum* (510)

*Aconitum carmichaelii* Debx. (274,
　294, 377, 1046, 1609, 1993)
*A. chinense* Paxt. (294, 402, 687,
　1609, 1716, 1993)
*A. coreanum* (Lévl.) Rap. (676,
　972)
*A. delavayi* Franch. (1716g, 1864)
*A. flavum* Hand.-Mazz. (1577)
*A. hemsleyanum* Pritz (1716f)
*A. kusnezoffii* Reichb. (1716b)
*A. sungpanense* Hand.-Mazz. (1716c)
*A. szechenyianum* Gáy (1577)
*A. taipeicum* Hand.-Mazz. (1716e)
*A. transsectum* Diels (1716d)
*A. vilmorinianum* Komarov
*Adonis amurensis* Regel et Radde
　(375)
*Anemone altaica* C. A. Meyer (227)
*A. davidii* Franch. (1814)
*A. flaccida* F. Schmidt (1552)
*A. raddeana* Regel (739)
*A. tomentosa* (Maxim.) P'ei (1408)
*A. vitifolia* Buch.-Ham. ex DC. (2111)
*Aquilegia ecalcarata* Maxim. (2070)
*A. incurvata* Hsiao (2182)
*Beesia calthaefolia* (Maxim.) Ulbr.
　(1645)
*Caltha palustris* L. (841)

*Cimicifuga acerina* (Sieb. et Zucc.)
Tanaka (1128)
*C. dahurica* (Turcz.) Maxim. (1223)
*C. foetida* L. (1223)
*C. heracleifolia* Kom. (1223)
*C. simplex* Wormsk. (2126)
*Clematis armandii* Franch. (472)
*C. chinensis* Osbeck (737, 1927)
*C. florida* Thunb. (1568)
*C. montana* Buch.-Ham. ex D. Don
(532)
*C. paniculata* Thunb. (1565)
*Coptis chinensis* Franch. (073, 283,
553, 1702, 2260)
*C. deltodes* C. Y. Cheng (553b)
*C. teetoides* C. Y. Cheng (553a)
*Delphinium giraldii* Diels (2269)
*Dichocarpum fargesii* (Franch.) Wang
et Hsiao (2094)
*Helleborus thibetanus* Franch. (1572)
*Paeonia lactiflora* Pall. (159, 202, 863,
1007, 1099, 1204)
*P. obovata* Maxim. (159, 202)
*P. suffruticosa* Andr. (525, 893, 954,
1470, 1474)
*P. veitchii* Lynch (159, 202)
*Pulsatilla chinensis* (Bunge) Regel
(1016)
*Ranunculus sceleratus* L. (1263)

*R. sieboldii* Miq. (2012)
*Semiaquilegia adoxoides* (DC.) Makino
(1614)
*Thalictrum angustifolium* L. (1313)
*T. baicalense* Turcz. (843)
*T. contortum* L. (1313)
*T. delavayi* Franch. (843)
*T. faberi* Ulbr. (1443)
*T. foliolosum* DC. (843)
*T. omeiense* W. T. Wang (1496)
*T. ramosum* Boivin (1313)
*T. thunbergii* DC. (2161)
*Trollius chinensis* Bunge (181)

### LARDIZABALACEAE 92

*Akebia quinata* (Thunb.) Dcne. (382,
909, 957, 2212)
*A. trifoliata* (Thunb.) Koidz. (998,
2212)
*Sargentodoxa cuneata* (Oliver) Rehd.
(1404)
*Stauntonia hexaphylla* Dcne. (2114)

### BERBERIDACEAE 93

*Berberis anhweiensis* Ahrendt (1884)
*B. brachypoda* Maxim. (1126)
*B. gagnepainii* Schneider (1769)
*B. julianae* Schneider (1769)
*B. sargentiana* Schneider (1126)
*B. soulieana* Schneider (1883)

*Epimedium acumbinatum* Franch.
(2045, 2187c)
*E. brevicornum* Maxim. (2045, 2187b)
*E. grandiflorum* Morr. (2045, 2187)
*E. sagittatum* (Sieb. et Zucc.) Maxim.
(2045, 2187a)
*Mahonia beali* (Fort.) Carr. (1276)
*M. fortunei* (Lindl.) Fedde (1276,
1884)
*M. ganpinensis* (Lévl.) Fedde (1884)
*M. gracilipes* (Oliver) Fedde (1884)
*M. japonica* (Thunb.) DC. (1276)
*Nandina domestica* Thunb. (921, 1601)

### PODOPHYLLACEAE 93a

*Diphylleia grayi* Fr. Schmidt (1171)
*D. sinensis* Li (1171)
*Dysosma pleiantha* (Hance) Woodson
(953)
*Podophyllum hexandrum* P. emodi
Wall. var. *chinense* Sprague (691A,
1500A)

### MENISPERMACEAE 94

*Arcangelisia loureiroi* (Pierre) Diels
(656)
*Cissampelos pareira* L. (438)
*Cocculus orbiculatus* (L.) DC. (895)
*C. sarmentosus* Diels (188)
*Cyclea barbata* (Wall.) Miers (2184)

*Cyclea hypoglauca* (Schauer) Diels
(2185)
*Diploclisia glaucescens* (Blume) Diels
(1679)
*Fibraurea tinctoria* Lour. (558)
*Hypserpa nitida* Miers ex Benth.
(2093)
*Menispermum dauricum* DC. (394,
1053)
*Sinomenium acutum* (Thunb.) Rehd.
et Wils. (212, 223)
*Stephania brachyandra* Diels (1542)
*S. cepharantha* Hayata (176, 1023)
*S. delavayi* Diels (1542)
*S. hernandifolia* (Willd.) Walper
(138)
*S. japonica* (Thunb.) Miers (138)
*S. longa* Lour. (333)
*S. sinica* Diels (186)
*S. tetrandra* S. Moore (324d, 1269)
*Tinospora capillipes* Cagnep. (180)
*T. sinensis* (Lour.) Merr. (678)

## MAGNOLIACEAE 95

*Magnolia amoena* Cheng (1621)
*M. coco* (Lour.) DC. (2083)
*M. denudata* Desr. (2222)
*M. liliflora* Desr. (302, 492)

*Magnolia officinalis* Rehd. et Wils.
(275, 289, 424, 425, 426, 1037,
1101, 1109)
*Michelia alba* DC. (988)

## ILLICIACEAE 95c

*Illicium difengpi* K.I.B. et K.I.M. ex
B. N. Chang (1518)
*I. henryi* Diels (1782a)
*I. verum* Hook. f. (951)
*I. yunnanensis* Franch. (1782b)

## SCHISANDRACEAE 95d

*Kadsura coccinea* (Lem.) A. C. Sm.
(405)
*K. heteroclita* (Roxb.) Craib (1437,
1521)
*K. longipedunculata* Finet et Gagnep.
(349, 1951)
*K. peltigera* Rehd. et Wils. (200)
*Schisandra chinensis* (Turcz.) Baill.
(1057, 1998)
*S. sphenanthera* Rehd. et Wils.
(1951)

## CALYCANTHACEAE 96

*Chimonanthus praecox* (L.) Link
(710, 1573)

## ANONACEAE 98

*Desmos cochinchinensis* Lour. (273)
*Fissistigma glaucescens* (Hance) Merr.
(1961)
*Polyalthia nemoralis* A. DC. (408)

## MYRISTICACEAE 99

*Myristica fragrans* Houtt. (603, 1656)

## LAURACEAE 102

*Actinodaphne chinensis* (Blume) Nees
(022)
*Cassytha filiformis* L. (1958, 2003)
*Cinnamomum burmannii* (Nees) Blume
(2176)
*C. camphora* (L.) Presl (028, 030-035)
*C. cassia* Presl (300, 690, 696)
*C. loureiroi* Nees (602, 674, 698)
*C. obtusifolia* Nees (1446)
*C. tamala* (Ham.) Nees et Eberm.
(1137)
*C. wilsonii* Gamble (282)
*Laurus nobilis* L. (2254)
*Lindera aggregata* (Sims) Kosterm.
(2000)
*Lindera chunii* Merr. (147, 2000)
*L. glauca* (Sieb. et Zucc.) Blume
(1173)

*Lindera obtusiloba* Blume (1120)
*L. strychnifolia* (Sieb. et Zucc.)
Villar = L. aggregata
*Litsea auriculata* Chien et Cheng
(1620)
*L. cubeba* (Lour.) Pers. (1193, 1662)
*L. glutinosa* (Lour.) C. B. Rob. (025)
*L. rotundifolia Hemsl.* var. *oblongifolia*
(Nees) Allen ≡ (022)
*Machilus leptophylla* Hand.-Mazz.
(1444)
*Phoebe sheareri* (Hemsl.) Gamble
(1849)
*Sassafras tsumu* Hemsl. (337)
(*Pseudosassafras laxiflora* (Hemsl.)
Nakai)

PAPAVERACEAE 104

*Chelidonium majus* L. (970)
*Corydalis ambigua* Cham. et Schlect.
(2159)
*C. decumbens* (Thunb.) Pers. (448)
*C. edulis* Maxim. (1827, 1828)
*C. hamosa* Migo (2159)
*C. incisa* (Thunb.) Pers. (1844)
*C. linarioides* Maxim. (1820)
*C. remota* Fischer ex Maxim. (2159)
*C. stenantha* Franch. (1997)

*Corydalis yanhusuo* W. T. Wang
(2159, 2244)
*Dactylicapnos scandens* (D. Don)
Hutchins. (1830)
*Macleaya cordata* (Willd.) R. Br.
(1098)
*Meconopsis quintuplinervia* Regel
(1976)
*Papaver nudicaule* L. (2150)
*P. somniferum* L. (004, 1360, 2018,
2196)

CRUCIFERAE 105

*Brassica campestris* L. var. *oleifera*
DC. (2206, 2267, 2268)
*B. hirta Moench* (099, 964)
*B. juncea* (L.) Coss. (098)
*Capsella bursa-pastoris* (L.) Medic.
(078)
*Cardamine leucantha* (Tausch.) O.E.
Schulz (1669)
*Draba nemorosa* L. (1647)
*Erysimum cheiranthoides* L. (1486)
*Isatis tinctoria* L. and *I. indigotica*
Fortune ex Lindley (222d, 1033,
1381, 1392)
*Lepidium apetalum* Willd. (1647)
*Malcolmia africana* (L.) R. Br. (1842)

*Raphanus sativus* L. (711, 765, 1110,
1528)
*Rorippa indica* (L.) Hiern. (1612)
(*Nasturtium montanum* (L.) DC.)
*Thlaspi arvense* L. (435, 962)

CAPPARIDACEAE 107

*Capparis membranacea* Gardn. et
Champ. (1747)
*Cleome gynandra* L. (981)

NEPENTHACEAE 111

*Nepenthes mirabilis* (Lour.) Druce
(248)

DROSERACEAE 112

*Drosera burmannii* Vahl (189)
*D. spathulata* Labill. (1509)

CRASSULACEAE 115

*Bryophyllum pinnatum* (Lam.) Kurz
(768)
*Kalanchoe laciniata* (L.) Pers. (061)
*Orostachys erudescens* (Maxim.)
Ohwi (1913)
*O. fimbriatus* (Turcz.) Berger (1913)

Sedum aizoon L. (204)
S. elatinoides Franch. (2028)
S. lineare Thunb. (359)
S. sarmentosum Bunge (298, 1229)

### SAXIFRAGACEAE 117

Astilbe chinensis (Maxim.) Franch. et Sav. (761)
A. rivularis Buch.-Ham. ex D. Don (2098)
Bergenia crassifolia (L.) Fritsch. and B. purpurascens (HK. f. et Thomas) Engler (2163A)
Cardiandra moellendorffii (Hance) Li (1695)
Dichroa febrifuga Lour. (039)
Hydrangea paniculata Sieb. (1756)
H. strigosa Rehd. (1591, 1756)
H. umbellata Rehd. (1591, 1756)
Penthorum chinense Pursh (1338)
Philadelphus sericanthus Koehne (1182)
Ribes alpestre Wall. ex Dcne. (1892)
R. mandschuricum (Maxim.) Kom. (1504)
R. tenue Jancz. (1134)
Saxifraga stolonifera (L.) Meerb. (515)

### PITTOSPORACEAE 118

Pittosporum glabratum Lindl. (594, 1160)

### HAMAMELIDACEAE 123

Liquidambar formosana Hance (339, 350, 351, 963, 1027, 1450, 2257)
L. orientalis Miller (1355)
Loropetalum chinense (R. Br.) Oliver (067)

### EUCOMMIACEAE 123a

Eucommia ulmoides Oliver (1743)

### ROSACEAE 126

Agrimonia pilosa Ledeb. (484, 819)
Chaenomeles cathayensis (Hemsl.) Schneid. (880A, 901, 2221)
 (C. sinensis (Thouin) Koehne
Chamaerhodos erecta (L.) Bunge (1510)
Cotoneaster coriaceus Franch. (2100)
C. horizontalis Dcne. (1320, 1526)
Crataegus cuneata Sieb. et Zucc. (1153)
C. pinnatifida Bunge (016, 017, 1153)
Cydonia oblonga Miller (1779A, 1932A)
Dasiphora davurica (Nestl.) Kom. et Klob.-Alis (2181)
D. fruticosa (L.) Rydb. (2064)
 (Potentilla fruticosa L.)

Duchesnea indica (Andr.) Focke (1212)
Eriobotrya japonica (Thunb.) Lindl. (956, 1076)
Geum aleppicum Jacq. (1938)
 (G. strictum Soland. ex. Ait.)
G. japonicum Thunb. (1344)
Photinia serrulata Lindl. (1265)
Potentilla chinensis Ser. (1928)
P. discolor Bunge (322)
P. freyniana Bornm. (1132)
Prinsepia uniflora Batal. (607, 911, 1375)
Prunus armeniaca L. (495, 662, 1607)
P. brachypoda Batalin var. eglandulosa Cheng (1953)
P. discadenia Koehne (2151)
P. humilis Bge. (2223)
P. japonica Thunb. (727, 2223, 2224)
P. mume (Sieb.) Sieb. et Zucc. (489, 867, 993, 994, 1977)
P. padus L. (2191)
P. persica (L.) Batsch (1072, 1501)
P. pseudocerasus Lindl. (2197)
P. tomentosa Thunb. (1201)
Pyracantha fortuneana (Maxim.) Li (233)

Pyrus betulaefolia Bunge (728)
P. calleryana Decne. (2104)
P. serrulata Rehd. (728)
Rosa chinensis Jacq. (2252)
R. davurica Pall. (1897)
R. graciliflora Rehd. et Wils. (1894)
R. laevigata Michx. (192-195)
R. mutiflora Thunb. (111)
R. omeiensis Rolfe (1908)
R. roxburghii Tratt. (1893)
R. rugosa Thunb. (869)
Rubus alceaefolius Poir. (1447)
R. blinii Lévl. (1936)
R. cochinchinensis Tratt. (2002)
R. coreanus Miq. (1494)
R. delavayi Franch. (1490)
R. hirsutus Thunb. (1903)
R. pacificus Hance (1462)
R. palmatus Thunb. (372)
R. parvifolius (372, 1213)
R. pungens Camb. (1500)
R. rosaefolius Smith (1489)
R. tephrodes Hance (1975)
R. xanthocarpus Bur. et Franch. (1535)
Sanguisorba officinalis L. (1555)
Sorbus alnifolia Sieb. et Zucc. (1346)
S. tianschanica Rupr. (1625)
S. unguiculata Koehne (1732)

LEGUMINOSAE 128

Abrus cantoniensis Hance (070)
A. precatorius L. (463)
Acacia catechu (L. f.) Willd. (313)
A. farnesiana Willd. (2023)
A. senegal (L.) Willd. (003)
A. suma Kurz ex Brandis (313)
Aeschynomene indica L. (1631)
Albizzia julibrissin Durazz. (415)
Alhagi pseudalhagi Desv. (1898)
Apios fortunei Maxim. (1778)
Astragalus adsurgens Pall. (1152, 1915)
A. bhotanensis Baker (1537)
A. chinensis L. (1152, 1915)
A. complanatus R. Br. (1152, 1809, 1915)
A. floridus Bentham (543b)
A. membranaceus (Fischer) Bunge (268, 543a, 961, 1560)
A. mongholicus Bunge (268, 543b, 1045)
A. sinicus L. (1875)
A. tongolensis Ulbr. (543a)
Bauhinia championii Benth. (231, 811)
B. pernervosa L. (1442)
Caesalpinia crista L. (1888)
C. minax Hance (918, 1258)
C. pulcherrima Swartz (342)
C. sappan L. (1361)

C. sepiaria Roxb. (1493, 2265)
Campylotropis delavayi (Franch.) Schindler (1650)
Canavalia ensiformis DC. (1450)
C. gladiata (Jacq.) DC. (1450)
Caragana franchetiana Kom. (2040)
C. sinica (Buc'hoz) Rehd. (164)
Cassia acutifolia Del. (318, 483)
C. angustifolia Vahl (318, 483)
C. mimosoides L. (1187)
C. nodosa Buch.-Ham. ex Roxb. (1221)
C. nomame (Sieb.) Kitagawa (1337)
C. occidentalis L. (1921)
C. tora L. (297, 1691, 2092)
Cercis chinensis Bunge (1835)
Craspedolobium schochii Harms (1586)
Crotalaria mucronata Desv. (253)
C. sessiliflora L. (2117)
Cullen corylifolia (L.) Medicus (Psoralea corylifolia L.) (651, 658, 1103)
Dalbergia odorifera T. Chen (102)
D. parviflora Roxb. (102)
D. sissoo Roxb. (102)
D. yunnanensis Franch. (2035)
Delanda umbellata (Thunb.) S. Y. Hu (158)
Derris elliptica Benth. (2238)
Desmodium pulchellum L. (1028)

*D. racemosum* (Thunb.) DC. (1181)
*D. styracifolium* (Osbeck) Merr. (167)
*D. triquetrum* L. (519)
　(*Pteroloma triquetrum* (L.) Benth.)
*Dolichos lablab* L. (1004, 1088, 1089)
*Dunbaria villosa* (Thunb.) Makino
　(2118)
*Entada phaseoloides* (L.) Merr. (705)
*Eriosma chinense* Vogel (618)
*Erythrina indica* Lam. (392)
*E. variegata* L. var. *orientalis* (L.)
　Merr. (1910)
*Gleditsia sinensis* Lam. (114, 578,
　1683, 1684, 1686, 1902, 2022)
*Glycine max* (L.) Merr. (800, 1425,
　1651)
*G. soja* Sieb. et Zucc. (1477, 1653,
　1661, 2105, 2129)
*Glycyrrhiza uralensis* Fischer (617,
　1561)
*Gueldenstaedtia multiflora* Bunge
　(1551b)
*G. pauciflora* Fischer ex DC. (1551b)
*Gymnocladus chinensis* Baill. (331)
*Haematoxylon campechianum* L.
　(1361)
*Hedysarum polybotrys* Hand.-Mazz.
　(543c)
*Indigofera bungeana* Steud. (1580)

*I. decora* Lindl. (1817)
*I. hancockii* Craib (1682)
*I. tinctoria* L. (222c)
*Kummerowia striata* (Thunb.)
　Schindler (079)
*Lespedeza cuneata* (Dum.) G. Don
　(2101)
*L. floribunda* Bunge (1579)
*L. pilosa* (Thunb.) Sieb. et Zucc.
　(1575)
*Lotus corniculatus* L. (1553)
*Medicago falcata* L. (2113)
*Melilotus suaveolens* Ledeb. (1706)
*Millettia dielsiana* (066)
*M. lasiopetala* (Hayata) Merr. (1022,
　1754)
*M. reticulata* Benth. (066)
*M. speciosa* Champ. ex Benth. (939)
*Mimosa pudica* L. (396)
*Moghania philippinensis* (Merr. et
　Rolfe) Li (137)
*Oxytropis glabra* DC. (1726)
*Pachyrhizus erosus* (L.) Urban (1530)
*Phaseolus calcaratus* Roxb. (158, 469)
*P. mungo* L. (797, 798, 801)
*Pongamia pinnata* (L.) Merr. (1321)
*Psoralea corylifolia* L. (651, 658,
　1103)
*Pterocarpus indicus* Willd. (1859)

*Pueraria edulis* Pamp. (634)
*P. lobata* (Willd.) Ohwi (633, 635)
*Pueraria thomsonii* Benth. (334, 634)
*Robinia pseudoacacia* L. (1881)
*Shuteria pampaniniana* Hand.-Mazz.
　(1576)
*S. sinensis* Hemsl. (1810)
*Smithia sensitiva* Ait. (1603)
*Sophora flavescens* Ait (668)
*S. japonica* L. (536, 538, 540)
*S. mairei* Pamp. (1992)
*S. tonkinensis* Gagnep (1192, 1655)
*Spatholobus suberectus* Dum. (066)
*Tamarindus indica* L. (1367)
*Tephrosia purpurea* (L.) Pers. (564)
*Thermopsis lupinoides* Link (2078)
　(*T. lanceolata* R. Br.)
*Trifolium repens* L. (1122)
*Trigonella foenum-graecum* L. (520,
　790)
*Vicia faba* L. (1672)
*V. sativa* L. (1385)
*Vigna cylindrica* (L.) Skeels (1014)
*Wisteria sinensis* Sweet (1861)
*Zornia diphylla* Pers. (601, 1642, 1646)

GERANIACEAE 129

*Geranium pratense* L. (1717)

*Geranium sibiricum* L. (717)
*G. wilfordii* Maxim. (717)
*Pelargonium graveolens* (Thunb.)
 L'Hérit. (1255)

OXALIDACEAE 130

*Averrhoa carambola* L. (1125, 2053)
*Oxalis corniculata* L. (1368, 1723)
*O. corymbosa* DC. (1812)

LINACEAE 132

*Linum usitatissimum* L. (521, 1405,
 2017)

ERYTHROXYLACEAE 134

*Erythroxylon coca* Lam. (654)

ZYGOPHYLLACEAE 135

*Tribulus terrestris* L. (072, 960,
 1876)

RUTACEAE 137

*Acronychia pedunculata* (L.) Miq.
 (1202)
*Atalantia buxifolia* (Poir.) Oliver
 (1800)
*Citrus aurantium* L. (154, 1453)
*C. erythrocarpa* Tanaka (118, 260)

*Citrus grandis* (L.) Osbeck (2201)
*C. medica* (L.) Osbeck (465)
*C. medica* (L.) Osbeck var.
 *sarcodactylis* (Noot.) Swingle
 (362, 1284)
*C. nobilis* Lour. (257, 612, 614)
*C. reticulata* Blanco (053, 054,
 121, 122, 123, 262, 263, 680,
 1377)
*C. sinensis* (L.) Osbeck (221, 257,
 261, 265, 1592)
*C. wilsonii* Tanaka (154, 465)
*Clausena dentata* (Willd.) Roem.
 (2095)
*C. lansium* (Lour.) Skeels (557)
*Dictamnus dasycarpus* Turcz. (437,
 488, 976)
*Evodia lepta* (Spreng.) Merr. (1138)
*E. trichotoma* (Lour.) Pierre (1946)
*Fortunella margarita* (Lour.) Swingle
 (165, 172)
*Glycosmis parviflora* (Sims) Little
 (1167) (*G. citrifolia* Lindl.)
*Micromelum falcatum* (Lour.)
 Tanaka (996)
*Murraya paniculata* (L.) Jack (084,
 229)
*Orixa japonica* Thunb. (039)
*Phellodendron amurense* Rupr. (556)

*Poncirus trifoliata* (L.) Raf. (154,
 156, 643)
*Tetradium rutaecarpum* (Juss.) Hartley
 (1947, 2005)
*Ruta graveolens* L. (2258)
*Skimmia reevesiana* Fortune (2188)
*Toddalia asiatica* (L.) Lam. (329)
*Zanthoxylum avicennae* (Lam.) DC.
 (2193)
*Z. bungeanum* Maxim. (528)
*Z. dimorphophyllum* Hemsl. (2050)
*Z. dissitum* Hemsl (1440)
*Z. multijugum* Franch. (1967)
*Z. nitidum* (Roxb.) DC. (529, 738)
*Z. schinifolium* Sieb. et Zucc. (2027)
*Z. simulans* Hance (270, 528)
*Z. tibetanum* Huang (2091)

SIMAROUBACHEAE 138

*Ailanthus altissima* (Miller) Swingle
 (303, 346, 358, 1290)
*Brucea javanica* (L.) Merr. (2021)

BURSERACEAE 139

*Boswellia bhau-dajiana* Birdw. (605)
*B. carteri* Birdw. (605, 631)
*B. neglecta* S. Moore (605)

*Canarium album* (Lour.) Raeusch. (613)

*C. pimela* Koenig. (712, 1969)

*Commiphora myrrha* (Nees) Engler (910)

### MELIACEAE 140

*Melia azedarach* L. (667)

*M. toosendan* Sieb. et Zucc. (284)

*Munronia delavayi* Franch. (1525e)

*M. hainanensis* How et T. Chen (1525b)

*M. henryi* Harms (1525)

*M. heterotricha* H. S. Lo (1525c)

*M. hunanensis* H. S. Lo (1525d)

*M. sinica* Diels (1525a)

*Toona sinensis* (A. Juss.) Roem. (452)

(*Cedrela sinensis* A. Juss.)

### POLYGALACEAE 145

*Polygala chinensis* Lour. (1391)

*P. crotalarioides* Koenig ex DC. (530, 1522)

*P. sibirica* L. (1637, 2242)

*P. telephioides* Willd. (183)

*P. tenuifolia* Willd. (2242)

### EUPHORBIACEAE 147

*Acalypha australis* L. (508a, 1569)

*Aleurites fordii* Hemsl. (1823, 1824, 2209)

*A. moluccana* (L.) Willd. (1257)

*A. montana* (Lour.) Wilson (1824)

*Breynia fruticosa* Hook. f. (406)

*Claoxylon polot* (Burm. f.) Merr. (1648)

*Croton crassifolius* Geisel. (069)

*C. lachnocarpus* Benth. (478)

*C. tiglium* L. (107, 287, 955, 1654)

*Endospermum chinense* Benth. (1421)

*Euphorbia antiquorum* L. (585)

*E. fischeriana* Steud. (714)

*E. helioscopia* L. (1718)

*E. heterophylla* L. (2087)

*E. hirta* L. (1399)

*E. humifusa* Willd. (1515)

*E. kansui* Liou (615)

*E. lathyris* L. (139, 272, 500)

*E. milii* Ch. des Moulins (1566)

*E. pekinensis* Rupr. (203, 1386a)

*E. pilulifera* L. (332)

*E. prolifera* Buch.-Ham. ex D. Don (1774)

*E. thymifolia* L. (467)

*Glochidion eriocarpum* Champ. ex Benth. (087)

*Glochidion puberum* (L.) Hutch. (1370)

*Mallotus apelta* (Lour.) Muell.-Arg. (1003)

*M. japonicus* Muell.-Arg. (2144)

*M. nepalensis* Muell.-Arg. (1194)

*Pedilanthus tithymaloides* (L.) Poit. (2237)

*Phyllanthus emblica* L. (2203, 2220)

*P. urinaria* L. (050)

*Ricinus communis* L. (1050, 1070, 1705)

*Sapium discolor* (Champ. ex Benth.) Muell.-Arg. (576, 1197)

*S. sebiferum* (L.) Roxb. (1945)

*Sauropus spatblifolius* Beitte (815) (*S. changianus* S. Y. Hu)

*Securinega suffruticosa* (Pall.) Rehd. (2131)

*Speranskia tuberculata* (Bunge) Baill. (1665)

### DAPHNIPHYLLACEAE 147a

*Daphniphyllum calycinum* Benth. (929)

### BUXACEAE 149

*Buxus microphylla* Sieb. et Zucc. var. *sinica* Rehd. et Wils. (560)

*Pachysandra terminalis* Sieb. et Zucc. (509)
*Sarcococca ruscifolia* Stapf (2122)

## CORIARIACEAE 151

*Coriaria sinica* Maxim. (836)

## ANACARDIACEAE 153

*Choerospondias axillaris* (Roxb.) Burtt et Hill (2004)
*Cotinus coggygria* Scop. (554)
*Hovenia dulcis* Thunb. (152)
*Mangifera indica* L. (856)
*Pistacia vera* L. (1979)
*P. weinmannifolia* Poiss. (1873)
*Rhus chinensis* Miller (1054, 1983, 1984, 2158)
*R. potaninii* Maxim. (1054, 1983)
*R. sylvestris* Sieb. et Zucc. (2068)
*R. verniciflua* Stokes (083, 610)

## AQUIFOLIACEAE 157

*Ilex asprella* (Hook. et Arn.) Champ. ex Benth. (620)
*I. chinensis* Sims (1798)
*I. cornuta* Lindl. (703, 704)
*I. franchetiana* Loes. (1186)
*I. pubescens* Hook. et Arn. (865)
*I. rotunda* Thunb. (232)

## CELASTRACEAE 158

*Celastrus flagellaris* Rupr. (1900)
*C. orbiculatus* Thunb. (919)
*Euonymus alatus* (Thunb.) Sieb. (689, 700)
*E. bungeanus* Maxim. (1350)
*E. grandiflorus* Wall. (2138)
*E. wilsonii* Sprague (1889)
*Tripterygium hypoglaucum* (Lévl.) Hutch. (1832)
*T. wilfordii* Hook. f. (807)

## STAPHYLLEACEAE 161

*Euscaphis japonica* (Thunb.) Dippel (2145)

## ACERACEAE 163

*Acer sinense* Pax (1943)
*A. trifidum* Kom. (2014)
*Dobinea delavayi* (Baill.) Engler (1397)

## HIPPOCASTANACEAE 164

*Aesculus chinensis* Bunge (1628)

## SAPINDACEAE 165

*Cardiospermum halicacabum* L. (1497)

*Euphoria longan* (Lour.) Steud. (821)
*Koelreuteria paniculata* Laxm. (806)
*Litchi chinensis* Sonn. (153, 726)
*Sapindus mukorossi* Gaertn. (900, 1956)
*Xanthoceras sorbifolia* Bunge (1932)

## BALSAMINACEAE 168

*Impatiens balsamina* L. (065, 341)
*I. textori* Miq. (2079)
*I. uliginosa* Franch. (1299)

## RHAMNACEAE 169

*Berchemia hypochrysa* Schneider (1260)
*B. kulingensis* Schneider (1837)
*B. lineata* DC. (1578)
*Paliurus ramosissimus* Poir. (823, 1574)
*Ventilago leiocarpa* Benth. (208)
*Zizyphus jujuba* Miller (575, 877, 1429, 1687)
*Z. jujuba* var. *spinosa* Hu (1374)

## VITACEAE 170

*Ampelocissus artemisiaefolia* Planch. (1396)

*Ampelopsis brevipedunculata* Koehne (1214)

*A. cantoniensis* (Hook. et Arn.) Planch. (1996)

*A. japonica* (Thunb.) Makino (989)

*Cayratia japonica* (Thunb.) Gagnep. (1970)

*Cissus modeccoides* Planch. (1742)

*Parthenocissus heterophylla* (Blume) Merr. (1118)

*P. tricuspidata* (Sieb. et Zucc.) Planch. (1514)

*Tetrastigma hypoglaucum* Planch. (1935)

*T. planicaule* (Hook. f.) Gagnep. (1087)

*Vitis quinquangularis* Rehd. (1944, 2121)

*V. romanetii* Roman. (2120)

*V. thunbergii* Sieb. et Zucc. (2199)

*V. wilsonae* Veitch (2120)

### TILIACEAE 174

*Microcos paniculata* L. (1104)

*Tilia tuan* Szyszyl. (2125)

### MALVACEAE 175

*Abelmoschus moschatus* Medicus (1941) (*A. sagittifolius* (Kurz) Merr.)

*Abutilon indicum* (L.) Swartz (889)

*A. theophrastii* Medic (889)

*Althaea rosea* (L.) Cav. (1846)

*Gossypium herbaceum* L. (879)

*Hibiscus mutabilis* L. (368, 369, 896)

*H. rosa-sinensis* L. (301, 361)

*H. syriacus* L. (271, 894, 1390)

*H. trionum* L. (2084)

*Malva neglecta* Wallr. (1358)

*M. parviflora* L. (1775)

*M. verticillata* L. (701, 1803)

*Sida rhombifolia* L. (550)

*Urena procumbens* L. (644)

### BOMBACACEAE 177

*Bombax ceiba* L. (902)

### STERCULIACEAE 178

*Firmiana simplex* Wight (1995)

*Helicteres angustifolia* L. (1161)

*H. isora* L. (583)

*Pterospermum heterophyllum* Hance (1030)

*Scaphium affine* (Mast.) Pierre (1042, 1065, 1403)

### DILLENIACEAE 180

*Actinidia callosa* Lindl. (1318)

*A. chinensis* Planch. (1508)

*Saurauia tristyla* DC. (1328)

*Tetracera asiatica* (Lour.) Hoogland (444)

### THEACEAE 186

*Camellia japonica* L. (1154)

*C. oleifera* Abel (019)

*C. sinensis* (L.) O. Ktze. (018, 020, 881)

*Eurya obtusifolia* H. T. Chang (2066)

### GUTTIFERAE 187

*Calophyllum membranaceum* Gardn. et Champ. (411)

*Cratoxylon ligustrinum* (Spach.) Blume (555)

*Garcinia hanburyi* Hook f. and *G. morella* Desr. (1507)

*G. multiflora* Champ. ex Benth. (1164)

*Hypericum ascyron* L. (568)

*H. bellum* L. (1777)

*H. japonicum* Thunb. (1517, 1593)

*H. perforatum* L. (150)

*Hypericum przewalskii* Maxim. (1432)
*H. sampsonii* Hance (2247)

## DIPTEROCARPACEAE 188

*Balanocarpus heimii* King (1413)
*Dryobalanops aromatica* Gaertn. f.
  (1094)
*Hopea micrantha* Hook. f. (1413)
*Shorea hypochra* Hance (1413)
*S. robusta* Gaertn. f. (1413)
*S. wiesneri* Schiffn. (1413)

## TAMARICACEAE 191

*Myricaria germanica* (L.) Desv.
  (1325)
*Tamarix chinensis* Lour. (058, 299,
  677)

## VIOLACEAE 198

*Viola chinensis* G. Don (1551c)
*V. diffusa* Ging. (1539)
*V. grypocera* A. Gray (1524)
*V. inconspicua* Blume (1551c)
*V. patrinii* DC. (1551c)
*V. tricolor* L. (1133)
*V. vaginata* Maxim. (1986)
*V. yedoensis* Makino (1551c)

## FLACOURTIACEAE 199

*Hydnocarpus anthelmintica* Pierre Ex
  Gagnep. and H. kurzii (King) Warb.
  (1400)

## STACHYURACEAE 200

*Stachyurus himalaicus* Hook. f. et
  Thoms. (328, 1822a)

## PASSIFLORACEAE 203

*Passiflora altebilobata* Hemsl. (2056)
*P. cochinchinensis* Spreng. (1217)

## CARICACEAE 205

*Carica papaya* L. (320)

## BEGONIACEAE 208

*Begonia aptera* Blume (2081)
*B. fimbristipulata* Hance (1851)
*B. wilsonii* Gagnep. (593)

## CACTACEAE 210

*Hylocereus undatus* (Haw.) Britton et
  Rose (738A, 955B)
*Opuntia dillenii* Haw. (490, 2216)

## THYMELAEACEAE 214

*Daphne genkwa* Sieb. et Zucc. (2245)
*Stellera chamaejasme* L. (436)
*Thymus mongolicus* L. (1511)
*Thymus serpyllum* L. (1511)
*Wikstroemia chamaedaphne* Meissner
  (562)
*W. dolichantha* Diels (1759)
*W. indica* (L.) C. A. Meyer (741)

## AQUILARIACEAE 214a

*Aquilaria agallocha* Roxb. (052)
*A. sinensis* (Lour.) Gilg (1757)

## ELAEAGNACEAE 215

*Elaeagnus angustifolia* L. (1151)
*E. glabra* Thunb. (852)
*E. pungens* Thunb. (852)
*E. umbellata* Thunb. (852)
*Hippophae rhamnoides* L. (1144A)

## LYTHRACEAE 216

*Ammannia baccifera* L. (1308)
*Lagerstroemia indica* L. (1868)

## PUNICACEAE 218

*Punica granatum* L. (757, 1259, 1627)

213

## NYSSACEAE 220a

Camptotheca acuminata Dcne. (397, 439)

## ALANGIACEAE 220b

Alangium chinense (Lour.) Harms (952)

## COMBRETACEAE 221

Quisqualis indica L. (128, 1238, 1302)
Terminalia chebula Retz. (416, 421, 638, 1674)

## MYRTACEAE 222

Baeckea frutescens L. (623)
Cleistocalyx operculata (Roxb.) Merr. et Perry (1341)
Eucalyptus globulus Labill. (015)
E. robusta Sm. (1436)
Melaleuca leucadendron L. (966)
Psidium guajava L. (323)
Rhodomyrtus tomentosa (Ait.) Hassk. (621)
Syzygium aromaticum (L.) Merr. et
Perry (905, 1639, 1640) (Eugenia caryophyllata Thunb.)
S. brachyantherum Merr. et Perry (2139)
S. cuminii (L.) Skeels (2139)

## MELASTOMATACEAE 223

Melastoma candidum D. Don (2115)
M. dodecandrum Lour. (1536)
M. sanguineum Sims (861)
Osbeckia chinensis L. (1604)

## ONAGRACEAE 224

Chamaenerion angustifolium (L.) Scop. (756)
Epilobium palustre L. (1330)
Jussiaea linifolia Vahl (1704)
J. repens L. (708)
J. suffruticosa L. (1307)
Ludwigia prostrata Roxb. (1336)
Oenothera erythrosepala Borbás (2253)
O. odorata Jacq. (2253)

## HYDROCARYACEAE 224a

Trapa incisa Sieb. et Zucc. var. quadricaudata Gluck (1895)

## CYNOMORIACEAE 226

Cynomorium coccineum L. (1347)
C. songaricum Rupr. (1347)

## ARALIACEAE 227

Acanthopanax = Eleutherococcus
Aralia armata (Wall.) Seem. (2195)
A. cordata Thunb. (281, 1748a, 1791)
A. decaisneana Hance (1896)
A. elata (Miq.) Seem. (1890)
Dendropanax proteus (Champ.) Benth. (1001)
Eleutherococcus evodiifolius (Franch.) S. Y. Hu (1939a)
E. giraldii (Harms) Nakai (1939b)
E. gracilistylus (W. W. Sm.) S. Y. Hu (1939h)
E. henryi Oliv. (1939f)
E. leucorrhizus Oliv. (1939e)
E. senticosus (Rupr. & Maxim.) Maxim. (096, 1911A, 1939g)
E. sessiliflorus (Rupr. et Maxim.) S. Y. Hu (1939i)
E. setchuenensis (Harms) Nakai (1939d)
E. trifoliatus (L.) S. Y. Hu (1117, 1939j, 1904)
E. verticillatus Hoo (1939c)
Hedera helix L. (037)

*Hedera nepalensis* K. Koch
var. *sinensis* (Tobl.) Rehd. (037)
*Heteropanax fragrans* (Roxb.) Seem.
(1420)
*Kalopanax pictus* (Thunb.) Nakai
(392, 926, 1877) (*Kalopanax
septemlobus* (Thunb.))
*Oplopanax elatus* (Nakai) Nakai
(1885)
*Panax bipinnatifidus* Seem (2240)
*P. ginseng* C. A. Meyer (599)
*P. japonicus* C. A. Meyer (1222)
*P. major* (Burk.) Ting (241)
*P. notoginseng* (Burk.) F. H.
Chen (1115, 1594)
*P. quinquefolium* L. (443)
*Schefflera arboricola* Hayata (092)
*S. delavayi* (Franch.) Harms (1417)
*S. heterophylla* (L.) Frodin (2011)
(*S. octophylla* (Lour.) Hassk)
*Tetrapanax papyrifer* (Hook.) K.
Koch (328, 1353, 1822b)

UMBELLIFERAE 228

*Anethum graveolens* L. (1261)
(*Peucedanum graveolens* S. Wats.)
*Angelica anomala* Lallem. (459, 967)
*A. citriodora* Hance (163)

*A. dahurica* (Fischer ex Hoffm.)
Franch. et Sav. (967)
*A. gigas* Nakai (1791a)
*A. porphyrocaulis* Nakai (281, 1748e)
*Angelica pubescens* Maxim. (281,
1748c)
*A. sinensis* (Oliver) Diels (699, 1483)
*Anthriscus sylvestris* (L.) Hoffm.
(947A)
*Bupleurum chinense* DC. (021a)
*B. falcatum* L. (021)
*B. scorzoneraefolium* Willd. (021)
*Carum carvi* L. (1675)
*Centella asiatica* (Linn.) Urb. (769,
1066)
*Changium smyrnioides* Wolff (884)
*Cicuta virosa* L. (1733)
*Cnidium monnieri* (L.) Cusson
(1205)
*Coriandrum sativum* L. (524, 2250)
*Cryptotaenia japonica* Hassk. (2013)
*Daucus carota* L. (1047)
*Eryngium foetidum* L. (2154)
*Ferula assafoetida* L. (005)
F. borealis Kuan (1146)
F. conocaula Korovin (005)
*F. sinkiangensis* K. M. Shen (005)
*Foeniculum vulgare* Miller (468, 537,
563)

*Glehnia littoralis* (A. Gray) F.
Schmidt (1052)
*Heracleum hemsleyanum* Diels (281,
1748d)
*H. lanatum* Michx. (281, 1748b)
*Hydrocotyle sibthorpioides* Lam.
(1061, 1246, 1610)
*Ledebouriella seseloides* (Hoffm.)
Wolff (325, 344) (see
*Saposhnikovia*)
*Ligusticum brachylobum* Franch.
(325a)
*L. jeholense* Nakai et Kitagawa (627)
*L. sinense* Oliver (627)
*L. wallichii* Franch. (279, 433, 496)
*Notopterygium forbesii* Boiss. (109b)
*N. franchetii* Boiss. (109a, 269)
*Notopterygium incisium* Ting (109,
269, 1315)
*Oenanthe javanica* (Blume) DC. (1300)
*Peucedanum decursivum* (Miq.)
Maxim. (1843)
*P. praeruptorum* Dunn (140)
*P. terebinthaceum* (Fischer) Fischer et
Turcz. (1240)
*Pimpinella diversifolia* DC. (944)
*Pleurospermum giraldii* Diels (2062)
*Pternopetalum vulgare* (Dunn) Hand.-
Mazz. (1834)

*Sanicula astrantifolia* Wolff ex
Kretschmer (1710)
*Saposhnikovia divaricata* (Turcz.)
Schinsch (325, 344) (*Ledebouriella
seseloides* (Hoffm.) Wolff)
*Tongoloa dunnii* (Boiss.) Wolff
(1460)

### CORNACEAE 229

*Aucuba chinensis* Benth. (1602)
*Cornus kousa* Hance var. *angustata*
Chun (2103)
*C. macrophylla* Wall. (1644)
*C. officinalis* Sieb. et Zucc. (254, 1165, 2219)
*Helwingia japonica* (Thunb.) Willd.
(2124)

### PYROLACEAE 231

*Monotropa uniflora* L. (1301)
*Pyrola rotundifolia* L. (783)

### ERICACEAE 233

*Gaultheria forrestii* Diels (1427)
*Rhododendron anthopogonoides*
Maxim. (477)

*Rhododendron dauricum* L. (853)
*R. mariae* Hance (1865)
*R. molle* G. Don (923, 2031)
*R. simsii* Planch. (1739)
*Vaccinium bracteatum* Thunb. (912)
*V. dunalianum* Wight var. *urophyllum*
Rehd. et Wils. (1428)
*V. fragile* Franch. (1760, 1949)

### MYRSINACEAE 236

*Ardisia crenata* Sims (1412)
*A. crispa* (Thunb.) A. DC. (470)
*A. gigantifolia* Stapf (837, 1725)
*A. japonica* (Hornsted) Blume (1831)
*A. mamillata* Hance (523)
*Embelia laeta* (L.) Mez. (606, 1373)
*Maesa japonica* (Thunb.) Mor. et
Zoll. (1734)
*Myrsine africana* L. (1407)

### PRIMULACEAE 237

*Androsace aizoon* Dubu ex DC.
(1589)
*A. umbellata* (Lour.) Merr. (1589)
*Lysimachia christinae* Hance (706)
*L. clethroides* Duby (171)

*Lysimachia foenum-graecum* Hance
(747, 749)
*L. fortunei* Maxim. (494)
*L. insignis* Hemsl. (1114, 1797)
*Primula patens* Turcz. (2198)
*P. sinodenticulata* Balf. (2146)

### PLUMBAGINACEAE 238

*Ceratostigma minus* Stapf (1833)
*C. plumbaginoides* Bunge (1829)
*C. willmottianum* Stapf (1829)
*Plumbago indica* L. (1841)
*P. zeylanica* L. (980)

### EBENACEAE 240

*Diospyros ebenum* Koenig (1980)
*D. kaki* L. f. (1253, 1254, 1273, 1277)
*D. lotus* L. (410)

### STYRACACEAE 241

*Styrax benzoin* Dryand. (014)
*S. hypoglaucus* Perkins (014)
*S. macrothyrsus* Perkins (014)
*S. subniveus* Merr. et Chun (014)
*S. tonkinensis* Craib (014)

## SYMPLOCACEAE 242

*Symplocos caudata* Wall. (1168)
*S. racemosa* Roxb. (1168)

## OLEACEAE 243

*Forsythia suspensa* (Thunb.) Vahl (743)
*Fraxinus bungeana* DC. (197)
*F. chinensis* Roxb. (987)
*F. rhynchophylla* Hance (197)
*Jasminum amplexicaule* Buch.-Ham. ex G. Don (935)
*J. officinale* L. (1357)
*J. polyanthum* Franch. (2127)
*J. sambac* (L.) Ait. (888)
*Ligustrum japonicum* Thunb. (942)
*L. lucidum* Ait. (942)
*L. quihuoi* Carr. (1327)
*L. sinense* Lour. var. *nitidum* Rehd. (1327)
*Osmanthus fragrans* (Thunb.) Lour. (692)
*O. matsumuranus* Hayata (2051)
*Syringa persica* L. (2134)
*S. pinnatifolia* Hemsl. (2241)
*S. reticulata* (Blume) Hara (1044)

## LOGANIACEAE 245

*Buddleia asiatica* Lour. (1026)
*B. lindleyana* Fortune ex Lindl. (1727)
*B. officinalis* Maxim. (872, 874)
*Gelsemium elegans* Benth. (649, 1384)
*Strychnos ignatii* Berg. (665)
*S. nux-vomica* L. (321, 824)
*S. wallichiana* Benth. (824)

## GENTIANACEAE 246

*Gentiana dahurica* Fischer (196)
*G. loureiroi* (D. Don) Griesb. (1551a)
*G. macrophylla* Pall. (196)
*G. scabra* Bunge (818, 1479)
*G. urnula* H. Sm. (1981)
*Nymphoides peltatum* (Gmel.) O. Ktze. (1317)
   (*Limnanthemum nymphoides* (L.) Hoffmgg. et Link)
*Swertia diluta* (Turcz.) Benth. et Hook. f. (1480)
*S. heterantha* Ling (1942)
*S. mileensis* Ho et Shih (224)
*S. pseudochinensis* Hara (1485)

## APOCYNACEAE 247

*Alstonia scholaris* (L.) R. Br. (1506)
*Apocynum venetum* L. (766)
*Catharanthus roseus* (L.) G. Don (36)
*Ervatamia hainanensis* Tsiang (1471)
*Melodinus suaveolens* Champ. ex Benth. (1155)
*Nerium oleander* L. (093)
   (*N. indicum* Miller)
*Parabarium micranthum* (A. DC.) Pierre (1744)
*Rauvolfia verticillata* (Lour.) Baill. (759)
*Strophanthus divaricatus* (Lour.) Hook. et Arn. (2036)
*Thevetia peruviana* (Pers.) K. Schum. (549)
*Trachelospermum jasminoides* (Lindl.) Lem. (767)
*Wrightia pubescens* R. Br. (1499)

## ASCLEPIADACEAE 248

*Cynanchum atratum* Bunge (1020)
*C. auriculatum* Royle ex Wight (1009)
*C. bungei* Dcne. (1009)

*Cynanchum paniculatum* (Bunge)
Kitagawa (499, 1557)
(*Pycnostelma paniculatum*
(Bunge) Schum.)

*C. stauntonii* (Dcne.)
Schlecht. ex Lévl. (965)

*C. wilfordii* (Maxim.) Hemsl. (937)
(*C. caudatum* Maxim. non Vell.)

*Hoya pandurata* Tsiang (1587)

*H. pottsii* Traill. (1587)

*Marsdenia tenacissima* (Roxb.) Wight
et Arn. (1816)

*Metaplexis japonica* (Thunb.) Makino
(764, 1595)

*Periploca calophylla* (Wight) Falc.
(1987)

*P. forrestii* Schlecht. (404)

*P. sepium* Bunge (450, 619, 1058)

*Pycnostelma paniculatum* (Bunge) K.
Schum ≡ (499, 1557)

*Streptocaulon griffithii* Hook. f. (660)

*Tylophora ovata* (Lindl.) Hook. et
Steud. (1135)

## CONVOLVULACEAE 249

*Argyreia acuta* Lour. (975)

*A. seguinii* (Lévl.) Vaniot (1183)

*Calystegia hederacea* Wall. (1434)

*Convolvulus arvensis* L. (1608)

*Cuscuta chinensis* Lam. (1789)

*C. japonica* Choisy (1789)

*Dichondra repens* Forster (839)

*Erycibe obtusifolia* Benth. (1643)

*Evolvulus alsinoides* L. (1793)

*Ipomoea cairica* (L.) Sweet (1937)

*I. hederacea* Jacq. (240, 315, 401,
407, 969)

*I. hungaiensis* Lingelsh. et Borza
(1773)

*I. nil* (L.) Roth (145, 240, 315, 401,
407, 969)
(*Pharbitis nil* (L.) Choisy)

*I. pes-caprae* (L.) Sweet (822)

## BORAGINACEAE 252

*Arnebia euchroma* (Royle) Johnst.
(1862a)

*A. guttata* Bunge (1862a)

*A. saxatilis* (Pall.) Benth. et Hook. f.
(1867) (*Slenoselenium saxatile*
(Pall.) Turcz.)

*Bothriospermum secundum* Maxim.
(2123)

*Cynoglossum amabile* Stapf et Drumm.
(1498)

*C. lanceolatum* Forsk. (2026)

*Cynoglossum officinale* L. (2061)

*C. zeylanicum* (Vahl) Thunb. (1571)

*Heliotropium indicum* L. (1435)

*Lithospermum erythrorhizon* Sieb. et
Zucc. (1091, 1698, 1862c)

*L. zollingeri* DC. (1520)

*Onosma hookeri* C. B. Clarke (1862b)

*O. paniculatum* Bur. et Franch.
(1862b)

*Symphytum officinale* L. (1302A)

## VERBENACEAE 253

*Callicarpa longissima* (Hemsl.) Merr.
(135)

*C. macrophylla* Vahl (1448)

*C. pedunculata* R. Br. (1838)

*Caryopteris incana* (Thunb.) Miq.
(2200)

*Clerodendrum cyrtophyllum* Turcz.
(1393)

*C. fortunatum* L. (669, 697)

*C. fragrans* Vent. (239)

*C. inerme* (L.) Gaertn. (666, 1312)

*C. kaempferi* (Jack.) Sieb. (059)

*C. serratum* (L.) Spreng. (1136)

*C. trichotomum* Thunb. (381, 1755)

*C. yunnanense* Hu (2001)

*Lantana camara* L. (845, 1988)
*Lippia nodiflora* (L.) Rich. (1398)
  (*Phyla nodiflora* (L.) Greene)
*Stachytarpheta jamaicensis* (L.)
  Vahl (2226)
*Verbena officinalis* L. (834)
*Vitex cannabifolia* Sieb. et Zucc. (547)
*V. negundo* L. (547, 891)
*V. rotundifolia* L. f. (851)
*V. trifolia* L. (205, 851)


LABIATAE 254

*Agastache rugosa* (Fischer et Meyer)
  O. Ktze. (413, 581b, 914)
*Ajuga decumbens* Thunb. (991)
*Anisomeles indica* (L.) O. Ktze. (326)
*Dracocephalum ruyschiana* L. (217)
*Elsholtzia ciliata* (Thunb.) Hyland.
  (456)
*E. haichowensis* Sun ex C. Y. Wu
  (456)
*E. rugulosa* Hemsl. (2116)
*E. splendens* Nakai ex E. Naekauwa
  (456)
*Glechoma hederacea* L. (1664)
*Isodon coetsa* (Buch.-Ham. ex D. Don)
  Kudo (2128) (*Plectranthus coetsa*
  Buch.-Ham. ex D. Don)

*Lamium barbatum* Sieb. et Zucc.
  (2071)
*Leonurus artemisia* (Lour.) S. Y. Hu
  (307, 312, 590, 591)
*L. tartarica* L. (307, 312, 591)
*Leucas zeylanica* (L.) R. Br. (356)
*Lycopus lucidus* Turcz. (1531, 1548,
  1721)
*Mentha arvensis* L. and *M. haplocalyx*
  Briq. (816, 1096)
*Mesona chinensis* Benth. (736)
*Microtoena insuavis* (Hance) Prain
  ex Dunn (2096)
*Mosla chinensis* Maxim. (1242)
*M. scabra* (Thunb.) C. Y. Wu (1230)
*M. soochouensis* Matsuda (1952)
*Nepeta cataria* L. (614A)
*Ocimum basilicum* L. (235, 684, 763)
*Origanum vulgare* L. (1768)
*Orthodon diantherus* (Buch.-Ham. ex
  Roxb.) Hand-Mazz (596, 1439)
*Orthosiphon aristatus* (Blume) Miq.
  (859)
*Perilla frutescens* (L.) Britt. (1012)
*P. frutescens* var. *crispa* (Thunb.)
  Dcne. (1858)
*P. ocymoides* L. (1359, 1362, 1363)
*Phlomis rotata* Benth. ex Hook. f.
  (1749)

*Plectranthus striatus* Benth. (82)
*Pogostemon cablin* (Blanco) Benth.
  (414, 581a, 682, 2046)
*P. patchouli* Pellet (682)
*Prunella vulgaris* L. (446)
*Rabdosia rubescens* (Hemsley) Hara
  (1804A)
*Salvia bowleygna* Dunn (919A)
*Salvia cavaleriei* Lévl. (2130)
*S. chinensis* Benth. (1233)
*S. miltiorrhiza* Bunge (1476)
*S. przewalskii* Maxim. (1476)
*Schizonepeta tenuifolia* (Benth.) Briq.
  (199)
*Scutellaria baicalensis* Georgi (545)
*S. barbata* D. Don (1029)
*S. indica* L. (395)
*Stachys baicalensis* Fischer (1331)
*S. neglecta* Klok. (1331)
*S. oblongifolia* Benth. (2152)
*S. recta* L. (1331)
*S. sieboldii* Miq. (1712)
*Teucrium viscidum* Blume (508b, 1176)
*Thymus mongolicus* Ronn. (1511)
*T. serpyllum* L. (1511)
*T. vulgaris* L. (1208)


SOLANACEAE 256

*Anisodus luridus* Link et Otto (1121)

*Anisodus tanguticus* (Maxim.) Pascher
  (1673)
  (*Scopolia tangutica* Maxim.)
*Atropa belladonna* L. (1588)
*Capsicum annuum* L. (709)
*Datura innoxia* Miller (2034b)
*D. metel* L. (335, 854, 2034a)
*Hyoscyamus niger* L. (713, 1606)
*Lycium barbarum* L. and *L. chinense*
  Miller (090, 134, 640, 641, 642,
  655, 1060, 1529A)
*Nicotiana tabacum* L. (2167)
*Physalis alkekengi* L. (1364, 1365)
*P. minima* L. (1505, 1623)
*P. peruviana* L. (1505)
*Scopola acutangula* C. Y. Wu et
  C. Chen (1121)
  (*Anisodus Iuridus* Link et Otto)
*Solanum capsicastrum* Link ex Schau
  (2080)
*S. indicum* L. (1597)
*S. khasianum* C. B. Clarke (1909)
*S. lyratum* Thunb. (1024)
*S. melongena* L. (124)
*S. nigrum* L. (814)
*S. pseudo-capsicum* L. (2232)
*S. surattense* Burm. f. (2132)
*S. torvum* Swartz (184, 1296)

*Solanum tuberosum* L. (2060)
*S. verbascifolium* L. (2149)


### SCROPHULARIACEAE 257

*Adenosma glutinosum* (L.) Druce
  (857, 864)
*A. indianum* (Lour.) Merr. (1426)
*Buchnera cruciata* Buch.-Ham. ex
  D. Don (2211)
*Digitalis purpurea* L. (2054)
*Limnophila aromatica* (Lam.) Merr.
  (1304)
*Lindernia anagallis* (Burm. f.)
  Pennell (1638)
*L. angustifolia* (Benth.) Wettst.
  (2039)
*L. antipoda* (L.) Alston (1305)
*L. crustacea* (L.) F. Muell. (907)
*L. ruellioides* (Colsm.) Pennell
  (2024)
*Paulownia fortunei* (Seem.) Hemsl.
  (1819)
*P. tomentosa* (Thunb.) Steud.
  (1819)
*Pedicularis davidii* Franch. (1461)
*P. resupinata* L. (827)

*Pedicularis rex* C. B. Clarke ex
  Maxim. (1950)
*Phtheirospermum japonicum*
  (Thunb.) Kanitz. (1380)
*P. tenuisectum* Bur. et Franch.
  (1708)
*Picrorrhiza kurrooa* Royle ex Benth.
  (516)
*P. scrophulariaeflora* Pennell (516)
*Rehmannia glutinosa* Libosch.(1225,
  1291, 1523)
*Ruellia drymophila* (Diels) Hand.-
  Mazz. (1541)
*Scoparia dulcis* L. (2097)
*Scrophularia ningpoensis* Hemsl.
  (505, 2248)
*Siphonostegia chinensis* Benth.
  (2178)
*Striga asiatica* (L.) O. Ktze. (1741)
*Veronica anagallis-aquatica* L.
  (1316)
*V. serpyllifolia* L. (1543)
*Veronicastrum axillare* (Sieb. et
  Zucc.) Yamazuki (1558)

### BIGNONIACEAE 258

*Campsis grandiflora* (Thunb.)
  Loisel. (748, 1869)

*Oroxylum indicum* (L.) Vent. (136, 899)
*Radermachera sinica* Hemsl. (1667)

PEDALIACEAE 259

*Sesamum indicum* L. (400)

OROBANCHACEAE 261

*Aeginetia indica* Roxb. (2099)
*Boschniakia rossica* (Cham. et Schltdl.) Fedtsch. et Flerov. (1714)
*Cistanche deserticola* Ma (640)
*Cistanche salsa* (C. A. Meyer) Benth. et Hook. f. (604, 1449, 1730)

GESNERIACEAE 262

*Didissandra sesquifolia* C. B. Clarke (1410)
*Lysionotus pauciflora* Maxim (1278)

ACANTHACEAE 266

*Acanthus ilicifolius* L. (720)
*Adhatoda vasica* Nees (1418)
*A. ventricosa* (Wall.) Nees (1418)
  (*Justicia ventricosa* Wall.
  *Gendarussa ventricosa* (Wall.)

Nees)
*Andrographis paniculata* (Burm. f.) Nees (278)
*Baphicacanthus cusia* (Nees) Bremek. (222b)
*Championella sarcorrhiza* C. Ling (1668)
*Dicliptera chinensis* (L.) Nees (645)
*Gendarussa ventricosa* (Wall.) Nees ≡ (1418)
*G. vulgaris* Nees (474)
  (*Justicia gendarussa* Burm. f.)
*Hygrophila salicifolia* (Vahl) Nees (1394)
*Hypoestes poilanei* Benoist (2102)
*Justicia procumbens* L. (778)
*Peristrophe bivalvis* (L.) Merr. (2133)
*P. roxburghiana* (Schultes) Bremek. (573)
*Rhinacanthus nasutus* (L.) Kurz (974)
*Thunbergia grandiflora* Roxb. (1815)

PLANTAGINACEAE 269

*Plantago asiatica* L. (046, 047)
*P. major* L. (046, 047)

RUBIACEAE 270

*Adina pilulifera* (Lam.) Franch. (1340)
*Cephaelis ipecacuanha* (Brot.) A. Rich. (1772)
*Cephalanthus occidentalis* L. (340)
*Cinchona calisaya* Wedd. (169)
*C. officinalis* L. (169)
*Coffea arabica* L. (095)
*Damnacanthus indicus* Gaertn. (527, 1880)
*Gardenia jasminoides* Ellis (125, 157, 544, 1162, 1175, 1298)
*Hedyotis auricularia* L. (316)
*H. cantonensis* How (1632)
*H. corymbosa* (L.) Lam. (1309)
*H. diffusa* Willd. (979)
  (*Oldenlandia diffusa* (Willd.) Roxb.)
*H. hedyotidea* (DC.) Merr. (1000)
*H. uncinella* Hook. et Arn. (2016)
*Ixora chinensis* Lam. (810)
*Knoxia corymbosa* Willd. (1386)
*K. valerianoides* Thorel ex Pitard (577)
*Luculia intermedia* Hutch. (2135)

*Morinda officinalis* How (060, 068, 950)

*M. umbellata* L. (2038)

*Mussaenda erosa* Champ. ex Benth. (1383)

*M. pubescens* Ait. f. (968, 1177)

*Nauclea officinalis* Pierre ex Pitard (1473)

*Ophiorrhiza succirubra* King ex Hook. f. (1532)

*Paederia scandens* (Lour.) Merr. (077)

*Pavetta hongkongensis* Brem. (1419)

*Psychotria rubra* (Lour.) Poir. (1189)

*Rubia cordifolia* L. (142, 148)

*R. yunnanensis* Diels (2262)

*Serissa foetida* Commers. ex Juss. (758)

*S. serissoides* (DC.) Druce (990)

*Uncaria gambir* (Hunt.) Roxb. (314)

*U. macrophylla* Wall. (1441)

*U. rhynchophylla* (Miq.) Jacks. (648)

*U. sinensis* (Oliver) Havil. (648)

CAPRIFOLIACEAE 271

*Abelia engleriana* (Graebn.) Rehd. (1836)

*Lonicera confusa* DC. (1796)

*L. japonica* Thunb. (190, 191, 600, 878, 1200, 2179)

*Sambucus chinensis* Maxim. (1724) (*S. javanica* auct., non Reinw.)

*S. williamsii* Hance (120) (*S. racemosa* auct., non L.)

*Triosteum fargesii* Franch. (1948)

*T. pinnatifidum* Maxim. (1635)

*Viburnum utile* Hemsl. (2052)

VALERIANACEAE 273

*Nardostachys chinensis* Batal. (616)

*Valeriana officinalis* L. (481)

DIPSACACEAE 274

*Dipsacus asper* Wall. (280, 293)

*D. chinensis* Batal. (264, 280, 293)

*D. japonicus* Miq. (501)

*Morina betonicoides* Benth. (1899)

*M. coulteriana* Royle (1899)

*M. delavayi* Franch. (1906)

CUCURBITACEAE 275

*Benincasa hispida* (Thunb.) Cogn. (1802)

*Bolbostemma paniculatum* (Maxim.) Franq. (1786)

*Citrullus lanatus* (Thunb.) Matsum et Nakai (433) (*C. vulgaris* Schrad.)

*Cucumis melo* L. (664, 672, 1613)

*C. melo* var. *conomon* Makino (1666)

*Cucurbita moschata* Duch. (915, 916)

*Lagenaria siceraria* (Molina) Standl. (518)

*Luffa acutangula* (L.) Roxb. (1348, 1616)

*L. agyptica* Miller (1348, 1616) (*L. cylindrica* (L.) Roem.)

*Momordica charantia* L. (663)

*M. cochinchinensis* (Lour.) Spreng. (903)

*Siraitia grosvenori* (Swingle) C. Jeffrey (760) (Momordica grosvenori Swingle)

*Solena amplexcaulis* (Lam.) Gandhi (1784)

*Trichosanthes cucumeroides* (Ser.) Maxim. (1922)

*T. kirilowii* Maxim. (671, 771, 772, 1611)

*Zehneria indica* (Lour.) Keran Dren (Melothria indica Lour.) (719)

CAMPANULACEAE 276

*Adenophora axilliflora* Borb. (917c)
*A. bulleyana* Diels (917i)
*A. capillaris* Hemsl. (917b)
*A. lilifolioides* Pax ex Hoffm. (917a)
*A. pereskiaefolia* (Fischer) G. Don (917d)
*A. polyantha* Nakai (917h)
*A. polymorpha* Ledeb. (1150)
*A. potaninii* Korsh. (917f)
*A. stricta* Miq. 867 (917g)
  (*A. polymorpha* var. *stricta* (Miq.) Makino)
*A. tetraphylla* (Thunb.) Fischer (917e, 1150)
  (*A. verticillata* (Pall.) Fischer)
*Campanumoea javanica* Blume (1792)
*Codonopsis convolvulacea* Kurz (1156)
*C. lanceolata* Benth. et Hook. f. (1169)
*C. pilosula* (Franch.) Nannf. (327, 441, 794, 1484)
*C. tangshen* Oliver (292, 327, 441, 794, 1484)
*Lobelia chinensis* Lour. (1036)
  (*L. radicans* Thunb.)
*L. hybrida* C. Y. Wu (1871)

*Lobelia seguinii* Lévl. et Vant. (2148)
*Platycodon grandiflorum* (Jacq.) A. DC. (119)
*Pratia begonifolia* (Wall.) Lindl. (1512, 1813)

COMPOSITAE 280

*Achillea alpina* L. (1227)
*A. millefolium* L. (2033)
*A. wilsoniana* Heimerl. (1770)
*Ainsliaea latifolia* (D. Don) Sch.-Bip. (1488)
*A. pertyoides* Franch. (2086)
*A. triflora* (Buch.-Ham. ex D. Don) Druce (1492)
*A. yunnanensis* Franch. (2162)
*Anaphalis margaritacea* (L.) Benth. (1445)
*Arctium lappa* L. (930, 936, 1411)
*Artemisia annua* L. (548)
*A. anomala* S. Moore (075, 751)
*A. apiacea* Hance (213, 1477)
*A. argyi* Lévl. et Vant. (006, 008, 010, 011, 2007)
*A. capillaris* Thunb. (2172)
*A. cina* Berg (418, 1191)
*A. lactiflora* Wall. (977, 2010)

*Artemisia monogyna* Waldst. (418)
*A. vulgaris* L. (006, 008, 010, 011, 2007)
*Aster ageratoides* Turcz. (1185)
*A. flaccidus* Bunge (1455)
*A. oreophilus* Franch. (2140)
*A. scaber* Thunb. (1801)
*A. tataricus* L. (1874)
*Atractylodes chinensis* (Bunge) Koidz. (862, 1286c, 1292, 1680b)
*A. japonica* Koidz. ex Kitam. (862c, 1286c, 1292, 1680c)
*A. lancea* (Thunb.) DC. (862, 1286c, 1292, 1680a)
*A. macrocephala* Koidz. (306, 742, 1010, 1224, 1286b, 2234, 2249)
*Aucklandia lappa* Dcne. (897)
  (*Saussurea lappa* (Dcne.) C. B. Clarke)
*Bidens pilosa* L. (691)
*Blumea balsamifera* (L.) DC. (007, 009, 012, 1094)
*Carpesium abrotanoides* L. (374, 1619)
*Carthamus tinctorius* L. (569, 2061)
*Centipeda minima* (L.) A. Br. et Ascher (947, 1107)

*Cephalanoplos segetum* (Bunge) Kitam. (466)

*Chrysanthemum boreale* (Makino) Makino (2077)

*C. cinerariaefolium* Vis. (255)

*C. indicum* L. (2076, 2077)

*C. lavandulaefolium* (Fischer) Makino (2077)

*C. morifolium* Ramat. (259)

*Cirsium belingschanicum* Petrak. (1886)

*C. eriophoroideum* (Hook. f.) Lévl. (1433)

*C. japonicum* DC. (1387)

*Cremanthodium hookerii* C. B. Clarke (1456)

*C. plantagineum* Maxim. (1590)

*Crepis lignea* (Vant.) Babc. (1916)

*Crossostephium chinense* (L.) Makino (080, 451)

*Dolomiaea souliei* (Franchet) Shih (867A)

*Echinops gmelinii* Turcz. (1149)

*Eclipta prostrata* L. (398, 866, 886)

*Elephantopus scaber* L. (1550)

*Emilia sonchifolia* (L.) DC. (2057)

*Erigeron breviscapus* (Vant.) Hand.-Mazz. (1502)

*Eupatorium fortunei* Turcz. (1059, 1720)

*Eupatorium japonicum* Thunb. (043, 1059, 1720)

*E. lindleyanum* DC. (2107)

*Gnaphalium adnatum* Wall. (1527)

*G. affine* D. Don (360)

*G. hypoleucum* DC. (1629)

*G. japonicum* Thunb. (1598)

*G. multiceps* Wall. (1287)

*Gynura divaricata* (L.) DC. (1002)

*G. segetum* (Lour.) Merr. (572, 1116, 1788a)

*Inula britannica* L. (175, 367, 503)

*I. cappa* (Buch.-Ham. ex D. Don) DC. (999, 2042)

*I. helenium* L. (1779)

*I. nervosa* Wall. (1715)

*I. racemosa* Hook. f. (1779)

*Ixeris chinensis* (Thunb.) Nakai (1178)

*I. denticulata* (Houtt.) Nakai (906)

*Kalimeris indica* (L.) Sch.-Bip. (830)
   (*Aster indicus* L.)

*Lactuca elata* Hemsl. (2147)
   (*L. raddeana* Maxim.)

*Laggera alata* (Roxb.) Sch.-Bip. (780, 789)

*Leibnitzia anandria* (L.) Nakai (1424)

*Ligularia lapathifolia* (Franch.) Hand.-Mazz. (1431)

*Pentanema indicum* (L.) Ling (1690)

*Petasites japonicus* (Sieb. et Zucc.) F. Schmidt (353)

*Rhaponticum uniflorum* (L.) DC. (774)

*Saussurea japonica* (Thunb.) DC. (347)

*S. lappa* (Dcne.) C. B. Clarke (685, 897b)

*Scorzonera austriaca* Willd. (2025)

*Senecio chrysanthemoides* DC. (1788b)

*S. nudicaulis* Buch.-Ham. ex C. B. Clarke (1852)

*S. orgzetorum* Diels (1416)

*S. scandens* Buch.-Ham. ex D. Don (143, 230)

*Siegesbeckia orientalis* L. (430, 434)

*Solidago virgo-aurea* L. (588)

*Sonchus brachyotus* DC. (962)

*Spilanthes acmella* (L.) Murr. (1636)

*Tagetes erecta* L. (1920)

*Tanacetum variifolium* (Chang) Ling (1454)

*Taraxacum mongolicum* Hand.-Mazz. (1112)
*T. officinale* L. (1112)
*Tussilago farfara* L. (131, 679)
*Vernonia andersonii* C. B. Clarke

(707)
*Vernonia cinera* (L.) Less. (2089)
*Vladimiria souliei* (Franch.) Ling (285, 897a)
*Wedelia chinensis* (Osbeck) Merr.

(1062)
*Wedelia prostrata* Hemsl. (796)
*Xanthium sibiricum* Patrin (1677)
*X. strumarium* L. (1677)
*Youngia japonica* (L.) DC. (561)

# ANIMALS

## SPONGE and SEA-URCHIN

Fresh water sponge (1855)
Sea urchin (389)

## MOLLUSKS

Bivalves:
   Clam shell (630, 636, 1040, 1931)
   Cockle shell (1912)
   Mother-of-pearl (049)
   Mussel (dried) (1478)
   Oyster shell (730, 892)
   Pearls (048)
Gastropods:
   Abalone shell (1236)
   Fresh water snail (1615)
   Spiral univalve shell (762)
Cowry:
   Cowry shell (1056, 1850)

Cephalopods:
   Cuttle-fish (1994)
   — bone (387, 1472)
   — egg (2006)
   squid bone (890)

## SEGMENTED WORMS

Earthworms (237, 1533)
Leeches (1297)

## CRUSTACEANS

King-crab shell (423)

## CENTIPEDES

Centipedes (1018, 1962)

## SCORPIONS and SPIDERS

Grass spiders (1689)

Scorpions (296, 479)
Wall spider egg mass (1069)

## INSECTS

Beetles:
   Blue-back beetle (1549)
   Cantharides (1034)
   Dried bean beetle (220)
   Dung beetle (110)
   Giant water beetle (817)
   Grubs of June beetle (089, 1794)
   Lady-bird beetle (1079)
   Long-horn beetle larva in
      Caesalpinia (2266)
   — in mulberry (1142)
   Rhinoceros beetle (1735)
Cicada with fungus growth (162)
Cockroach excrete (308)
Crickets (440)

Damselfly nymph (1529)
Exuviae of cicada (026)
Gadfly (871, 934)
Gall insects (1985)
Maggots (653, 1310, 1960)
Mole crickets (773)
Praying mantis egg case on mulberry
    branch (1143)
Red cicade (571)
Silkworm:
    Silk wool (1349)
    Silkworm cocoon (1670)
    — excreta (1670)
    — pupa (1670)
    — sick and dead (101, 106)
    — slough (1670)
Stinkbug (228)
Wasp and larva (1764)
Wingless cockroach (1082, 1787)
Wood louse (1288)
Other insects:
    Exotic worm (2041)
    Gall insect in Cocklebur (1678)

### FISHES

Bones in fish head (2233)
Fish and egg (1765)

Fish swim bladder (2231)
Flying fish (1934)
Glassfish (2189)
Pipe-fish (384)
Sea horse (385)
Spring-fish (2210)

### AMPHIBIANS

Frog (378, 447)
Frog oviduct (637)
Toads (023, 027, 310)

### REPTILES

Gecko (629, 1209)
Hooked-jaw turtle (2180)
Lizard (1264)
Snakes:
    Agkistrodon (085, 978)
    Black-striped snake (1989)
    Cobra (2156)
    Dried snake (1086)
    Paipu snake (1006)
    White-band Krait (978)
Products from snake:
    Cobratoxin (2156a)
    Python skin (595)
    Snake skin (812)

Snake slough (1210, 1216)
Tortoise:
    Fresh water turtle shell (1080)
    Glue from tortoise shell (688)
    Land tortoise shell (695)
    Rim of fresh water turtle shell
        (1081)
    Tortoise shell (1452)
Tree lizard (2164)

### BIRDS

All parts of crow (1999)
Black-bone fowl (1959)
Crow's gall bladder (1999a)
Duck egg and shell (2020)
Eagle bone (2192)
— beak & claw (2192)
— head (2192)
Eyes of eagle (2192)
Indian cuckoo (1738)
Inner shell of fowls' egg (343)
Lining of chicken gizzard (074, 924)
Mandarin duck (2251)
Oriole (2190)
Whole duck (2008)

## MAMMALS

Ambergris (820)
Antelope horn (750)
Ass-hide glue (001, 198, 943, 1073, 1090)
Bat dung (746, 2112)
Bear's gall (498)
Cave bat dung (746, 1971)
Deer blood (784)
— fetus (793)
— horn (608, 775, 777, 786, 1180)
— penis (791)
— sinew (776)
— tail (802)
Dog's penis & testicle (552, 647)
Donkey hide glue (808)
Donkey penis (804)
Elephant hide (461)
Goat or sheep (2030)
— bladder (1959a)
— blood (1959b)
— bone (1959c)
— bone marrow (1959d)

Goat or sheep
— brain (1959e)
— fat (1959f)
— fetus (1959g)
— heart (1959h)
— kidney (1959i)
— liver (1959j)
— lung (1959k)
— meat (1959l)
— milk (1959m)
— pancreas (1959n)
— penis and testis (2049)
— skin (1959o)
— stomach (1959p)
— stomach nodule (2044)
— thyroid gland (1959r)
Goat sinew (1198)
— whisker (1959s)
Hedgehog skin (1911)
Leopard bone (1043)
Musk deer (navel gland secretion) (1207)
Otter liver (1334, 1451)
Ox gall (940)

Ox horn (928)
Ox or buffalo penis (938)
Pangolin scales (097, 291, 1157)
— skin (1158)
Rhinoceros horn (429)
Seal penis & testis (383)
Tiger bone (517)
Tiger bone glue (514)
Water buffalo:
— bone (933)
— horn (928, 1324)
Whale spit ambergris (820)
Wild horse meat (2108)
Wild pig:
— feet (2073)
— gall bladder (1163)
— head bone (2073)
— hide (2073)
— testis (2073)

### MAN

Charred human hair (511)
Human placenta (412, 1840)

## MINERALS

### A

Actinolite (086, 2032)

Agate (832)
Alum (White vitriol) (971)

Ammonium chloride (792)
Arsenic (1077)

Arsenolite (493)
Arsenopyrite (493)
Auripigment (1882)

### B — C

Borax (1064, 2256)
Bornite copper ore (1866)
Calamine (787)
Calomel (211)
Chlorite-schist (218, 873)
Cinnabar (1475)
   Artificial — (Vermilion) (2174)
   High grade — (055)
Copper rust (1818)
Coral (1124)

### F — G

Ferric ammonium sulphate (210)
Fluorite (1857)
Fossil bone (813)
Fossil crab (1243)
Fossil shell of spirifer (1282)
Fossil teeth (809)
Fossilized resin (Amber) (522)
Glauber's salt (473, 1074, 1102;
   sulfate of soda)

Gold leaf (185)
Gypsum (502, 1252)
— & calcite (399, 1329)

### H

Halite (Salt rock) (225, 922, 1395)
Halloysite (160, 1234)
Hematite (045, 1562a)

### I — K

Iron ores:
   Black ferric oxide (1562c)
   Hematite (045, 1562a)
   Iron rust (1562d)
   Limonite (1206, 1562b, 2225)
   Magnetic oxide of iron (1215)
   Magnetite (1215, 1562e, 1907)
Kaolinite (535, 626)

### L

Lapis Chloritii (218)
— Lazuli (207)
Lead (White) (1303)
Lime (1250)
Limonite (1206, 1562b, 2225)
Litharge (Galena) (876, 1649)
Lye or Potash (133)

### M

Magnesium sulphate (855)
Magnetite (1215, 1562e, 1907)
Mercuric oxide (1226)
Mercury (Quicksilver) (1345)
   Red oxide of — (567, 1123)
Mica:
   Brown — (207, 218)
   Common — (2261)
   Pink-speckled — (149)
   Silvery colored mica-schist (2173)
Mica-schist (873)
Mirabilita (473, 504, 1074, 1102)

### N — O

Nepherite grains (2217)
Ophicalcite (531)
Orpiment (Auripigment) (1882)

### P — R

Potash (133)
Pumice (363)
Pyrite (1845)
Pyrolusite (883, 1978)
Quartz (723, 1008, 1025)
   Crystallized — (1283)
Realgar (Red arsenic sulfide) (497)

Realgar, High grade (882)
Residual brine (2165)

S

Sal ammoniac (922)
Salty tea (2166)
Selenite (2243)
Silver (2183)
Smithsonite (787)
Soda of sulphate containing
  $MgSO_4$ (1102)

Sodium sulfate (Mirabilita) (473, 504,
  1074, 1102)
Stalactite (305)
—, Tubular (945)
Sulfur (755)
— preparation (002)

T

Talc (534)

Powder of talc (Kaolinite) (535)

V

Vermiculite (170)
Vermilion (252, 2174)
Vitriols:
  —, Blue (Copper sulfate) (1468)
  —, Green (Ferrous sulfate) (781)
  —, White (Zinc sulfate) (971)

# MISCELLANEOUS

Amber (fossilized resin) (522)
Beeswax (345)
Bezoars:
  Dog — (646)
  Horse — (833)
  Monkey — (427)
  Nodules in goat stomach (2044)
  Ox or buffalo gall stone (932)
Bird nest (1795, 2169)
Deposite in tobacco pipe (2170)
Furnace soil (371)
Gelatin (206)
Honey (348, 875)
Hornet nest (336, 782)
Human faeces preparation (597)
Human urine sediment (598)
Imitation cinnabar (309)

Imitation dragon's blood (670)
Indigo mold (216)
Insect secretions:
  On Dalbergia (1863)
  On Ficus (1863)
Insect white wax (986)
Juice of ginger & garlic (063)
Maltose (850)
Mud or soil:
  — from furnace (371)
  — from swallow nest (2160)
Nodules in goat stomach (2044)
Old liquid manure (168)
Paste of tangerine peels (054)
Petroleum (1267)
Plant ashes (1707)

Potash from grass ashes (1694)
Powder of Liquorice, radish treated
  with sodium sulfate (2246)
Preparation from chalk (1745)
Preserved Citrus peels (151)
Rabbit dung (1703, 1925, 2255)
Residual salt (2165)
Solidified oily mass from smoke of
  tannery (2155)
Soot from tanning factory (1078)
Soot from the bottom of a boiler
  (1017)
Sparrow excrement (1013)
Tabasheer from bamboo (244, 1600)
Urine deposit preparation (236)
Wens from monkey (428)

# APPENDICES

I.  A. A guide to the syllables of the Wade system of romanization

   B. A table for the conversion of Pinyin to the Wade system

II. Alphabetic lists of families and genera of plants.

   A.  A list of families with reference numbers or abbreviations

   B.  A generic list with family numbers or abbreviations indicating the position of each genus in Part II

III. The conversion of simplified Chinese characters into classical form

IV. An index of Chinese names

## A guide to the syllables of the Wade system of romanization

|  |  |  |  |  |  |  |  |
|---|---|---|---|---|---|---|---|
| A | 阿 | Chi | 鷄 | Chiung | 局 | Chü | 橘 |
| Ai | 艾 | Ch'i | 漆 | Ch'iung | 瓊 | Ch'ü | 去 |
| An | 安 | Chia | 加 | Cho | 酌 | Chüan | 娟 |
| Ang | 昂 | Ch'ia | 卡 | Ch'o | 戳 | Ch'üan | 全 |
| Ao | 奥 | Chiang | 薑 | Chou | 州 | Chüeh | 腳 |
| Cha | 槎 | Ch'iang | 羌 | Ch'ou | 臭 | Ch'üeh | 雀 |
| Ch'a | 叉 | Chiao | 茭 | Chu | 竹 | Chün | 菌 |
| Chai | 齋 | Ch'iao | 蕎 | Ch'u | 楮 | Ch'ün | 羣 |
| Ch'ai | 柴 | Chieh | 桔 | Chua | 抓 | Ên | 恩 |
| Chan | 占 | Ch'ieh | 茄 | Chuai | 拽 | Êrh | 兒 |
| Ch'an | 闡 | Chien | 建 | Ch'uai | 揣 | Fa | 髮 |
| Chang | 章 | Ch'ien | 千 | Chuan | 專 | Fan | 番 |
| Ch'ang | 昌 | Chih | 枳 | Ch'uan | 川 | Fang | 防 |
| Chao | 朝 | Ch'ih | 赤 | Chuang | 狀 | Fei | 榧 |
| Ch'ao | 潮 | Chin | 金 | Ch'uang | 牀 | Fên | 粉 |
| Chê | 浙 | Ch'in | 秦 | Chui | 錐 | Fêng | 楓 |
| Ch'ê | 車 | Ching | 荆 | Ch'ui | 吹 | Fo | 佛 |
| Chên | 珍 | Ch'ing | 青 | Chun | 准 | Fou | 否， |
| Ch'ên | 陳 | Chio | 角 | Ch'un | 椿 | Fu | 浮 |
| Chêng | 正 | Chiu | 酒 | Chung | 終 | Ha | 芙哈 |
| Ch'êng | 呈 | Ch'iu | 秋 | Ch'ung | 蟲 | Hai | 海 |

233

| | | | | | | | |
|---|---|---|---|---|---|---|---|
| Han | 漢 | Hui | 茴 | K'ao | 考 | La | 辣 |
| Hang | 杭 | Hun | 昏 | Kên | 根 | Lai | 來 |
| Hao | 好 | Hung | 紅 | K'ên | 肯 | Lan | 欖 |
| Hei | 黑 | Huo | 活 | Kêng | 庚 | Lang | 莨 |
| Hên | 很 | I | 一 | K'êng | 坑 | Lao | 牢 |
| Hêng | 亨 | Jan | 蚋 | Ko | 葛 | Lê | 笁 |
| Ho | 合 | Jang | 嚷 | K'o | 柯 | Lei | 雷 |
| Hou | 侯 | Jao | 繞 | Kou | 枸 | Lêng | 冷 |
| Hsi | 西 | Jê | 熱 | K'ou | 口 | Li | 李 |
| Hsia | 下 | Jên | 人 | Ku | 古 | Lia | 倆 |
| Hsiang | 香 | Jêng | 仍 | K'u | 苦 | Liang | 茛 |
| Hsiao | 小 | Jih | 日 | Kua | 瓜 | Liao | 蓼 |
| Hsieh | 瀉 | Jo | 若 | K'ua | 夸 | Lieh | 列 |
| Hsien | 鮮 | Jou | 肉 | Kuai | 乖 | Lien | 蓮 |
| Hsin | 心 | Ju | 乳 | K'uai | 快 | Lin | 林 |
| Hsing | 杏 | Juan | 軟 | Kuan | 貫 | Ling | 靈 |
| Hsiu | 修 | Jui | 枘 | K'uan | 寬 | Liu | 柳 |
| Hsiung | 雄 | Jun | 閏 | Kuang | 廣 | Lo | 羅 |
| Hsü | 徐 | Jung | 茸 | K'uang | 匡 | Lou | 蔞 |
| Hsüan | 玄 | Ka | 尬 | Kuei | 桂 | Lu | 鹵 |
| Hsüeh | 血 | Kai | 該 | K'uei | 葵 | Luan | 欒 |
| Hsün | 熏 | K'ai | 揩 | Kun | 棍 | Lun | 侖 |
| Hu | 胡 | Kan | 甘 | K'un | 昆 | Lung | 龍 |
| Hua | 花 | K'an | 刊 | Kung | 工 | Lü | 呂 |
| Huai | 槐 | Kang | 杠 | K'ung | 孔 | Lüan | 孿 |
| Huan | 幻 | K'ang | 亢 | Kuo | 過 | Ma | 麻 |
| Huang | 黃 | Kao | 高 | K'uo | 蛄 | Mai | 麥 |

| | | | | | | | |
|---|---|---|---|---|---|---|---|
| Man | 滿 | Nien | 年 | P'ên | 盆 | Sêng | 僧 |
| Mang | 芒 | Nin | 您 | Pêng | 崩 | Sha | 沙 |
| Mao | 毛 | Ning | 寧 | P'êng | 捧 | Shai | 篩 |
| Mei | 梅 | Niu | 牛 | Pi | 必 | Shan | 山 |
| Mên | 門 | No | 糯 | P'i | 枇 | Shang | 傷 |
| Mêng | 夢 | Nou | 耨 | Piao | 標 | Shao | 少 |
| Mi | 密 | Nu | 奴 | P'iao | 瓢 | Shê | 蛇 |
| Miao | 苗 | Nuan | 暖 | Pieh | 別 | Shên | 申 |
| Mieh | 乜 | Nui | 內 | P'ieh | 撇 | Shêng | 生 |
| Mien | 棉 | Nun | 嫩 | Pien | 蔫 | Shih | 石 |
| Min | 民 | Nung | 農 | P'ien | 片 | Shou | 手 |
| Ming | 茗 | Nü | 女 | Pin | 賓 | Shu | 朮 |
| Miu | 繆 | O (Ngo) | 鵝 | P'in | 貧 | Shua | 耍 |
| Mo | 蘑 | Ou (Ngou) | 藕 | Ping | 兵 | Shuai | 甩 |
| Mo | 茉 | Pa | 巴 | P'ing | 屏 | Shuan | 拴 |
| Mou | 牡 | P'a | 扒 | Po | 葡 | Shuang | 雙 |
| Mu | 木 | Pai | 白 | P'o | 朴 | Shui | 水 |
| Na | 納 | P'ai | 排 | P'ou | 抔 | Shun | 吮 |
| Nai | 奈 | Pan | 半 | Pu | 不 | Shuo | 說 |
| Nan | 南 | P'an | 判 | P'u | 蒲 | So | 鎖 |
| Nang | 囊 | Pang | 邦 | Sa | 颯 | Sou | 梭 |
| Nao | 腦 | P'ang | 旁 | Sai | 賽 | Ssŭ | 絲 |
| Nêng | 能 | Pao | 包 | San | 三 | Su | 素 |
| Ni | 你 | P'ao | 拋 | Sang | 桑 | Suan | 酸 |
| Niang | 娘 | Pei | 北 | Sao | 騷 | Sui | 碎 |
| Niao | 尿 | P'ei | 佩 | Sê | 色 | Sun | 孫 |
| Nieh | 捏 | Pên | 本 | Sên | 森 | Sung | 松 |

235

|  |  |  |  |  |  |
|---|---|---|---|---|---|
| Ta | 大 | Tou | 豆 | Tso | 左 |
| T'a | 他 | T'ou | 偸 | Ts'o | 挫 |
| Tai | 玳 | Tu | 杜 | Tsou | 走 |
| T'ai | 太 | T'u | 土 | Ts'ou | 湊 |
| Tan | 丹 | Tuan | 端 | Tsu | 足 |
| T'an | 檀 | T'uan | 團 | Ts'u | 粗 |
| Tang | 當 | Tui | 堆 | Tsuan | 攢 |
| T'ang | 糖 | T'ui | 推 | Ts'uan | 竄 |
| Tao | 刀 | Tun | 敦 | Tsui | 嘴 |
| T'ao | 桃 | T'un | 吞 | Ts'ui | 崔 |
| Tê | 得 | Tung | 冬 | Tsun | 尊 |
| T'ê | 特 | T'ung | 同 | Ts'un | 存 |
| Têng | 登 | Tsa | 雜 | Tsung | 宗 |
| T'êng | 藤 | Ts'a | 擦 | Ts'ung | 蔥 |
| Ti | 地 | Tsai | 哉 | Tzǔ | 子 |
| T'i | 提 | Ts'ai | 榮 | Tz'ǔ | 莿 |
| Tiao | 刁 | Tsan | 贊 | Wa | 瓦 |
| T'iao | 條 | Ts'an | 鼉 | Wai | 外 |
| Tieh | 跌 | Tsang | 藏 | Wan | 萬 |
| T'ieh | 鉄 | Ts'ang | 蒼 | Wang | 王 |
| Tien | 點 | Tsao | 糟 | Wei | 威 |
| T'ien | 天 | Ts'ao | 草 | Wên | 文 |
| Ting | 丁 | Tsê | 澤 | Wêng | 翁 |
| T'ing | 尊 | Ts'ê | 側 | Wo | 我 |
| Tiu | 丟 | Tsên | 怎 | Wu | 五 |
| To | 多 | Tsêng | 增 | Ya | 牙 |
| T'o | 佗 | Ts'êng | 層 | Yai | 崖 |

|  |  |
|---|---|
| Yang | 洋 |
| Yao | 藥 |
| Yeh | 葉 |
| Yen | 眼 |
| Yin | 銀 |
| Ying | 櫻 |
| Yu | 油 |
| Yung | 榕 |
| Yü | 郁 |
| Yüeh | 月 |
| Yüan | 元 |
| Yün | 雲 |

# APPENDIX I–B

## A table for the conversion of Pinyin to Wade system

| Pinyin | Wade | Pinyin | Wade | Pinyin | Wade | Pinyin | Wade |
|--------|------|--------|------|--------|------|--------|------|
| a | a | cai | ts'ai | chuang | ch'uang | die | tieh |
| ai | ai | can | ts'an | chui | ch'ui | ding | ting |
| an | an | cang | ts'ang | chun | ch'un | diu | tiu |
| ang | ang | cao | ts'ao | chuo | ch'o | dong | tung |
| ao | ao | ce | ts'ê | ci | tz'ŭ (ts'ŭ) | dou | tou |
| ba | pa | cen | ts'ên | cong | ts'ung | du | tu |
| bai | pai | ceng | ts'êng | cou | ts'ou | duan | tuan |
| ban | pan | cha | ch'a | cu | ts'u | dui | tui |
| bang | pang | chai | ch'ai | cuan | ts'uan | dun | tun |
| bao | pao | chan | ch'an | cui | ts'ui | duo | to |
| bei | pei | chang | ch'ang | cun | ts'un | e | ê, o |
| ben | pên | chao | ch'ao | cuo | ts'o | en | ên |
| beng | pêng | che | ch'ê | da | ta | eng | êng |
| bi | pi | chen | ch'ên | dai | tai | er | êrh |
| bian | pien | cheng | ch'êng | dan | tan | fa | fa |
| biao | piao | chi | ch'ih | dang | tang | fan | fan |
| bie | pieh | chong | ch'ung | dao | tao | fang | fang |
| bin | pin | chou | ch'ou | de | tê | fei | fei |
| bing | ping | chu | ch'u | deng | têng | fen | fên |
| bo | po | chua | ch'ua | di | ti | feng | fêng |
| bu | pu | chuai | ch'uai | dian | tien | fo | fo |
| ca | ts'a | chuan | ch'uan | diao | tiao | fou | fou |

237

| Pinyin | Wade | Pinyin | Wade | Pinyin | Wade | Pinyin | Wade |
|--------|------|--------|------|--------|------|--------|------|
| fu | fu | hei | hei | jun | chün | leng | lêng |
| ga | ka | hen | hên | ka | k'a | li | li |
| gai | kai | heng | hêng | kai | k'ai | lia | lia |
| gan | kan | hong | hung | kan | k'an | lian | lien |
| gang | kang | hou | hou | kang | k'ang | liang | liang |
| gao | kao | hu | hu | kao | k'ao | liao | liao |
| ge | kê, ko | hua | hua | ke | k'ê, k'o | lie | lieh |
| gei | kei | huai | huai | ken | k'ên | lin | lin |
| gen | kên | huan | huan | keng | k'êng | ling | ling |
| geng | kêng | huang | huang | kong | k'ung | liu | liu |
| gong | kung | hui | hui | kou | k'ou | long | lung |
| gou | kou | hun | hun | ku | k'u | lou | lou |
| gu | ku | huo | huo | kua | k'ua | lu | lu |
| gua | kua | ji | chi | kuai | k'uai | lü | lü |
| guai | kuai | jia | chia | kuan | k'uan | luan | luan |
| guan | kuan | jian | chien | kuang | k'uang | lüe | lüeh |
| guang | kuang | jiang | chiang | kui | k'uei | lun | lun |
| gui | kui | jiao | chiao | kun | k'un | luo | lo |
| gun | kun | jie | chieh | kuo | k'uo | ma | ma |
| guo | kuo | jin | chin | la | la | mai | mai |
| ha | ha | jing | ching | lai | lai | man | man |
| hai | hai | jiong | chiung | lan | lan | mang | mang |
| han | han | jiu | chiu | lang | lang | mao | mao |
| hang | hang | ju | chü | lao | lao | me | me |
| hao | hao | juan | chüan | le | lê, lo | mei | mei |
| he | hê, ho | jue | chüeh, chüo | lei | lei | men | mên |

| Pinyin | Wade | Pinyin | Wade | Pinyin | Wade | Pinyin | Wade |
|--------|------|--------|------|--------|------|--------|------|
| meng | mêng | niu | niu | pu | p'u | rui | jui |
| mi | mi | nong | nung | qi | ch'i | run | jun |
| mian | mien | nou | nou | qia | ch'ia | ruo | jo |
| miao | miao | nu | nu | qian | ch'ien | sa | sa |
| mie | mieh | nü | nü | qiang | ch'iang | sai | sai |
| min | min | nuan | nuan | qiao | ch'iao | san | san |
| ming | ming | nüe | nüeh | qie | ch'ieh | sang | sang |
| miu | miu |  | nüo | qin | ch'in | sao | sao |
| mo | mo |  | nio | qing | ch'ing | se | sê |
| mou | mou | nuo | no | qiong | ch'iung | sen | sên |
| mu | mu | o | o | qiu | ch'iu | seng | sêng |
| na | na | ou | ou | qu | ch'ü | sha | sha |
| nai | nai | pa | p'a | quan | ch'üan | shai | shai |
| nan | nan | pai | p'ai | que | ch'üeh | shan | shan |
| nang | nang | pan | p'an | qun | ch'ün | shang | shang |
| nao | nao | pang | p'ang | ran | jan | shao | shao |
| nei | nei | pao | p'ao | rang | jang | she | shê |
| nen | nên, nun | pei | p'ei | rao | jao | shei | shei |
| neng | nêng | pen | p'ên | re | jê | shen | shên |
| ni | ni | peng | p'êng | ren | jên | sheng | shêng |
| nian | nien | pi | p'i | reng | jêng | shi | shih |
| niang | niang | pian | p'ien | ri | jih | shou | shou |
| niao | niao | piao | p'iao | rong | jung | shu | shu |
| nie | nieh | pie | p'ieh | rou | jou | shua | shua |
| nin | nin | pin | p'in | ru | ju | shuai | shuai |
| ning | ning | ping | p'ing | ruan | juan | shuan | shuan |
|  |  | po | p'o |  |  |  |  |
|  |  | pou | p'ou |  |  |  |  |

| Pinyin | Wade | Pinyin | Wade | Pinyin | Wade | Pinyin | Wade |
|--------|------|--------|------|--------|------|--------|------|
| shuang | shuang | tu | t'u | xue | hsüeh, hsüo | zha | cha |
| shui | shui | tuan | t'uan | xun | hsün | zhai | chai |
| shun | shun | tui | t'ui | ya | ya, yai | zhan | chan |
| shuo | shuo | tun | t'un | yan | yen | zhang | chang |
| si | sŭ, szŭ, ssŭ | tuo | t'o | yang | yang | zhao | chao |
| song | sung | wa | wa | yao | yao | zhe | chê |
| sou | sou | wai | wai | ye | yeh | zhei | chei |
| su | su | wan | wan | yi | i, yi | zhen | chên |
| suan | suan | wang | wang | yin | yin | zheng | chêng |
| sui | sui | wei | wei | ying | ying | zhi | chih |
| sun | sun | wen | wên | yo | yo | zhong | chung |
| suo | so | weng | wêng | yong | yu | zhou | chou |
| ta | t'a | wo | wo | you | yung | zhu | chu |
| tai | t'ai | wu | wu | yu | yü | zhua | chua |
| tan | t'an | xi | hsi | yuan | yüan | zhuai | chuai |
| tang | t'ang | xia | hsia | yue | yüeh | zhuan | chuan |
| tao | t'ao | xian | hsien | yun | yün | zhuang | chuang |
| te | t'ê | xiang | hsiang | za | tsa | zhui | chui |
| teng | t'êng | xiao | hsiao | zai | tsai | zhun | chun |
| ti | t'i | xie | hsieh | zan | tsan | zhou | cho |
| tian | t'ien | xin | hsin | zang | tsang | zi | tzŭ (tsŭ) |
| tiao | t'iao | xing | hsing | zao | tsao | zong | tsung |
| tie | t'ieh | xiong | hsiung | ze | tsê | zou | tsou |
| ting | t'ing | xiu | hsiu | zei | tsei | zu | tsu |
| tong | t'ung | xu | hsü | zen | tsên | zuan | tsuan |
| tou | t'ou | xuan | hsüan | zeng | tsêng | zui | tsui |
| | | | | | | zun | tsun |
| | | | | | | zuo | tso |

A List of Families with Reference Numbers or Abbreviations

Acanthaceae 266
Aceraceae 163
Adiantaceae (F26)
Aizoaceae 84
Alangiaceae 220b
Algae (Alg)
Alismataceae 15
Amarantaceae 79
Amaryllidaceae 40
Anacardiaceae 153
Angiopteridaceae (F9)
Anonaceae 98
Apocynaceae 247
Aquifoliaceae 157
Aquilariaceae 214a
Araceae 23
Araliaceae 227
Aristolochiaceae 74
Asclepiadaceae 248
Ascomycetes (A-myc)
Aspleniaceae (F30)

Balsaminaceae 168

Basidiomycetes (B-myc)
Begoniaceae 208
Berberidaceae 93
Betulaceae 61
Bignoniaceae 258
Blechnaceae (F32)
Bombacaceae 177
Boraginaceae 252
Botrychiaceae (F7)
Bryophytes (Bryo)
Burmanniaceae 49
Burseraceae 139
Buxaceae 149

Cactaceae 210
Calycanthaceae 96
Campanulaceae 276
Cannaceae 47
Capparidaceae 107
Caprifoliaceae 271
Caricaceae 205
Caryophyllaceae 87
Celastraceae 158

Cephalotaxaceae 5b
Chenopodiaceae 78
Chloranthaceae 54
Combretaceae 221
Commelinaceae 33
Compositae 280
Convolvulaceae 249
Coriariaceae 151
Cornaceae 229
Crassulaceae 115
Cruciferae 105
Cucurbitaceae 275
Cupressaceae 6c
Cycadaceae 1
Cynomoriaceae 226
Cyperaceae 20

Daphniphyllaceae 147a
Davalliaceae (F21)
Dicksoniaceae (F18)
Dilleniaceae 180
Dioscoreaceae 43
Dipsacaceae 274

Dipteridaceae (F41)
Dipterocarpaceae 188
Dryopteridaceae (F37)

Ebenaceae 240
Elaeagnaceae 215
Ephedraceae 7
Equisetaceae (F5)
Ericaceae 233
Eriocaulaceae 30
Erythroxylaceae 134
Eucommiaceae 123a
Euphorbiaceae 147

Fagaceae 62
Flacourtiaceae 199

Gasteromycete (G-myc)
Gentianaceae 246
Geraniaceae 129
Gesneriaceae 262
Ginkgoaceae 4
Gnetaceae 7a
Gramineae 19

Guttiferae 187

Hamamelidaceae 123
Hippocastanaceae 164
Hydrocaryaceae 224a

Illiciaceae 95c
Iridaceae 44

Juglandaceae 60
Juncaceae 36

Labiatae 254
Lardizabalaceae 92
Lauraceae 102
Leguminosae 128
Lemnaceae 24
Lichens (Lich)
Liliaceae 38
Linaceae 132
Lindsaeaceae (F20)
Loganiaceae 245
Loranthaceae 67
Lygodiaceae (F12)
Lythraceae 216

Magnoliaceae 95

Malvaceae 175
Marantaceae 48
Marsileaceae (F48)
Melastomataceae 223
Meliaceae 140
Moraceae 64
Musaceae 45
Myricaceae 57
Myristicaceae 99
Myrsinaceae 236
Myrtaceae 222

Nepenthaceae 111
Nyctaginaceae 80
Nymphaeaceae 88
Nyssaceae 220a

Oleaceae 243
Onagraceae 224
Ophioglossaceae (F6)
Orchidaceae 50
Orobanchaceae 261
Osmundaceae (F10)
Oxalidaceae 130

Palmae 21
Pandanaceae 9
Papaveraceae 104

Passifloraceae 203
Pedaliaceae 259
Philydraceae 35
Phytolaccaceae 83
Pinaceae 6
Piperaceae 53
Pittosporaceae 118
Plantaginaceae 269
Plumbaginaceae 238
Podophyllaceae 93a
Polygalaceae 145
Polygonaceae 77
Polypodiaceae (F42)
Pontederiaceae 34
Portulacaceae 85
Potamogetonaceae 11
Primulaceae 237
Proteaceae 66
Psilotaceae (F1)
Pteridaceae (F24)
Punicaceae 218
Pyrolaceae 231

Ranunculaceae 91
Rhamnaceae 169
Rosaceae 126
Rubiaceae 270

Rutaceae 137

Salicaceae 56
Salviniaceae (F49)
Santalaceae 69
Sapindaceae 165
Saururaceae 52
Saxifragaceae 117
Schisandraceae 95d
Scrophulariaceae 257
Selaginellaceae (F3)
Simaroubaceae 138
Sinopteridaceae (F25)
Solanaceae 256
Sparganiaceae 10
Stachyuraceae 200
Staphyleaceae 161
Stemonaceae 37
Sterculiaceae 178
Styracaceae 241
Symplocaceae 242

Taccaceae 42
Tamaricaceae 191
Taxaceae 5
Taxodiaceae 6a
Theaceae 186

Thelypteridaceae (F31)      Ulmaceae 63         Valerianaceae 273      Woodsiaceae (F34)
Thymelaeaceae 214          Umbelliferae 228    Verbenaceae 253
Tiliaceae 174              Urticaceae 65       Violaceae 198          Zingiberaceae 46
Typhaceae 8                                    Vitaceae 170           Zygophyllaceae 135

# APPENDIX II–B

## A Generic List with Family Numbers or Abbreviations
## Indicating the Position of Each Genus in Part II

Abacopteris F31          Actinodaphne 102      Akebia 92            Amomum 46
Abelia 271               Adenophora 276        Alangium 220b        Amorphophallus 23
Abelmoschus 175          Adenosma 257          Albizzia 128         Ampelocissus 170
Abrus 128                Adhatoda 266          Aleurites 147        Ampelopsis 170
Abutilon 175             Adiantum F26          Aleuritopteris F25   Anaphalis 280
Acacia 128               Adina 270             Alhagi 128           Andrographis 266
Acalypha 147             Adonis 91             Alisma 15            Androsace 237
Acanthopanax 227         Aeginetia 261         Allium 38            Anemarrhena 38
Acanthus 266             Aeschynomene 128      Alocasia 23          Anemone 91
Acer 163                 Aesculus 164          Aloe 38              Anethum 228
Achillea 280             Agaricus (B-myc)      Alpinia 46           Angelica 228
Achnatherum 19           Agastache 254         Alstonia 247         Angiopteris F9
Achyranthes 79           Aglaonema 23          Alternanthera 79     Anisodus 256
Aconitum 91              Agrimonia 126         Althaea 175          Anisomeles 254
Acorus 23                Ailanthus 138         Amaranthus 79        Antenoron 77
Acronychia 137           Ainsliaea 280         Amitostigma 50       Antiaris 64
Actinidia 180            Ajuga 254             Ammannia 216         Apios 128
                                                                    Apluda 19

Apocynum 247
Aquilaria 214a
Aquilegia 91
Aralia 227
Arcangelisia 94
Arctium 280
Ardisia 236
Areca 21
Arenaria 87
Argyreia 249
Arisaema 23
Aristolochia 74
Armillaria (B-myc)
Arnebia 252
Artemisia 280
Artocarpus 64
Asarum 74
Asparagus 38
Asplenium F30
Aster 280
Astilbe 117
Astragalus 128
Atalantia 137
Atractylodes 280
Atropa 256
Aucklandia 280
Aucuba 229
Auricularia (B-myc)
Avena 19

Averrhoa 130

Baeckea 222
Balanocarpus 188
Bambusa 19
Baphicacanthus 266
Bauhinia 128
Beesia 91
Begonia 208
Belamcanda 44
Benincasa 275
Berberis 93
Berchemia 169
Bergenia 117
Beta 78
Betula 61
Bidens 280
Biota 6c
Blechnum F32
Bletilla 50
Blumea 280
Boehmeria 65
Bolbostemma 275
Bombax 177
Boschniakia 261
Boswellia 139
Bothriospermum 252
Botrychium F7
Bougainvillea 80

Brassica 105
Breynia 147
Broussonetia 64
Brucea 138
Bryophyllum 115
Bulbophyllum 50
Buchnera 257
Buddleia 245
Bupleurum 228
Burmannia 49
Buxus 149

Caesalpinia 128
Caladium 23
Callicarpa 253
Calligonum 77
Caloglossa (Alg)
Calophyllum 187
Caltha 91
Calvatia (G-myc)
Calystegia 249
Camellia 186
Campanumoea 276
Campsis 258
Camptandra 46
Camptotheca 220a
Campylotropis 128
Canarium 139

Canavalia 128
Canna 47
Cannabis 64
Capparis 107
Capsella 105
Capsicum 256
Caragana 128
Cardamine 105
Cardiandra 117
Cardiocrinum 38
Cardiospermum 165
Carex 20
Carica 205
Carpesium 280
Carthamus 280
Carum 228
Carya 60
Caryopteris 253
Cassia 128
Cassytha 102
Castanea 62
Catharanthus 247
Caulokaempferia 46
Cayratia 170
Celastrus 158
Celosia 79
Celtis 63
Centella 228
Centipeda 280

Cephaelis 270
Cephalanoplos 280
Cephalanthus 270
Cephalotaxus 5b
Ceratostigma 238
Cercis 128
Chaenomeles 126
Chamaenerion 224
Chamaerhodos 126
Championella 266
Changium 228
Chelidonium 104
Chenopodium 78
Chimonanthus 96
Chloranthus 54
Chlorophytum 38
Choerospondias 153
Chrysanthemum 280
Cibotium F18
Cicuta 228
Cimicifuga 91
Cinchona 270
Cinnamomum 102
Cirsium 280
Cissampelos 94
Cissus 170
Cistanche 261
Citrullus 275

Citrus 137
Cladonia (Lich)
Claoxylon 147
Clausena 137
Claviceps (A-myc)
Cleistocalyx 222
Clematis 91
Cleome 107
Clerodendrum 253
Clitocybe (B-myc)
Cnidium 228
Cocculus 94
Cocos 21
Codium (Alg)
Codonopsis 276
Coffea 270
Coix 19
Collen 128
Colocasia 23
Commelina 33
Commiphora 139
Convolvulus 249
Coptis 91
Cordyceps (A-myc)
Cordyline 38
Coriaria 151
Coriandrum 228
Coriolus (B-myc)
Cornus 229
Corydalis 104

Corylus 61
Costus 46
Cotinus 153
Cotoneaster 126
Craspedolobium 128
Crataegus 126
Cratoxylon 187
Cremanthodium 280
Cremastra 50
Crepis 280
Crinum 38
Crocus 44
Crossostephium 280
Crotalaria 128
Croton 147
Cryptotaenia 228
Cucumis 275
Cucurbita 275
Cudrania 64
Cunninghamia 6a
Curculigo 40
Curcuma 46
Cuscuta 249
Cyathula 79
Cycas 1
Cyclea 94
Cydonia 126
Cymbopogon 19
Cynanchum 248

Cynodon 19
Cynoglossum 252
Cynomorium 226
Cyperus 20
Cypripedium 50
Cyrtomium F37

Dactylicapnos 104
Daemonorops 21
Dalbergia 128
Damnacanthus 270
Daphne 214
Daphniphyllum 147a
Dasiphora 126
Datura 256
Daucus 228
Debregeasia 64
Delanda 128
Delphinium 91
Dendrobium 50
Dendropanax 227
Derris 128
Desmodium 128
Desmos 98
Dianthus 87
Dichocarpum 91
Dichondra 249
Dichroa 117
Dicliptera 266

Haematoxylon 128
Hedera 227
Hedychium 46
Hedyotis 270
Hedysarum 128
Helicia 66
Helicteres 178
Heliotropium 252
Helleborus 91
Helminthostachys F8
Helwingia 229
Hemerocallis 38
Hemipilia 50
Heracleum 228
Heteropanax 227
Heteropogon 19
Hibiscus 175
Hippophae 215
Hocquartia=Aristolochia
    74
Homalomena 23
Hopea 188
Hordeum 19
Hosta 38
Houttuynia 52
Hovenia 153
Hoya 248
Humata F41
Humulus 64
Hydnocarpus 199

Hydrangea 117
Hydrocotyle 228
Hygrophila 266
Hylocereus 210
Hyoscyamus 256
Hypericum 187
Hypoëstes 266
Hypoxis 40
Hypserpa 94

Ilex 157
Illicium 95c
Impatiens 168
Imperata 19
Indigofera 128
Inula 280
Iphigenia 38
Ipomoea 249
Iris 44
Isatis 105
Isodon 254
Ixeris 280
Ixora 270

Jasminum 243
Juglans 60
Juncus 36
Juniperus 6c
Jussiaea 224

Justicia 266

Kadsura 95d
Kaempferia 46
Kalanchoe 115
Kalimeris 280
Kalopanax 227
Knoxia 270
Kochia 78
Koelreuteria 165
Kummerowia 128
Kyllinga 20

Lactuca 280
Lagenaria 275
Lagerstroemia 216
Laggera 280
Laminaria (Alg)
Lamium 254
Lantana 253
Laportea 65
Lasiosphaera (G-myc)
Laurus 102
Ledebouriella 228
Leersia 19
Leibnitzia 280
Lemna 24
Lentinus (B-myc)
Leonurus 254

Lepidium 105
Lepisorus F42
Leptochloa 19
Lespedeza 128
Leucas 254
Ligularia 280
Ligusticum 228
Ligustrum 243
Lilium 38
Limnanthemum=Nymphoides
    246
Limnophila 257
Lindera 102
Lindernia 257
Linum 132
Liparis 50
Lippia 253
Liquidambar 123
Liriope 38
Litchi 165
Lithocarpus 62
Lithospermum 252
Litsea 102
Livistona 21
Lobaria (Lich)
Lobelia 276
Lodoicea 21
Lonicera 271
Lophatherum 19
Loranthus 67

247

Loropetalum 123
Lotus 128
Luculia 270
Ludisia 50
Ludwigia 224
Luffa 275
Luzula 36
Lychnis 87
Lycium 256
Lycoperdon (G-myc)
Lycopodium F2
Lycopus 254
Lycoris 40
Lygodium F12
Lysimachia 237
Lysionotus 262

Machilus 102
Macleaya 104
Maesa 236
Magnolia 95
Mahonia 93
Malcolmia 105
Mallotus 147
Malva 175
Mangifera 153
Marchantia (Bryo)
Marsdenia 248

Marsilea F48
Meconopsis 104
Medicago 128
Melaleuca 222
Melastoma 223
Melia 140
Melilotus 128
Melodinus 247
Melothria 275
Menispermum 94
Mentha 254
Mesona 254
Metaplexis 248
Michelia 95
Microcos 174
Micromelum 137
Microtoena 254
Millettia 128
Mimosa 128
Mirabilis 80
Mnium (Bryo)
Moghania 128
Mollugo 84
Momordica 275
Monascus (A-myc)
**Monochoria 34**
Monotropa 231
Morchella (A-myc)

Morina 274
Morinda 270
Morus 64
Mosla 254
Munronia 140
Murraya 137
Musa 45
Musella 45
Mussaenda 270
Myrica 57
Myricaria 191
Myristica 99
Myrsine 236

Nandina 93
Narcissus 40
Nardostachys 273
Nauclea 270
Nelumbo 88
Nepenthes 111
Nepeta 254
Nephrolepis F21
Nerium 247
Nicotiana 256
Nostoc (Alg)
Notopterygium 228
Nymphoides 246

Ocimum 254

Oenanthe 228
Oenothera 224
Oldenlandia 270
Omphalia (B-myc)
Onosma 252
Ophioglossum F6
Ophiopogon 38
Ophiorrhiza 270
Oplopanax 227
Opuntia 210
Origanum 254
Orixa 137
Orostachys 115
Oroxylum 258
Orthodon 254
Orthosiphon 254
Oryza 19
Osbeckia 223
Osmanthus 243
Osmunda F10
Oxalis 130
Oxyria 77
Oxytropis 128

Pachyrhizus 128
Pachysandra 149
Paederia 270
Paeonia 91

Rhododendron 233
Rhodomyrtus 222
Rhoeo 33
Rhus 153
Ribes 117
Ricinus 147
Robinia 128
Rohdea 38
Rorippa 105
Rosa 126
Roscoea 46
Rubia 270
Rubus 126
Ruellia 257
Rumex 77
Ruta 137

Saccharum 19
Sagittaria 15
Salix 56
Salsola 78
Salvia 254
Salvinia F49
Sambucus 271
Sanguisorba 126
Saposhnikovia 228
Santalum 69
Sapindus 165

Sapium 147
Saponaria 87
Saposhnikovia 228
Sarcandra 54
Sarcanthus 50
Sarcococca 149
Sargassum (Alg)
Sargentodoxa 92
Sassafras 102
Saurauia 180
Sauropus 147
Saururus 52
Saussurea 280
Saxifraga 117
Saxiglossum F42
Scaphium 178
Schefflera 227
Schisandra 95d
Schizocapsa 42
Schizonepeta 254
Scilla 38
Scirpus 20
Scoparia 257
Scopolia 256
Scorzonera 280
Scrophularia 257
Scurrula 67
Scutellaria 254
Securinega 147
Sedum 115

Selaginella F3
Semiaquilegia 91
Senecio 280
Serissa 270
Sesamum 259
Setaria 19
Shiraia (A-myc)
Shorea 188
Shuteria 128
Siegesbeckia 280
Sida 175
Silene 87
Sinomenium 94
Siphonostegia 257
Siraitia 275
Skimmia 137
Smilax 38
Smithia 128
Solanum 256
Solena 275
Solidago 280
Sonchus 280
Sophora 128
Sorbus 126
Sorghum 19
Sparganium 10
Spatholobus 128
Speranskia 147
Spilanthes 280
Spiranthes 50

Spirodela 24
Stachys 254
Stachytarpheta 253
Stachyurus 200
Stahlianthus 46
Stauntonia 92
Stellaria 87
Stellera 214
Stemona 37
Stenoloma F20
Stephania 94
Sterculia 178
Stereocaulon (Lich)
Streptocaulon 248
Striga 257
Strophanthus 247
Strychnos 245
Styrax 241
Swertia 246
Symphytum 252
Syringa 243
Symplocos 242
Syzygium 222

Tacca 42
Tagetes 280
Talinum 85
Tamarindus 128
Tamarix 191

Tanacetum 280
Taraxacum 280
Taxillus 67
Taxus 5
Tephrosia 128
Terminalia 221
Tetracera 180
Tetrapanax 227
Tetrastigma 170
Teucrium 254
Thalictrum 91
Thermopsis 128
Thesium 69
Thevetia 247
Thlaspi 105
Thuja 6c
Thunbergia 266
Thymus 214
Tilia 174
Tinospora 94
Toddalia 137
Tongoloa 228
Toona 140

Torreya 5
Trachelospermum 247
Trachycarpus 21
Tradescantia 33
Trapa 224a
Tremella (B-myc)
Tribulus 135
Tricholoma (B-myc)
Trichosanthes 275
Trifolium 128
Trigonella 128
Triosteum 271
Tripterygium 158
Triticum 19
Trollius 91
Tulipa 38
Tussilago 280
Tylophora 248
Typha 8
Typhonium 23

Ulmus 63

Ulva (Alg)
Umbilicaria (B-myc)
Uncaria 270
Undaria (Alg)
Urena 175
Urginea 38
Usnea (lich)

Vaccaria 87
Vaccinium 233
Valeriana 273
Ventilago 169
Veratrum 38
Verbena 253
Vernonia 280
Veronica 257
Veronicastrum 257
Viburnum 271
Vicia 128
Vigna 128
Viola 198
Viscum 67

Vitex 253
Vitis 170
Vladimiria 280

Wedelia 280
Wikstroemia 214
Wisteria 128
Woodsia F34
Woodwardia F32
Wrightia 247

Xanthium 280
Xanthoceras 165

Youngia 280

Zanthoxylum 137
Zea 19
Zehneria 257
Zingiber 46
Zizania 19
Zizyphus 169
Zornia 128

# APPENDIX III

# The Conversion of Simplified Chinese Characters

# into Classical Form

| | | | | | | | | | | | | | |
|---|---|---|---|---|---|---|---|---|---|---|---|---|---|
| 2畫 | 门[門] | 区[區] | 为[爲] | 戋[戔] | 叽[嘰] | [彙] | 发[發] | 扫[掃] | 划[劃] | 则[則] | 伪[僞] | 冲[衝] | 讶[訝] |
| 厂[廠] | 义[義] | 车[車] | 斗[鬥] | 扑[撲] | 叹[嘆] | 头[頭] | [髮] | 扬[揚] | 迈[邁] | 刚[剛] | 向[嚮] | 妆[妝] | 讷[訥] |
| 卜[蔔] | 卫[衛] | 【丨】 | 忆[憶] | 节[節] | 【丿】 | 汉[漢] | 圣[聖] | 场[場] | 毕[畢] | 网[網] | 后[後] | 庄[莊] | 许[許] |
| 儿[兒] | 飞[飛] | 冈[岡] | 订[訂] | 术[術] | 们[們] | 宁[寧] | 对[對] | 亚[亞] | 【丨】 | 【丿】 | 会[會] | 庆[慶] | 讹[訛] |
| 几[幾] | 习[習] | 贝[貝] | 计[計] | 龙[龍] | 仪[儀] | 讦[訐] | 台[臺] | 芗[薌] | 贞[貞] | 钆[釓] | 杀[殺] | 刘[劉] | 论[論] |
| 了[瞭] | 马[馬] | 见[見] | 讣[訃] | 厉[厲] | 丛[叢] | 讧[訌] | [檯] | 朴[樸] | 师[師] | 钇[釔] | 合[閤] | 齐[齊] | 讼[訟] |
| 3畫 | 乡[鄉] | 【丿】 | 认[認] | 灭[滅] | 尔[爾] | 讨[討] | [颱] | 机[機] | 当[當] | 朱[硃] | 众[衆] | 产[産] | 讽[諷] |
| 干[乾] | 4畫 | 气[氣] | 讥[譏] | 东[東] | 乐[樂] | 写[寫] | 纠[糾] | 权[權] | 尘[塵] | 迁[遷] | 爷[爺] | 闭[閉] | 农[農] |
| [幹] | 【一】 | 长[長] | 【一】 | 轧[軋] | 处[處] | 让[讓] | 驭[馭] | 过[過] | 吁[籲] | 乔[喬] | 伞[傘] | 问[問] | 设[設] |
| 亏[虧] | 丰[豐] | 仆[僕] | 丑[醜] | 【丨】 | 冬[鼕] | 礼[禮] | 丝[絲] | 协[協] | 吓[嚇] | 伟[偉] | 创[創] | 闯[闖] | 访[訪] |
| 才[纔] | 开[開] | 币[幣] | 队[隊] | 卢[盧] | 鸟[鳥] | 讪[訕] | 6畫 | 压[壓] | 虫[蟲] | 传[傳] | 杂[雜] | 关[關] | 诀[訣] |
| 万[萬] | 无[無] | 从[從] | 办[辦] | 业[業] | 务[務] | 讫[訖] | 【一】 | 厌[厭] | 曲[麯] | 伛[傴] | 负[負] | 灯[燈] | 【一】 |
| 与[與] | 韦[韋] | 仑[侖] | 邓[鄧] | 旧[舊] | 刍[芻] | 训[訓] | 玑[璣] | 库[庫] | 团[團] | 优[優] | 犷[獷] | 汤[湯] | 寻[尋] |
| 千[韆] | 专[專] | 仓[倉] | 劝[勸] | 帅[帥] | 饥[饑] | 议[議] | 动[動] | 页[頁] | [糰] | 伤[傷] | 犸[獁] | 忏[懺] | 尽[盡] |
| 亿[億] | 云[雲] | 风[風] | 双[雙] | 归[歸] | 【丶】 | 讯[訊] | 执[執] | 夸[誇] | 吗[嗎] | 伥[倀] | 凫[鳧] | 兴[興] | [儘] |
| 个[個] | 艺[藝] | 仅[僅] | 书[書] | 叶[葉] | 邝[鄺] | 记[記] | 巩[鞏] | 夺[奪] | 屿[嶼] | 价[價] | 邬[鄔] | 讲[講] | 导[導] |
| 么[麽] | 厅[廳] | 凤[鳳] | 5畫 | 号[號] | 冯[馮] | 【一】 | 圹[壙] | 达[達] | 岁[歲] | 伦[倫] | 饦[飥] | 讳[諱] | 孙[孫] |
| 广[廣] | 历[歷] | 乌[烏] | 【一】 | 电[電] | 闪[閃] | 辽[遼] | 扩[擴] | 夹[夾] | 回[迴] | 伧[傖] | 饧[餳] | 讴[謳] | 阵[陣] |
| | [曆] | 【丶】 | 击[擊] | 只[隻] | 兰[蘭] | 边[邊] | 扪[捫] | 轨[軌] | 岂[豈] | 华[華] | 【丶】 | 军[軍] | |
| | | 闩[門] | | [祇] | 汇[匯] | 出[齣] | | 尧[堯] | | 伙[夥] | 壮[壯] | | |

| | | | | | | | | | | | | | |
|---|---|---|---|---|---|---|---|---|---|---|---|---|---|
| 阳〔陽〕 | 寿〔壽〕 | 块〔塊〕 | 歼〔殲〕 | 听〔聽〕 | 邻〔鄰〕 | 这〔這〕 | 怆〔愴〕 | 陆〔陸〕 | 驴〔驢〕 | 茏〔蘢〕 | 码〔碼〕 | 黾〔黽〕 | 钏〔釧〕 |
| 阶〔階〕 | 麦〔麥〕 | 声〔聲〕 | 来〔來〕 | 呛〔嗆〕 | 肠〔腸〕 | 庐〔廬〕 | 穷〔窮〕 | 陇〔隴〕 | 纼〔紖〕 | 苹〔蘋〕 | 厕〔廁〕 | 鸣〔鳴〕 | 钦〔欽〕 |
| 阴〔陰〕 | 玛〔瑪〕 | 报〔報〕 | 欤〔歟〕 | 呜〔嗚〕 | 龟〔龜〕 | 闰〔閏〕 | 证〔證〕 | 陈〔陳〕 | 纽〔紐〕 | 茑〔蔦〕 | 奋〔奮〕 | 咛〔嚀〕 | 钧〔鈞〕 |
| 妇〔婦〕 | 进〔進〕 | 拟〔擬〕 | 轩〔軒〕 | 别〔彆〕 | 犹〔猶〕 | 闱〔闈〕 | 诂〔詁〕 | 坠〔墜〕 | 纾〔紓〕 | 范〔範〕 | 态〔態〕 | 咝〔噝〕 | 钫〔鈁〕 |
| 妈〔媽〕 | 远〔遠〕 | 㧑〔撝〕 | 连〔連〕 | 财〔財〕 | 狈〔狽〕 | 闲〔閑〕 | 诃〔訶〕 | 陉〔陘〕 | **8畫** | 荦〔犖〕 | 瓯〔甌〕 | 罗〔羅〕 | 刿〔劌〕 |
| 戏〔戲〕 | 违〔違〕 | 芜〔蕪〕 | 轫〔軔〕 | 囵〔圇〕 | 鸠〔鳩〕 | 间〔間〕 | 词〔詞〕 | 妫〔媯〕 | 【一】 | 茎〔莖〕 | 殴〔毆〕 | 岽〔崬〕 | 侠〔俠〕 |
| 观〔觀〕 | 韧〔韌〕 | 苇〔葦〕 | 【丨】 | 帏〔幃〕 | 岛〔島〕 | 闵〔閔〕 | 评〔評〕 | 妩〔嫵〕 | 玮〔瑋〕 | 枢〔樞〕 | 垄〔壟〕 | 帜〔幟〕 | 侥〔僥〕 |
| 欢〔歡〕 | 划〔劃〕 | 芸〔蕓〕 | 卤〔鹵〕 | 岗〔崗〕 | 邹〔鄒〕 | 闷〔悶〕 | 诅〔詛〕 | 妪〔嫗〕 | 环〔環〕 | 枥〔櫪〕 | 郏〔郟〕 | 岭〔嶺〕 | 侦〔偵〕 |
| 买〔買〕 | 运〔運〕 | 苈〔藶〕 | 〔滷〕 | 岘〔峴〕 | 饨〔飩〕 | 灿〔燦〕 | 识〔識〕 | 妊〔姙〕 | 责〔責〕 | 柜〔櫃〕 | 轰〔轟〕 | 岖〔嶇〕 | 侧〔側〕 |
| 纡〔紆〕 | 抚〔撫〕 | 苋〔莧〕 | 邺〔鄴〕 | 帐〔帳〕 | 饧〔餳〕 | 灶〔竈〕 | 诈〔詐〕 | 驱〔驅〕 | 现〔現〕 | 㭎〔棡〕 | 顷〔頃〕 | 凯〔凱〕 | 凭〔憑〕 |
| 红〔紅〕 | 坛〔壇〕 | 苁〔蓯〕 | 坚〔堅〕 | 岚〔嵐〕 | 饪〔飪〕 | 炀〔煬〕 | 诉〔訴〕 | 纯〔純〕 | 表〔錶〕 | 枧〔梘〕 | 转〔轉〕 | 峄〔嶧〕 | 侨〔僑〕 |
| 纣〔紂〕 | 〔罎〕 | 苍〔蒼〕 | 时〔時〕 | 【丿】 | 饫〔飫〕 | 沣〔灃〕 | 诊〔診〕 | 纰〔紕〕 | 玱〔瑲〕 | 枨〔棖〕 | 轭〔軛〕 | 败〔敗〕 | 侩〔儈〕 |
| 驮〔馱〕 | 抟〔摶〕 | 严〔嚴〕 | 旷〔曠〕 | 针〔針〕 | 饬〔飭〕 | 沤〔漚〕 | 诒〔詒〕 | 纱〔紗〕 | 规〔規〕 | 板〔闆〕 | 斩〔斬〕 | 账〔賬〕 | 货〔貨〕 |
| 纤〔縴〕 | 坏〔壞〕 | 芦〔蘆〕 | 旸〔暘〕 | 钉〔釘〕 | 饭〔飯〕 | 沥〔瀝〕 | 诎〔詘〕 | 纲〔綱〕 | 匦〔匭〕 | 枞〔樅〕 | 轮〔輪〕 | 贩〔販〕 | 侪〔儕〕 |
| 〔纖〕 | 抠〔摳〕 | 劳〔勞〕 | 呒〔嘸〕 | 钊〔釗〕 | 饮〔飲〕 | 沦〔淪〕 | 诏〔詔〕 | 纳〔納〕 | 拢〔攏〕 | 松〔鬆〕 | 软〔軟〕 | 贬〔貶〕 | 侬〔儂〕 |
| 纥〔紇〕 | 坜〔壢〕 | 克〔剋〕 | 县〔縣〕 | 钋〔釙〕 | 系〔係〕 | 沧〔滄〕 | 译〔譯〕 | 纴〔紝〕 | 拣〔揀〕 | 枪〔槍〕 | 鸢〔鳶〕 | 贮〔貯〕 | 质〔質〕 |
| 驯〔馴〕 | 扰〔擾〕 | 苏〔蘇〕 | 里〔裏〕 | 钌〔釕〕 | 〔繫〕 | 沨〔渢〕 | 灵〔靈〕 | 驳〔駁〕 | 垆〔壚〕 | 枫〔楓〕 | 【丨】 | 图〔圖〕 | 征〔徵〕 |
| 纨〔紈〕 | 坝〔壩〕 | 极〔極〕 | 呓〔囈〕 | 乱〔亂〕 | 【丶】 | 沟〔溝〕 | 层〔層〕 | 纵〔縱〕 | 担〔擔〕 | 构〔構〕 | 齿〔齒〕 | 购〔購〕 | 径〔徑〕 |
| 约〔約〕 | 贡〔貢〕 | 杨〔楊〕 | 园〔園〕 | 体〔體〕 | 冻〔凍〕 | 沩〔溈〕 | 迟〔遲〕 | 纶〔綸〕 | 顶〔頂〕 | 丧〔喪〕 | 虏〔虜〕 | 【丿】 | 舍〔捨〕 |
| 级〔級〕 | 抡〔掄〕 | 两〔兩〕 | 呖〔嚦〕 | 佣〔傭〕 | 状〔狀〕 | 沪〔滬〕 | 张〔張〕 | 纷〔紛〕 | 拥〔擁〕 | 画〔畫〕 | 肾〔腎〕 | 钍〔釷〕 | 刽〔劊〕 |
| 纩〔纊〕 | 折〔摺〕 | 丽〔麗〕 | 围〔圍〕 | 彻〔徹〕 | 亩〔畝〕 | 沈〔瀋〕 | 际〔際〕 | 纸〔紙〕 | 势〔勢〕 | 枣〔棗〕 | 贤〔賢〕 | 钎〔釺〕 | 郐〔鄶〕 |
| 纪〔紀〕 | 抢〔搶〕 | 医〔醫〕 | 吨〔噸〕 | 余〔餘〕 | 庑〔廡〕 | 怀〔懷〕 | | 纹〔紋〕 | 拦〔攔〕 | 卖〔賣〕 | 昙〔曇〕 | 钐〔釤〕 | 怂〔慫〕 |
| 驰〔馳〕 | 坞〔塢〕 | 励〔勵〕 | 邮〔郵〕 | 佥〔僉〕 | 库〔庫〕 | 忧〔憂〕 | | 纺〔紡〕 | 㧟〔擓〕 | 郁〔鬱〕 | 国〔國〕 | 钓〔釣〕 | 籴〔糴〕 |
| 纫〔紉〕 | 坟〔墳〕 | 还〔還〕 | 困〔睏〕 | 谷〔穀〕 | 疗〔療〕 | 忾〔愾〕 | | | 拧〔擰〕 | 矾〔礬〕 | 畅〔暢〕 | 钒〔釩〕 | 觅〔覓〕 |
| **7畫** | 护〔護〕 | 矶〔磯〕 | 员〔員〕 | | 应〔應〕 | 怅〔悵〕 | | | 拨〔撥〕 | 矿〔礦〕 | 咙〔嚨〕 | 钔〔鍆〕 | 贪〔貪〕 |
| 【一】 | 壳〔殼〕 | | 呗〔唄〕 | | | | | | 择〔擇〕 | 砀〔碭〕 | 虮〔蟣〕 | | 贫〔貧〕 |
| | 奁〔奩〕 | | | | | | | | | | | | |

| | | | | | | | | | | | | | |
|---|---|---|---|---|---|---|---|---|---|---|---|---|---|
| 戗〔戧〕 | 闸〔閘〕 | 诓〔誆〕 | 肃〔肅〕 | 绡〔綃〕 | 挠〔撓〕 | 荮〔葤〕 | 面〔麵〕 | 眬〔矓〕 | 贴〔貼〕 | 钯〔鈀〕 | 鸲〔鴝〕 | 亲〔親〕 | 浇〔澆〕 |
| 肤〔膚〕 | 闹〔鬧〕 | 诔〔誄〕 | 隶〔隸〕 | 驻〔駐〕 | 赵〔趙〕 | 药〔藥〕 | 牵〔牽〕 | 哑〔啞〕 | 贶〔貺〕 | 毡〔氈〕 | 狭〔狹〕 | 飒〔颯〕 | 浈〔湞〕 |
| 䏝〔膞〕 | 郑〔鄭〕 | 试〔試〕 | 录〔錄〕 | 绊〔絆〕 | 贲〔賁〕 | 标〔標〕 | 轺〔軺〕 | 鸥〔鷗〕 | 贻〔貽〕 | 氢〔氫〕 | 狮〔獅〕 | 闻〔聞〕 | 浉〔溮〕 |
| 肿〔腫〕 | 单〔單〕 | 诖〔詿〕 | 弥〔彌〕 | 驼〔駝〕 | 挡〔擋〕 | 栈〔棧〕 | 轻〔輕〕 | 哗〔嘩〕 | 【丿】 | 适〔適〕 | 独〔獨〕 | 闼〔闥〕 | 浊〔濁〕 |
| 胀〔脹〕 | 炜〔煒〕 | 诘〔詰〕 | 〔瀰〕 | 绍〔紹〕 | 垲〔塏〕 | 栉〔櫛〕 | 鸦〔鴉〕 | 响〔響〕 | 钙〔鈣〕 | 种〔種〕 | 狯〔獪〕 | 闽〔閩〕 | 测〔測〕 |
| 肮〔骯〕 | 炝〔熗〕 | 诚〔誠〕 | 陕〔陝〕 | 驿〔驛〕 | 挢〔撟〕 | 栊〔櫳〕 | 虿〔蠆〕 | 哙〔噲〕 | 钚〔鈈〕 | 秋〔鞦〕 | 狱〔獄〕 | 闾〔閭〕 | 浍〔澮〕 |
| 胁〔脅〕 | 炉〔爐〕 | 郓〔鄆〕 | 驽〔駑〕 | 绎〔繹〕 | 挤〔擠〕 | 栋〔棟〕 | 【丨】 | 哝〔噥〕 | 钛〔鈦〕 | 复〔復〕 | 孙〔孫〕 | 阀〔閥〕 | 浏〔瀏〕 |
| 迳〔逕〕 | 浅〔淺〕 | 衬〔襯〕 | 驾〔駕〕 | 经〔經〕 | 挥〔揮〕 | 栌〔櫨〕 | 战〔戰〕 | 哟〔喲〕 | 钝〔鈍〕 | 〔複〕 | 贸〔貿〕 | 阁〔閣〕 | 济〔濟〕 |
| 鱼〔魚〕 | 泷〔瀧〕 | 袆〔褘〕 | 参〔參〕 | 骀〔駘〕 | 挦〔撏〕 | 栎〔櫟〕 | 觇〔覘〕 | 峡〔峽〕 | 钞〔鈔〕 | 笃〔篤〕 | 饵〔餌〕 | 阂〔閡〕 | 浐〔滻〕 |
| 狞〔獰〕 | 泸〔瀘〕 | 视〔視〕 | 艰〔艱〕 | 绐〔紿〕 | 荐〔薦〕 | 栏〔欄〕 | 点〔點〕 | 峣〔嶢〕 | 钟〔鐘〕 | 俦〔儔〕 | 饶〔饒〕 | 养〔養〕 | 浑〔渾〕 |
| 备〔備〕 | 泺〔濼〕 | 诛〔誅〕 | 线〔線〕 | 贯〔貫〕 | 荚〔莢〕 | 柠〔檸〕 | 临〔臨〕 | 帧〔幀〕 | 钠〔鈉〕 | 俨〔儼〕 | 蚀〔蝕〕 | 姜〔薑〕 | 浒〔滸〕 |
| 枭〔梟〕 | 泞〔濘〕 | 话〔話〕 | 绀〔紺〕 | **9畫** | 荛〔蕘〕 | 桠〔椏〕 | 览〔覽〕 | 罚〔罰〕 | 钡〔鋇〕 | 俩〔倆〕 | 饷〔餉〕 | 类〔類〕 | 浓〔濃〕 |
| 饯〔餞〕 | 泻〔瀉〕 | 诞〔誕〕 | 绁〔紲〕 | 【一】 | 荜〔蓽〕 | 树〔樹〕 | 竖〔豎〕 | 峤〔嶠〕 | 钢〔鋼〕 | 俪〔儷〕 | 饸〔餄〕 | 娄〔婁〕 | 浔〔潯〕 |
| 饰〔飾〕 | 泼〔潑〕 | 诟〔詬〕 | 绂〔紱〕 | 贰〔貳〕 | 贳〔貰〕 | 郦〔酈〕 | 尝〔嘗〕 | 贱〔賤〕 | 钣〔鈑〕 | 俭〔儉〕 | 饹〔餎〕 | 总〔總〕 | 浕〔濜〕 |
| 饱〔飽〕 | 泽〔澤〕 | 诠〔詮〕 | 练〔練〕 | 帮〔幫〕 | 荞〔蕎〕 | 砖〔磚〕 | 眍〔瞘〕 | 贵〔貴〕 | 钤〔鈐〕 | 贷〔貸〕 | 饺〔餃〕 | 娈〔孌〕 | 恸〔慟〕 |
| 饲〔飼〕 | 泾〔涇〕 | 诡〔詭〕 | 组〔組〕 | 珑〔瓏〕 | 荟〔薈〕 | 砗〔硨〕 | 哒〔噠〕 | 虾〔蝦〕 | 钥〔鑰〕 | 顺〔順〕 | 饼〔餅〕 | 弯〔彎〕 | 恹〔懨〕 |
| 饳〔飿〕 | 怜〔憐〕 | 询〔詢〕 | 驵〔駔〕 | 顸〔頇〕 | 荠〔薺〕 | 砚〔硯〕 | 哓〔嘵〕 | 蚁〔蟻〕 | 钦〔欽〕 | 剑〔劍〕 | | 孪〔孿〕 | 恺〔愷〕 |
| 饴〔飴〕 | 怆〔愴〕 | 诣〔詣〕 | 绅〔紳〕 | 垭〔埡〕 | 荡〔蕩〕 | 砜〔碸〕 | 哔〔嗶〕 | 蚂〔螞〕 | 钧〔鈞〕 | 鸽〔鴿〕 | | 将〔將〕 | 恻〔惻〕 |
| 【丶】 | 学〔學〕 | 诤〔諍〕 | 细〔細〕 | 挝〔撾〕 | 垩〔堊〕 | 残〔殘〕 | 贵? | 虽〔雖〕 | 钨〔鎢〕 | 须〔須〕 | | 奖〔獎〕 | 恼〔惱〕 |
| 变〔變〕 | 宝〔寶〕 | 该〔該〕 | 驶〔駛〕 | 项〔項〕 | 荤〔葷〕 | 殇〔殤〕 | | 骂〔罵〕 | 钩〔鉤〕 | 胧〔朧〕 | | 炼〔煉〕 | 恽〔惲〕 |
| 庞〔龐〕 | 宠〔寵〕 | 详〔詳〕 | 驸〔駙〕 | 挞〔撻〕 | 荥〔滎〕 | 轲〔軻〕 | | 哕〔噦〕 | 钪〔鈧〕 | 胨〔腖〕 | | 炽〔熾〕 | 举〔舉〕 |
| 庙〔廟〕 | 审〔審〕 | 诧〔詫〕 | 驷〔駟〕 | 挟〔挾〕 | 荦〔犖〕 | 轳〔轤〕 | | 剐〔剮〕 | 钫〔鈁〕 | 胪〔臚〕 | | 烁〔爍〕 | 觉〔覺〕 |
| 疟〔瘧〕 | 帘〔簾〕 | 诨〔諢〕 | 终〔終〕 | | 荧〔熒〕 | 轴〔軸〕 | | 郧〔鄖〕 | 钬〔鈥〕 | 胆〔膽〕 | | 烂〔爛〕 | 宪〔憲〕 |
| 疠〔癘〕 | 实〔實〕 | 诩〔詡〕 | 织〔織〕 | | 荨〔蕁〕 | 轶〔軼〕 | | 勋〔勳〕 | 钭〔鈄〕 | 胜〔勝〕 | | 烃〔烴〕 | 窃〔竊〕 |
| 疡〔瘍〕 | | 【一】 | 驺〔騶〕 | | 荩〔藎〕 | 轷〔軤〕 | | | 钮〔鈕〕 | 胫〔脛〕 | | 洁〔潔〕 | 诫〔誡〕 |
| 剂〔劑〕 | | | | | 荫〔蔭〕 | 轸〔軫〕 | | | | | | 洒〔灑〕 | 诬〔誣〕 |
| 废〔廢〕 | | | | | 荭〔葒〕 | 轹〔轢〕 | | | | | | 疯〔瘋〕 | 语〔語〕 |

| | | | | | | | | | | | | | |
|---|---|---|---|---|---|---|---|---|---|---|---|---|---|
| 袄[襖] | 结[結] | 盏[盞] | 莺[鶯] | 毙[斃] | 觊[覬] | 铄[鑠] | 爱[愛] | 桨[槳] | 涟[漣] | 课[課] | 绥[綏] | 萚[蘀] | 殓[殮] |
| 诮[誚] | 绔[絝] | 捞[撈] | 鸪[鴣] | 致[緻] | 贼[賊] | 铅[鉛] | 鸰[鴒] | 浆[漿] | 润[潤] | 诿[諉] | 绦[縧] | 勋[勛] | 赉[賚] |
| 袮[襕] | 绕[繞] | 载[載] | 莼[蓴] | 【丨】 | 贿[賄] | 铆[鉚] | 颁[頒] | 症[癥] | 涢[溳] | 谀[諛] | 继[繼] | 萝[蘿] | 辄[輒] |
| 误[誤] | 骁[驍] | 赶[趕] | 桡[橈] | 龀[齔] | 赂[賂] | 铈[鈰] | 颂[頌] | 痈[癰] | 涡[渦] | 谁[誰] | 绨[綈] | 萤[螢] | 辅[輔] |
| 诰[誥] | 骄[驕] | 盐[鹽] | 桢[楨] | 鸬[鸕] | 赃[贓] | 铉[鉉] | 脏[臟] | 斋[齋] | 涂[塗] | 谂[諗] | 骏[駿] | 萦[縈] | 辆[輛] |
| 诱[誘] | 骅[驊] | 埘[塒] | 档[檔] | 虑[慮] | 赅[賅] | 铊[鉈] | 脐[臍] | 痉[痙] | 涤[滌] | 调[調] | 鸶[鷥] | 营[營] | 堑[塹] |
| 诲[誨] | 骆[駱] | 损[損] | 桤[榿] | 监[監] | 赆[贐] | 铋[鉍] | 脑[腦] | 准[準] | 润[潤] | 谄[諂] | **11畫** | 萨[薩] | 【丨】 |
| 诳[誆] | 骈[駢] | 埚[堝] | 桥[橋] | 紧[緊] | 【丿】 | 铌[鈮] | 胶[膠] | 离[離] | 涧[澗] | 谅[諒] | 【一】 | 萧[蕭] | 颅[顱] |
| 鸩[鴆] | 绞[絞] | 捡[撿] | 桦[樺] | 晒[曬] | 钰[鈺] | 铍[鈹] | 脓[膿] | 阃[閫] | 涨[漲] | 谆[諄] | 琎[璡] | 梦[夢] | 喷[噴] |
| 说[說] | 骇[駭] | 赍[賫] | 桧[檜] | 晓[曉] | 钱[錢] | 铎[鐸] | 玺[璽] | 阄[鬮] | 烫[燙] | 谇[誶] | 琏[璉] | 观[觀] | 悬[懸] |
| 诵[誦] | 统[統] | 挚[摯] | 桩[樁] | 唛[嘜] | 钲[鉦] | 氢[氫] | 鸱[鴟] | 阅[閱] | 涩[澀] | 谈[談] | 琐[瑣] | 觋[覡] | 啭[囀] |
| 【一】 | 绗[絎] | 热[熱] | 样[樣] | 唝[嗊] | 钳[鉗] | 牺[犧] | 鸲[鴝] | 阆[閬] | 悭[慳] | 谊[誼] | 麸[麩] | 检[檢] | 跃[躍] |
| 垦[墾] | 给[給] | 捣[搗] | 贾[賈] | 唠[嘮] | 钴[鈷] | 敌[敵] | 鸵[鴕] | 家[傢] | 悯[憫] | 诹[諏] | 掳[擄] | 棂[欞] | 啮[嚙] |
| 昼[晝] | 绚[絢] | 壶[壺] | 逦[邐] | 鸭[鴨] | 钵[鉢] | 积[積] | 袅[裊] | 宾[賓] | 宽[寬] | 诺[諾] | 掴[摑] | 啬[嗇] | 跄[蹌] |
| 费[費] | 绛[絳] | 聂[聶] | 砺[礪] | 唢[嗩] | 钶[鈳] | 称[稱] | 皱[皺] | 窍[竅] | 宾[賓] | 读[讀] | 鸷[鷙] | 匮[匱] | 蛎[蠣] |
| 逊[遜] | 络[絡] | 莱[萊] | 砾[礫] | 晔[曄] | 钷[鉕] | 笕[筧] | 饽[餑] | 窎[窵] | 剧[劇] | 诽[誹] | 掷[擲] | 酝[醞] | 蛊[蠱] |
| 阴[陰] | 绝[絕] | 莲[蓮] | 础[礎] | 晕[暈] | 钸[鈈] | 笔[筆] | 饾[餖] | 鸾[鸞] | 娲[媧] | 袜[襪] | 掸[撣] | 厣[厴] | 蛏[蟶] |
| 险[險] | **10畫** | 莳[蒔] | 砻[礱] | 鸮[鴞] | 钹[鈸] | 债[債] | 饿[餓] | 烧[燒] | 娴[嫻] | 绡[綃] | 壸[壼] | 硕[碩] | 累[纍] |
| 贺[賀] | 【一】 | 莴[萵] | 硚[礄] | 唰[㕲] | 钺[鉞] | 倾[傾] | 馁[餒] | 烛[燭] | 难[難] | 骋[騁] | 悫[愨] | 硖[硤] | 啰[囉] |
| 怼[懟] | 艳[艷] | 获[獲] | 顾[顧] | 唢[嗩] | 钻[鑽] | 赁[賃] | 恋[戀] | 烨[燁] | 诸[諸] | 绢[絹] | 据[據] | 硗[磽] | 啸[嘯] |
| 垒[壘] | 顼[頊] | 恶[惡] | 轼[軾] | 圆[圓] | 钼[鉬] | 颀[頎] | | 烩[燴] | 诹[諏] | 绣[繡] | 掺[摻] | 硙[磑] | 帻[幘] |
| 娅[婭] | 珲[琿] | [噁] | 轾[輊] | | 钽[鉭] | 徕[徠] | | 烬[燼] | 读[讀] | 绤[綌] | 掼[摜] | 袭[襲] | 崭[嶄] |
| 娆[嬈] | 蚕[蠶] | 荛[蕘] | 轿[轎] | | 钾[鉀] | 舰[艦] | | 炼[煉] | 诼[諑] | 祯[禎] | 职[職] | 翚[翬] | 逻[邏] |
| 娇[嬌] | 顽[頑] | 莹[瑩] | 辂[輅] | | 铀[鈾] | 舱[艙] | | | 袜[襪] | 验[驗] | 聍[聹] | 殒[殞] | 帼[幗] |
| 绑[綁] | 莹[瑩] | | 鸫[鶇] | | 钿[鈿] | 耸[聳] | | | 涞[淶] | | 聋[聾] | | 赈[賑] |
| 绒[絨] | | | 顿[頓] | | 铁[鐵] | | | | | | 龚[龔] | | 婴[嬰] |
| | | | 趸[躉] | | 铂[鉑] | | | | | | | | 赊[賒] |
| | | | | | 铃[鈴] | | | | | | | | |

| | | | | | | | | | | | | | |
|---|---|---|---|---|---|---|---|---|---|---|---|---|---|
| 【丿】 | 铮〔錚〕 | 龛〔龕〕 | 阐〔闡〕 | 谎〔謊〕 | 婵〔嬋〕 | 绿〔綠〕 | 棱〔稜〕 | 喷〔噴〕 | 链〔鏈〕 | 筜〔簹〕 | 褒〔襃〕 | 裢〔褳〕 | 绱〔緔〕 |
| 铡〔鍘〕 | 铯〔銫〕 | 羟〔羥〕 | 谏〔諫〕 | 姊〔嫭〕 | 骖〔驂〕 | 椤〔欏〕 | 畴〔疇〕 | 铿〔鏗〕 | 筛〔篩〕 | 装〔裝〕 | 裣〔襝〕 | 缊〔縕〕 |
| 铐〔銬〕 | 铰〔鉸〕 | 盖〔蓋〕 | 谐〔諧〕 | 鞑〔韃〕 | 颀〔頎〕 | 赍〔齎〕 | 践〔踐〕 | 锓〔鋟〕 | 胺〔膾〕 | 蛮〔蠻〕 | 裤〔褲〕 | 缌〔緦〕 |
| 铑〔銠〕 | 铱〔銥〕 | 粝〔糲〕 | 谑〔謔〕 | 颈〔頸〕 | 缀〔綴〕 | 楦〔楥〕 | 销〔銷〕 | 锖〔鏿〕 | 傧〔儐〕 | 裔〔裔〕 | 裥〔襇〕 | 缎〔緞〕 |
| 铒〔鉺〕 | 铲〔鏟〕 | 断〔斷〕 | 谒〔謁〕 | 绩〔績〕 | 缁〔緇〕 | 楼〔樓〕 | 遗〔遺〕 | 锂〔鋰〕 | 储〔儲〕 | 痨〔癆〕 | 禅〔禪〕 | 缑〔緱〕 |
| 铓〔鋩〕 | 铳〔銃〕 | 脸〔臉〕 | 谓〔謂〕 | 绪〔緒〕 | 12畫 | 鹉〔鵡〕 | 蛱〔蛺〕 | 锃〔鋥〕 | 傩〔儺〕 | 庼〔廎〕 | 谠〔讜〕 | 猴〔緱〕 |
| 铕〔銪〕 | 铵〔銨〕 | 猎〔獵〕 | 谔〔諤〕 | 绫〔綾〕 | 【一】 | 觃〔覎〕 | 硷〔鹻〕 | 锄〔鋤〕 | 惩〔懲〕 | 廒〔廒〕 | 御〔禦〕 | 谡〔謖〕 |
| 铗〔鋏〕 | 银〔銀〕 | 逻〔邏〕 | 谕〔諭〕 | 续〔續〕 | 靓〔靚〕 | 硗〔磽〕 | 鹃〔鵑〕 | 锆〔鋯〕 | 锗〔鍺〕 | 颏〔頦〕 | 鹇〔鷳〕 | 谢〔謝〕 |
| 铙〔鐃〕 | 铷〔銣〕 | 弥〔獼〕 | 谖〔諼〕 | 绮〔綺〕 | 琼〔瓊〕 | 辇〔輦〕 | 喽〔嘍〕 | 锇〔鋨〕 | 锧〔鑕〕 | 领〔領〕 | 阑〔闌〕 | 谣〔謠〕 |
| 铛〔鐺〕 | 铷〔鉤〕 | 馃〔餜〕 | 谗〔讒〕 | 骑〔騎〕 | 鼋〔黿〕 | 弹〔彈〕 | 嵘〔嶸〕 | 锈〔銹〕 | 锓〔鋟〕 | 释〔釋〕 | 阒〔闃〕 | 谤〔謗〕 |
| 铝〔鋁〕 | 矫〔矯〕 | 馄〔餛〕 | 谘〔諮〕 | 绯〔緋〕 | 颊〔頰〕 | 趋〔趨〕 | 嵝〔嶁〕 | 锉〔銼〕 | 歆〔歆〕 | 鹆〔鵒〕 | 阕〔闋〕 | 谦〔謙〕 |
| 铜〔銅〕 | 鸪〔鴣〕 | 馆〔館〕 | 谙〔諳〕 | 绰〔綽〕 | 雳〔靂〕 | 辊〔輥〕 | 锋〔鋒〕 | 锌〔鋅〕 | 腊〔臘〕 | 腭〔腭〕 | 阔〔闊〕 | 谥〔謚〕 |
| 锦〔錦〕 | 秽〔穢〕 | 【丶】 | 诂〔詁〕 | 骤〔驟〕 | 辐〔輻〕 | 辋〔輞〕 | 锆〔鋯〕 | 锒〔鋃〕 | 鹏〔鵬〕 | 腌〔醃〕 | 阖〔闔〕 | 【一】 |
| 铟〔銦〕 | 笺〔箋〕 | 鸾〔鸞〕 | 渖〔瀋〕 | 绲〔緄〕 | 揿〔撳〕 | 椠〔槧〕 | 锐〔銳〕 | 鲀〔魨〕 | 类〔類〕 | 属〔屬〕 | 鹈〔鵜〕 | 耢〔耮〕 |
| 铠〔鎧〕 | 笾〔籩〕 | 颜〔顏〕 | 滗〔潷〕 | 绳〔繩〕 | 揽〔攬〕 | 暂〔暫〕 | 锑〔銻〕 | 鲁〔魯〕 | 审〔審〕 | 屡〔屢〕 | 鹐〔鵮〕 | 鹋〔鶓〕 |
| 铡〔鍘〕 | 债〔債〕 | 痪〔瘓〕 | 渗〔滲〕 | 雅〔雅〕 | 蛰〔蟄〕 | 赏〔賞〕 | 赌〔賭〕 | 鲂〔魴〕 | 窝〔窩〕 | 骘〔騭〕 | 鹑〔鶉〕 | 鹊〔鵲〕 |
| 铢〔銖〕 | 偾〔僨〕 | 痒〔癢〕 | 谛〔諦〕 | 维〔維〕 | 絷〔縶〕 | 辌〔輬〕 | 赎〔贖〕 | 锐〔銳〕 | 誉〔譽〕 | 愤〔憤〕 | 鹒〔鶊〕 | 辋〔輞〕 |
| 铣〔銑〕 | 偿〔償〕 | 惭〔慚〕 | 谜〔謎〕 | 绵〔綿〕 | 搁〔擱〕 | 翘〔翹〕 | 赐〔賜〕 | 锓〔鋟〕 | 琉〔瑠〕 | 慑〔懾〕 | 鹔〔鷫〕 | 骛〔鶩〕 |
| 铥〔銩〕 | 偻〔僂〕 | 惧〔懼〕 | 谝〔諞〕 | 绶〔綬〕 | 搂〔摟〕 | 【丨】 | 赒〔賙〕 | 锔〔鋦〕 | 颍〔潁〕 | 滞〔滯〕 | 骝〔騮〕 | 摄〔攝〕 |
| 铤〔鋌〕 | 躯〔軀〕 | 旋〔鏇〕 | 谞〔諝〕 | 【一】 | 搅〔攪〕 | 辈〔輩〕 | 赔〔賠〕 | 锒〔鋃〕 | 飐〔颭〕 | 湿〔濕〕 | 缝〔縫〕 | 摅〔攄〕 |
| 铧〔鏵〕 | 皑〔皚〕 | 惊〔驚〕 | 惮〔憚〕 | 弹〔彈〕 | 绸〔綢〕 | 凿〔鑿〕 | 喷〔噴〕 | 锓〔鋟〕 | 馉〔餶〕 | 溃〔潰〕 | 缏〔緶〕 | 摆〔擺〕 |
| 铨〔銓〕 | 衅〔釁〕 | 阈〔閾〕 | 惨〔慘〕 | 堕〔墮〕 | 绺〔綹〕 | 辏〔輳〕 | 【丿】 | 锛〔錛〕 | 馈〔饋〕 | 溅〔濺〕 | 缃〔緗〕 | 辐〔輻〕 |
| 铩〔鎩〕 | 鸺〔鵂〕 | 阉〔閹〕 | 惯〔慣〕 | 随〔隨〕 | 卷〔綣〕 | 辉〔輝〕 | 铸〔鑄〕 | 锘〔鍩〕 | 馊〔餿〕 | 湾〔灣〕 | 缄〔緘〕 | 鹜〔鶩〕 |
| 铪〔鉿〕 | 衔〔銜〕 | 阇〔闍〕 | 祷〔禱〕 | 粜〔糶〕 | 综〔綜〕 | 蒋〔蔣〕 | 锊〔鋝〕 | 鹅〔鵝〕 | 颐〔頤〕 | 溇〔漊〕 | 缂〔緙〕 | 摁〔摁〕 |
| 铫〔銚〕 | 舻〔艫〕 | 阆〔閬〕 | 谌〔諶〕 | 隐〔隱〕 | 绽〔綻〕 | 萎〔萎〕 | 锎〔鐦〕 | 颒〔頮〕 | 【丶】 | 漠〔漠〕 | 缇〔緹〕 | 缂〔緙〕 |
| 铭〔銘〕 | 盘〔盤〕 | 阊〔閶〕 | 谋〔謀〕 | 绾〔綰〕 | 婳〔嫿〕 | 韩〔韓〕 | 睐〔睞〕 | 铽〔鋱〕 | 筑〔築〕 | 【丶】 | 缈〔緲〕 | |
| 铬〔鉻〕 | 鸼〔鵃〕 | 阋〔鬩〕 | 谍〔諜〕 | 婵〔嬋〕 | | 睑〔瞼〕 | 铽〔鋱〕 | | | | | |

13畫
【一】

| | | | | | | | | | | | | | |
|---|---|---|---|---|---|---|---|---|---|---|---|---|---|
| 〔羆〕 | 殡〔殯〕 | 锛〔錛〕 | 腻〔膩〕 | 瘅〔癉〕 | 谨〔謹〕 | 瑗〔瑗〕 | 觜〔齜〕 | 锻〔鍛〕 | 鲙〔鱠〕 | 谰〔讕〕 | 聪〔聰〕 | 嘱〔囑〕 | 鲤〔鯉〕 |
| 赪〔赬〕 | 雾〔霧〕 | 锝〔鍀〕 | 鹏〔鵬〕 | 瘆〔瘮〕 | 谩〔謾〕 | 赘〔贅〕 | 龈〔齦〕 | 锼〔鎪〕 | 鲚〔鱭〕 | 谱〔譜〕 | 觏〔覯〕 | 颢〔顥〕 | 鲦〔鰷〕 |
| 摈〔擯〕 | 辌〔輬〕 | 锞〔錁〕 | 鹒〔鶊〕 | 瘗〔瘞〕 | 谪〔謫〕 | 觏〔覯〕 | 鹍〔鶤〕 | 锽〔鍠〕 | 鲛〔鮫〕 | 谲〔譎〕 | 辚〔轔〕 | 颐〔頤〕 | 皖〔皖〕 |
| 毂〔轂〕 | 辑〔輯〕 | 锟〔錕〕 | 鲆〔鮃〕 | 阃〔閫〕 | 谬〔謬〕 | 韬〔韜〕 | 颗〔顆〕 | 锇〔鋨〕 | 鲟〔鱘〕 | 【一】 | 蕲〔蘄〕 | 颙〔顒〕 | 卿〔卿〕 |
| 摊〔攤〕 | 输〔輸〕 | 锡〔錫〕 | 鲇〔鮎〕 | 阄〔鬮〕 | 谫〔譾〕 | 叇〔靆〕 | 䁖〔瞜〕 | 锒〔鋃〕 | 镀〔鍍〕 | 嫱〔嬙〕 | 鹕〔鶘〕 | 蕴〔蘊〕 | 徼〔徼〕 |
| 鹊〔鵲〕 | 【丨】 | 锣〔鑼〕 | 鲈〔鱸〕 | 阅〔閱〕 | 辟〔闢〕 | 墙〔牆〕 | 鹍〔鶤〕 | 镁〔鎂〕 | 鏊〔鏊〕 | 鹜〔鶩〕 | 樯〔檣〕 | 镍〔鎳〕 | 馔〔饌〕 |
| 蓝〔藍〕 | 频〔頻〕 | 锤〔錘〕 | 鲊〔鮓〕 | 粮〔糧〕 | 媛〔媛〕 | 蔷〔薔〕 | 跷〔蹺〕 | 镂〔鏤〕 | 馒〔饅〕 | 缥〔縹〕 | 樱〔櫻〕 | 镎〔鎿〕 | 【丶】 |
| 蓨〔蓨〕 | 龃〔齟〕 | 锥〔錐〕 | 稣〔穌〕 | 数〔數〕 | 嫱〔嬙〕 | 嵝〔嶁〕 | 踊〔踴〕 | 镃〔鎡〕 | 【丶】 | 骠〔驃〕 | 飘〔飄〕 | 锋〔鋒〕 | 瘿〔癭〕 |
| 鹋〔鶓〕 | 龄〔齡〕 | 锦〔錦〕 | 鲋〔鮒〕 | 滗〔潷〕 | 缙〔縉〕 | 蔹〔蘞〕 | 蜡〔蠟〕 | 锎〔鐦〕 | 銮〔鑾〕 | 骡〔騾〕 | 履〔履〕 | 镏〔鎦〕 | 瘤〔癟〕 |
| 蓟〔薊〕 | 龅〔齙〕 | 锧〔鑕〕 | 鲍〔鮑〕 | 滟〔灧〕 | 缜〔縝〕 | 蔺〔藺〕 | 蝇〔蠅〕 | 锏〔鐧〕 | 瘗〔瘞〕 | 缧〔縲〕 | 魇〔魘〕 | 镐〔鎬〕 | 颜〔顏〕 |
| 蒙〔矇〕 | 龆〔齠〕 | 锫〔錇〕 | 鲅〔鮁〕 | 滤〔濾〕 | 缚〔縛〕 | 蔼〔藹〕 | 蝉〔蟬〕 | 鹙〔鶖〕 | 瘘〔瘻〕 | 缨〔纓〕 | 餍〔饜〕 | 镑〔鎊〕 | 鹣〔鶼〕 |
| 〔濛〕 | 鉴〔鑒〕 | 锭〔錠〕 | 鲐〔鮐〕 | 滥〔濫〕 | 缛〔縟〕 | 鹛〔鶥〕 | 鹗〔鶚〕 | 稳〔穩〕 | 阔〔闊〕 | 【丿】 | 霉〔黴〕 | 镒〔鎰〕 | 鲨〔鯊〕 |
| 〔懞〕 | 嗟〔嗟〕 | 键〔鍵〕 | 鲑〔鮭〕 | 滗〔潷〕 | 辔〔轡〕 | 榿〔榿〕 | 槚〔檟〕 | 箦〔簀〕 | 鲞〔鯗〕 | 缫〔繅〕 | 辎〔輜〕 | 镓〔鎵〕 | 澜〔瀾〕 |
| 颐〔頤〕 | 跶〔躂〕 | 锯〔鋸〕 | 鲔〔鮪〕 | 滢〔瀅〕 | 缝〔縫〕 | 槛〔檻〕 | 嘤〔嚶〕 | 箧〔篋〕 | 糁〔糝〕 | 【丨】 | 【一】 | 镔〔鑌〕 | 额〔額〕 |
| 献〔獻〕 | 跷〔蹺〕 | 锰〔錳〕 | 鲒〔鮚〕 | 溧〔溧〕 | 骝〔騮〕 | 槟〔檳〕 | 罴〔羆〕 | 箨〔籜〕 | 鹚〔鶿〕 | 龉〔齬〕 | 题〔題〕 | 镉〔鎘〕 | 谳〔讞〕 |
| 蓣〔蕷〕 | 跸〔蹕〕 | 锱〔錙〕 | 颖〔穎〕 | 滦〔灤〕 | 缢〔縊〕 | 槠〔櫧〕 | 嗳〔噯〕 | 箪〔簞〕 | 潇〔瀟〕 | 龊〔齪〕 | 颗〔顆〕 | 篑〔簣〕 | 谶〔讖〕 |
| 榄〔欖〕 | 跻〔躋〕 | 辞〔辭〕 | 鹐〔鵮〕 | 漓〔灕〕 | 缟〔縞〕 | 酽〔釅〕 | 赙〔賻〕 | 箩〔籮〕 | 潋〔瀲〕 | 觑〔覷〕 | 踬〔躓〕 | 篓〔簍〕 | 谴〔譴〕 |
| 榇〔櫬〕 | 跹〔躚〕 | 颓〔頹〕 | 飔〔颸〕 | 溆〔漵〕 | 缠〔纏〕 | 酾〔釃〕 | 罂〔罌〕 | 箓〔籙〕 | 潍〔濰〕 | 觎〔覦〕 | 踯〔躑〕 | 鹥〔鷖〕 | 【一】 |
| 榈〔櫚〕 | 蜗〔蝸〕 | 辟〔闢〕 | 飕〔颼〕 | 滪〔澦〕 | 缡〔縭〕 | 酿〔釀〕 | 赚〔賺〕 | 箫〔簫〕 | | 觐〔覲〕 | 蹉〔蹉〕 | 蝾〔蠑〕 | 缬〔纈〕 |
| 楼〔樓〕 | 暖〔暖〕 | 辞〔辭〕 | 雏〔雛〕 | 添〔添〕 | 缢〔縊〕 | 霁〔霽〕 | 鹘〔鶻〕 | 【丿】 | 赛〔賽〕 | 【一】 | 颞〔顳〕 | 鹠〔鶹〕 | 鹤〔鶴〕 |
| 榉〔櫸〕 | 赗〔賵〕 | 颓〔頹〕 | 馎〔餺〕 | 慑〔懾〕 | 缣〔縑〕 | 愿〔願〕 | 膑〔臏〕 | 锲〔鍥〕 | 窦〔竇〕 | 耧〔耬〕 | 蹒〔蹣〕 | 鲮〔鯪〕 | 谵〔譫〕 |
| 赖〔賴〕 | 【丿】 | 筹〔籌〕 | 馍〔饃〕 | 慢〔慢〕 | 缤〔繽〕 | 殡〔殯〕 | 錯〔錯〕 | 锶〔鍶〕 | 谭〔譚〕 | 璎〔瓔〕 | 蹑〔躡〕 | 鲯〔鯕〕 | 【一】 |
| 碛〔磧〕 | 锗〔鍺〕 | 签〔簽〕 | 馏〔餾〕 | 誊〔謄〕 | 骟〔騸〕 | 殨〔殨〕 | 锠〔錩〕 | 锼〔鎪〕 | 谮〔譖〕 | 撵〔攆〕 | 蹓〔蹓〕 | 蝶〔蝶〕 | 屦〔屨〕 |
| 碍〔礙〕 | 错〔錯〕 | 〔籤〕 | 馐〔饈〕 | 寝〔寢〕 | | 殡〔殯〕 | 锷〔鍔〕 | 锘〔鍩〕 | 禚〔禚〕 | 撷〔擷〕 | 撄〔攖〕 | 鲭〔鯖〕 | 缭〔繚〕 |
| 碜〔磣〕 | 锘〔鍩〕 | 简〔簡〕 | 酱〔醬〕 | 窝〔窩〕 | **14畫** | 瘗〔瘞〕 | 锸〔鍤〕 | 鲖〔鮦〕 | 褛〔褸〕 | 聩〔聵〕 | 噜〔嚕〕 | 鲔〔鮪〕 | 缮〔繕〕 |
| 鹑〔鶉〕 | 锚〔錨〕 | 觎〔覦〕 | 颔〔頷〕 | 窨〔窨〕 | 【一】 | 锡〔錫〕 | 鲗〔鰂〕 | | 谯〔譙〕 | **15畫** | | 鲥〔鰣〕 | 缯〔繒〕 |
| 尴〔尷〕 | 锚〔錨〕 | 锚〔錨〕 | 鹑〔鶉〕 | 窦〔竇〕 | | | 鲣〔鰹〕 | | | | | | |

| | | | | | | | |
|---|---|---|---|---|---|---|---|
| **16畫** | 锾〔鍰〕 | 瘪〔癟〕 | 嗬〔噂〕 | 编〔編〕 | 雒〔雒〕 | 镣〔鐐〕 | 镵〔鑱〕 | **25畫** |
| | 锵〔鏘〕 | 斓〔斕〕 | 鹍〔鵾〕 | 【丶】 | 膯〔膯〕 | 颖〔穎〕 | 賸〔賸〕 | |
| **【一】** | 镛〔鏞〕 | 辩〔辯〕 | 赡〔贍〕 | 鹜〔鶩〕 | 鲭〔鯖〕 | 鳖〔鱉〕 | 鳏〔鰥〕 | 镢〔钁〕 |
| 糇〔糇〕 | 镜〔鏡〕 | 濑〔瀨〕 | 【丿】 | 辫〔辮〕 | 鲰〔鯫〕 | 鳝〔鱔〕 | 穰〔穰〕 |
| 撖〔撖〕 | 镝〔鏑〕 | 濒〔瀕〕 | 镞〔鏃〕 | 赢〔贏〕 | 鳃〔鰓〕 | 鳞〔鱗〕 | 戆〔戇〕 |
| 颏〔頦〕 | 镞〔鏃〕 | 懒〔懶〕 | 镣〔鐐〕 | 懑〔懣〕 | 鳊〔鯿〕 | 鳟〔鱒〕 | |
| 薮〔藪〕 | 鲁〔魯〕 | 黉〔黌〕 | 镤〔鏷〕 | 鹞〔鷂〕 | 鳋〔鰠〕 | **【一】** | |
| 颠〔顛〕 | 赞〔贊〕 | **【一】** | 镦〔鐓〕 | 骤〔驟〕 | 鳌〔鰲〕 | 骧〔驤〕 | |
| 橹〔櫓〕 | 篮〔籃〕 | 鹬〔鷸〕 | 镧〔鑭〕 | | **【丶】** | **21畫** | |
| 橼〔櫞〕 | 篱〔籬〕 | 颡〔顙〕 | 镨〔鐠〕 | **18畫** | 颤〔顫〕 | | |
| 鹭〔鷺〕 | 魉〔魎〕 | 缰〔繮〕 | 镝〔鐯〕 | | 癫〔癲〕 | 颦〔顰〕 | |
| 赝〔贗〕 | 鲭〔鯖〕 | 缱〔繾〕 | 错〔鐯〕 | **【一】** | 癣〔癬〕 | 躏〔躪〕 | |
| 飙〔飆〕 | 鲮〔鯪〕 | 缲〔繰〕 | 镩〔鑹〕 | 鳌〔鰲〕 | 谶〔讖〕 | 鳢〔鱧〕 | |
| 碛〔磧〕 | 鲰〔鯫〕 | 缳〔繯〕 | 镪〔鏹〕 | 鞯〔韉〕 | **【一】** | 鳣〔鱣〕 | |
| 鏊〔鏊〕 | 鲱〔鯡〕 | 缴〔繳〕 | 镫〔鐙〕 | 魇〔魘〕 | 骥〔驥〕 | 癞〔癩〕 | |
| 辙〔轍〕 | 鲲〔鯤〕 | **17畫** | 簖〔籪〕 | **【丨】** | 缵〔纘〕 | 赣〔贛〕 | |
| 辚〔轔〕 | 鲳〔鯧〕 | | 鹪〔鷦〕 | 戳〔戳〕 | | 灏〔灝〕 | |
| **【丨】** | 鲵〔鯢〕 | **【一】** | 鳝〔鱔〕 | 颢〔顥〕 | **19畫** | **22畫** | |
| 醭〔醭〕 | 鲶〔鯰〕 | 薛〔薛〕 | 鲽〔鰈〕 | 鹭〔鷺〕 | | | |
| 螨〔蟎〕 | 鲷〔鯛〕 | 鹩〔鷯〕 | 鲙〔鱠〕 | 器〔器〕 | **【一】** | 鹳〔鸛〕 | |
| 鹦〔鸚〕 | 鲸〔鯨〕 | **【丨】** | 鳃〔鰓〕 | 髅〔髏〕 | 攒〔攢〕 | 镶〔鑲〕 | |
| 赠〔贈〕 | 鲻〔鯔〕 | 龋〔齲〕 | 鳁〔鰛〕 | **【丿】** | 霭〔靄〕 | **23畫** | |
| **【丿】** | 獭〔獺〕 | 醒〔醒〕 | 鳄〔鱷〕 | 镀〔鍍〕 | **【丨】** | | |
| 镨〔鐠〕 | **【丶】** | 瞩〔矚〕 | 鳅〔鰍〕 | 镭〔鐳〕 | 蹙〔蹙〕 | 趱〔趲〕 | |
| 镖〔鏢〕 | 鹧〔鷓〕 | 踌〔躊〕 | 鳇〔鰉〕 | 镮〔鐶〕 | 巅〔巔〕 | 颧〔顴〕 | |
| 镗〔鏜〕 | 瘦〔瘦〕 | 蹑〔躡〕 | 鳍〔鰭〕 | 镱〔鐿〕 | 髋〔髖〕 | 躜〔躦〕 | |
| | | 蟥〔蟥〕 | 鳏〔鰥〕 | 镱〔鐿〕 | 骸〔骸〕 | | |
| | | | | | **【丿】** | | |
| | | | | | 镞〔鏃〕 | | |

# APPENDIX IV

## Index of Chinese Names

1. Entries are arranged in the order of the number of strokes of their first characters. For those with the same stroke count, structural forms in the order of 、一丨丿 of their first strokes are to be followed.
2. Numerals following the Chinese names are their entry numbers in Part I of this volume.
3. Horizontal stroke (一) includes: ㄱㄱㄱㄱㄱㄱ; vertical stroke ( 丨 ) includes: ㄴㄴ; slant stroke (丿) includes: ㄑㄥㄧ.
4. Stroke counts for the following radicals are: 辶 3, 衤 4, 礻 5, 阝 3, 艹 4.

一、詞目按第一字筆畫分先後，畫數相同的按起筆筆形、一丨丿順序排列。
二、詞目後的數字爲該詞目在本書第一部分的次序碼。
三、橫（一）的筆形包括ㄱㄱㄱㄱㄱㄱ等；豎（丨）包括ㄴㄴ；撇（丿）包括ㄑㄥㄧ。
四、辶爲三畫；衤爲四畫；礻爲五畫；阝爲三畫；艹爲四畫。

### 1 畫

**[ 一 ]**

一口血　1696
一支箭　587
一把傘　1718
一朵雲　594,2186
一葉萩　594A,2131
一點血　593
一點紅　2057
一支黃花　588

### 2 畫

**[ 一 ]**

二丑　240,315
刁竹　1557
十大功勞　1276
了刁竹　1557
了哥王　741
刀豆　1500
刀口藥　1492
刀豆子　1500
刀豆根　1500
七加皮　092
七里香　084
七指蕨　081
七葉蓮　092
七葉一枝花　091,1685
丁香　1639
丁力子　1647
丁公藤　920,1643
丁字草　1646
丁香油　1640
丁癸草　601,1642
丁榔皮　1644

**[ 丿 ]**

入地龍　606
人胞　1840
人參　599

259

| | | | | |
|---|---|---|---|---|
| 大泡桐　1417 | 大葉桉　1436 | 大葉紫珠　1448 | 小青皮　221 | 山蟹　1172 |
| 大青根　1393 | 大腹皮　1093,1401 | 大葉鈎藤　1441 | 小芙蓉　1525c | 山八角　2038 |
| 大青草　1394 | 大槿花　1390 | 大葉楠根　1444 | 小飛揚　467 | 山大刀　1189 |
| 大青葉　1392 | 大頭陳　1426 | 大葉鳳尾　1438 | 小紅豆　469 | 山大顏　1189 |
| 大青鹽　1395 | 大蕉皮　1388 | 大酸味草　1812 | 小通草　1822a | 山小橘　1167 |
| 大芸香　1027,1450, | 大獨活　1791a | 大駁骨丹　1418 | 小茴香　468,563 | 山火筒　1098 |
| 　　　2257 | 大羅傘　1412 | 大對經草　1432 | 小狼毒　1774 | 山牛膝　1781 |
| 大活血　1951 | 大一枝箭　1409 | 大樹跌打　1421 | 小黃芪　543b | 山甘草　1177 |
| 大胡麻　1405 | 大一面鑼　1410 | 大獨葉草　1431 | 小駁骨　474 | 山石榴　1908 |
| 大風茅　347 | 大二郎箭　1398 | 大蘭花生　1626 | 小銅錘　1813 | 山甲片　291 |
| 大風藤　2121 | 大九股牛　1397 | 大葉白頭翁　1445 | 小羅傘　470 | 山甲皮　1158 |
| 大紅袍　1407 | 大九節鈴　1396 | 大葉風沙藤　1437 | 小婆婆納　1543 | 山白芷　999,2042 |
| 大海子　1403 | 大火草根　1408 | 大葉馬尾蓮　1443 | 小葉枇杷　477 | 山白菊　1185 |
| 大浮萍　1402 | 大白頂草　1416 | 大葉蛇泡簕　1447 | 小葉買麻藤　476 | 山羊血　1198 |
| 大朗傘　1667 | 大汗淋草　568 | | 小葉雙眼龍　478 | 山羊角　1198 |
| 大馬勃　835b | 大地棕根　1423 | [丨] | 小蟬花　24a | 山羊筋　1198 |
| 大茴香　951 | 大豆黃捲　1425 | 上冰片　1094 | 山丹　1190,1190b | 山肉桂　1446 |
| 大茶根　1383 | 大夜關門　1442 | 口蘑　722,995 | 山甲　291,1156 | 山竹子　1164 |
| 大茶藥　649,1384 | 大刺兒棻　1433 | 小米　471 | 山奈　1130,1184 | 山竹根　1164 |
| 大草烏　1716d | 大金不換　1391 | 小皂　331 | 山參　599 | 山沉香　2241 |
| 大草蔻　1430 | 大飛揚草　1399 | 小茴　468 | 山椒　738 | 山豆根　394,1053, |
| 大麻仁　829,1414 | 大風沙藤　1521 | 小麥　364 | 山菰　1195 | 　　　1192,1655 |
| 大麥仁　1415 | 大透骨消　1427 | 小薊　466 | 山楂　1153 | 山牡丹　1183 |
| 大麥芽　1415 | 大透骨草　1428 | 小元參　2248 | 山稜　1127 | 山油柑　1202 |
| 大巢棻　1385 | 大楓子油　1400 | 小木通　472 | 山漆　1115 | 山枝茶　1160 |
| 大蛇藥　1420 | 大葉山桂　1446 | 小生地　1225 | 山蒟　1166 | 山枝仁　1160 |
| 大萍葉　366 | 大葉花椒　1440 | 小仙茅　2067 | 山蒜　1188 | 山枝根　1160 |
| 大楓子　1400 | 大葉香薷　1439 | 小白芨　543a | 山橙　1155 | 山枇杷　1186 |
| | | 小豆蔻　475,1015a | 山橘　1167 | 山刺柏　1196 |
| | | | 山藥　1199 | |

| | | | | |
|---|---|---|---|---|
| 山礬花 1168 | 山楂餅 017 | 千打錘 147 | 川木香 285,897 | 六月霜 758 |
| 山礬根 1168 | 山楂糕 1153 | 千年見 144 | 川太片 1048 | 六角英 778 |
| 山礬葉 1168 | 山葡萄 2199 | 千年健 927 | 川牛膝 276,286,931a | 六稜菊 789 |
| 山羌活 1758 | 山蒼子 1193 | 千里光 143,230,1788b | 川白芷 967 | 火麻 582 |
| 山扁豆 1187 | 山蒼樹 1662 | 千金子 139,500,2208 | 川朴花 289 | 火葱 480 |
| 山枳麻 1161 | 山慈菇 683,1195 | 千張紙 136,899 | 川防風 325a | 火殃簕 585 |
| 山胡椒 1173 | 山螞蝗 1181 | 千層紙 149 | 川貝母 288 | 火炭母 584 |
| 山苦荬 2147 | 山銀花 120,190 | 千層樓 150 | 川花楸 1732 | 火索麻 583 |
| 山苦蕒 1178 | 山薄荷 1768 | 川巴 287,955 | 川金子 272 | 火麻仁 582 |
| 山海螺 1169 | 山薑子 1159 | 川朴 275,424 | 川南星 1622a | 文旦 2201 |
| 山桐子 1194 | 山藥頭 1199 | 川芎 279 | 川厚朴 275 | 文甲 1983 |
| 山核桃 1170 | 山藿香 508b,1176 | 川貝 288,1051b | 川厚樸 275 | 文竹 1930 |
| 山茶花 1154 | 山櫻桃 1201 | 川羌 109a,269 | 川烏頭 1609 | 文蛤 1931 |
| 山荔枝 1179 | 山鷄蛋 1156 | 川松 616 | 川草薢 1048 | 文冠果 1932 |
| 山茱萸 1165 | 山蘿蔔 1203 | 川附 274,377 | 川楝子 284 | 文鰩魚 1934 |
| 山烏柏 576 | 山紅梔仁 1175 | 川芭 287 | 川練子 284 | 文殊蘭果 1933 |
| 山烏龜 1542 | 山馬角片 1180 | 川芪 268,543 | 川槿皮 271 | |
| 山梅根 1182 | 山烏柏根 1197 | 川活 281 | 川續斷 280 | [一] |
| 山野烟 1121 | 山道年蒿 1191 | 川桂 282 | 川藏沙參 917b | 丑牛 240,315 |
| 山荷葉 1171 | 山銀柴胡 2171 | 川連 283,553 | | 孔雀尾 178 |
| 山梔子 1162 | | 川烏 294,687 | **4畫** | 不食草 947,1107 |
| 山萸肉 2219 | [丿] | 川椒 270,528 | | 不留子 1106 |
| 山黃芪 1837 | | 川膝 276,286 | [、] | 牙皂 2022 |
| 山草薢 1048 | 久香虫 228 | 川鴻 277,1719 | 心葉淫羊藿 2187 | 牙皂莢 2022 |
| 山猪膽 1163 | 女貞 942 | 川歸 1483 | 方杞 324 | 牙痛草 2026 |
| 山楂片 1153 | 女貞子 942 | 川斷 293 | 方通 328 | 王瓜 1922 |
| 山楂肉 1153 | 千日紅 141 | 川芎 279 | 方通草 328,1822b | 王孫 1924 |
| 山楂乾 1153 | 千斤拔 137 | 川鬱 292,1484 | 六月雪 758 | 王瓜根 1922 |
| | 千斤藤 138 | | | |

水銀　1345
水蓼　1319
水龍　1322
水蘇　1331
水丁香　1336
水木草　1323
水牛角　1324
水田七　1335
水仙子　1310,1960
水仙花　1306
水仙根　1306
水仙桃　1307
水白臘　1327
水百合　1326
水防己　324b
水君子　1283,1302
水折耳　1294
水皂莢　1337
水松皮　1333
水松鬚　1333
水芙蓉　1304
水金鳳　1299
水枇杷　1328
水柏枝　1325
水胡滿　1312
水映草　1704
水苦蕒　1316
水飛廉　1302A
水流豆　1321

水案板　1293
水蓮沙　1320
水翁皮　1341
水翁花　1341
水梔子　544
水梔根　1298
水梔葉　1298
水莧菜　1308
水梨藤　1318
水黃連　2168
水黃蓮　1313
水晶蘭　1301
水榆果　1346
水楊枝　1343
水楊根　1343
水楊莓　1340,1344
水葫蘆　1311
水蜈蚣　1342
水慈菇　2143
水團花　1340
水綫草　1309
水蔗草　1295
水澤蘭　1338
水龍骨　1322
水獺肝　1334
水羅豆　1321
水鷄頭　1335
水鷄蘇　1331
水金雲母　170

水紅花子　1314
水蝦子草　1305
水楊木白皮　1343
水濕柳葉莕　1330

[ 丿 ]

手片　1284
勾藤　648
及己　62
片膠　1090
片紫草　1091
升麻　1223
升麻肉　1223
升麻頭　1223
丹皮　893,954,1474
丹砂　252,1475
丹根　525,1470
丹參　1476
丹鬚　1470
丹根鬚　1470
月石　2256
月砂　2255
月黃　1507
月見草　2253
月季花　2252
月桂子　2254
月季花根　2252

月季花葉　2252
牛子　936
牛房　930
牛虻　871,934
牛草　183,2207
牛黃　932
牛膝　931,1781
牛膽　940
牛鞭　938
牛大力　939
牛皮消　937
牛耳楓　929
牛角碎　928
牛角腮　928
牛旁子　930,936
牛骨碎　933
牛蒡子　936,1411
牛尾獨活　1748d
毛朮　862
毛芍　863
毛茶　999
毛栝　861
毛薑　1218
毛山朮　862
毛冬靑　865
毛披樹　865
毛草龍　1307
毛梨子　1508

毛將軍　857
毛膏菜　1509
毛獨活　1748c
毛薑黃　858
毛麝香　857,864
毛曼陀羅　2034b
毛麝香末　864
毛麝香葉　864
毛葉兎耳風　1976

**5 畫**

[ 丶 ]

玄參　505,2248
玄明粉　504,2246
玄精石　502,2243
牟夏　1031,1356
牟枝蓮　1029
牟夏片　1031
牟夏末　1031
牟夏麯　1031
牟楓荷　1030
牟邊旗　1035
牟邊蓮　1036

[ 一 ]

甘露子　1712

本杞　642,1060
布渣葉　1104
平朮　1010
平貝　1051d
功勞木　1276
功勞子　703
功勞葉　704,1276
打馬　1413
打碗花　1434
朮　1286
朮頭　1292
加皮　096
加冠　071
巨胥子　264
古山龍　656
古羊藤　660
古柯葉　654
瓦松　1913
瓦韋　1914
瓦楞子　1912
甘石　787
甘松　616
甘草　617,1561
甘陝荊芥　0614A
甘遂　615
甘葛　634
甘蔗　609
甘菊花　259
玉瓜　2221
玉米　2227
玉竹　2215
玉金　2213
玉柏　2229
玉屑　2217
玉米軸　2227
玉米鬚　2227
玉芙蓉　2216
玉珊瑚　2237
玉帶根　2237
玉蜀黍　2227
玉環釵　541
玉龍鞭　2226
玉簪花　2239
玉簪葉　2239
玉蘭花　2222
玉珊瑚根　2232
玉蜀黍根　2236
玉蜀黍葉　2236
石耳　1239
石灰　1250
石竹　266,1235
石松　1275
石花　1247
石活　1245
石英　1283
石栗　1257
石脂　160,1234
石斛　1245
石棗　1280
石楠　1265
石膏　1252
石榴　1627
石蒜　1274
石葦　1281
石蓮　1258
石蓴　1237
石燕　1282
石蕨　1681
石膽　1468
石蟹　1172,1243
石蠶　1279
石上柏　1271
石上藕　1279
石木耳　1239
石仙桃　1244
石吊蘭　1278
石決明　1236
石防風　1240
石見穿　1233
石伸筋　1711
石刷把　1272
石奇蛇　1711
石花菜　1248
石柑子　1251
石指甲　1229
石胡荽　1246
石南藤　1256,1266
石風丹　1241
石香薷　1242
石栗子　1257
石豇豆　1232
石寄生　1231
石黃皮　1249
石菖蒲　1228
石腊紅　1255
石楠葉　1265
石葦葉　1281
石腦油　1267
石榴皮　757,1259
石榴花　1259
石蓮子　1258
石澎子　1268
石龍子　1264
石龍芮　1263
石龍芻　1262
石蟬草　1270
石薺薴　1230
石蟾蜍　1269
石羅藤　1260
石蘭藤　1256
石榴樹皮　1259

[丨]

甲片　097,291
申薑　885,1218
凸粉　1745
母連　553
母草　907
母丁香　905
田七　1116,1594
田蔥　1633
田螺　1615
田字草　1095
田旋花　1608
田基黃　1517,1593
田葛菜　1612
田唇烏蠅翼　1603
北辛　432,1049
北山豆根　1192a
北味　1057
北芪　543a,1045
北五味　1057
北沙參　1052
北味子　1998
北柴胡　021a
北烏頭　1716b
北寄生　076,1140A
北細辛　1049
北蒼朮　1680b
北鶴虱　1047

| | | | |
|---|---|---|---|
| 安息香　014 | | 百足　1018 | 地蓉　1536 |
| 幷頭草　1029 | | 百部　1005 | 地筋　1513 |
| 米鈎　648 | | 百解　2185 | 地楡　1555 |
| 米洋參　1544 | | 百合粉　973 | 地稔　1536 |
| 羊　2030 | | 百里香　1511 | 地膚　1519 |
| 羊腎　2049 | | 百步蛇　85,1006 | 地錢　1546 |
| 羊蹄　2055 | | 百脉根　1553 | 地錦　1514 |
| 羊鞭　2049 | | 百草霜　1017 | 地龍　237,1533 |
| 羊藿　2045 | | 百蕊草　983 | 地膽　1549 |
| 羊山刺　2050 | | 西芎　279,433 | 地蘿　189 |
| 羊耳菊　2042 | | 西芪　543 | 地八角　1537 |
| 羊耳蒜　2043 | | 西連　553 | 地不容　1542 |
| 羊角豆　1921 | | 西歸　1483 | 地石榴　1545 |
| 羊角抝　2036 | | 西黨　441,1484 | 地皮消　1541 |
| 羊角草　2039 | | 西瓜霜　434 | 地白草　1539 |
| 羊角荣　981 | | 西河柳　299 | 地仙桃　1520 |
| 羊角參　2037 | | 西洋參　443 | 地瓜子　1530 |
| 羊角藤　2038 | | 西紅花　442 | 地瓜藤　1545 |
| 羊肚菌　2059 | | 西北狼毒　436 | 地羊鵲　1553 |
| 羊屎木　2051 | | 西寧大黃　1406a | 地耳草　1517 |
| 羊草結　2044 | | 西藏紅花　442 | 地血香　1521 |
| 羊胲子　2044 | | 地瓜　1530 | 地花生　1522 |
| 羊蹄草　2057 | | 地沙　1544 | 地芙蓉　1542 |
| 羊胡鬚草　2047 | | 地釘　1551 | 地肤子　1519 |
| 羊屎條根　2052 | | 地笋　1531,1548 | 地肤苗　1519 |
| 羊食子根　2052 | | 地烏　1552 | 地枯蔞　1528 |
| 羊蹄暗消　2056 | | 地黃　1225,1523 | 地柏枝　1538 |
| 羊躑躅根　2031 | | 地椒　1511 | 地柏葉　1540 |

[一]

| | |
|---|---|
| 夷花　492 | 地茄子　1512 |
| 戎鹽　225,1395 | 地骨皮　134,640,655 |
| 扣子花　1889 | 地牯牛　1529 |
| 吉林參　599 | 地毡草　1509 |
| 耳草　316 | 地涌蓮　1556 |
| 耳環石斛　541 | 地麻黃　1534 |
| 灰葉　564 | 地梭羅　1546 |
| 灰葉根　564 | 地莓子　1535 |
| 灰包馬勃　835a | 地黃瓜　1524 |
| 羽箭　2211 | 地黃花　1523 |
| 羽葉丁香　2241 | 地黃葉　1523 |
| 羽葉三七　2240 | 地黃蓮　1525 |
| 朴　1101 | 地棗子　880 |
| 朴花　425 | 地貴草　1532 |
| 朴根　426,1101 | 地楊梅　1554 |
| 朴硝　1074,1102 | 地楓皮　1518 |
| 老鴉　1999 | 地蜂子　1132 |
| 老君鬚　716 | 地精草　1516 |
| 老虎芋　393 | 地膏藥　1527 |
| 老虎扭　1462 | 地骷髏　1528 |
| 老鼠尾　1785a | 地錦草　1515 |
| 老鼠刺　720 | 地膽頭　1550 |
| 老龍皮　718 | 地澀澀　1543 |
| 老鶴草　717 | 地薔薇　1510 |
| 老蘿葡頭　1528 | 地蘇木　1547 |
| 老鼠拉冬瓜　719 | 地鱉虫　1082 |
| 百合　973 | 地瓜兒苗　1531,1548,<br>　　　　1721 |

| | | | | |
|---|---|---|---|---|
| 杜松實　1750 | 貝母　288,1051 | 佛手花　362 | 京子　205 | [一] |
| 杜果釘　1888 | 貝齒　1056,1850 | 佛手柑　362 | 京芍　159,202 | |
| 杜鵑花　1739 | 見山　132 | 佛手乾　362 | 京膠　198,943 | 門冬　870 |
| 豆仁　955,1654 | 見血封喉　130 | 佛甲草　359 | 京大戟　203,1386a | 武夷　1957 |
| 豆皮　1660 | 旱油荣　1612 | 佛耳草　360 | 京茅朮　1680a | 拉拉秧　805 |
| 豆衣　800 | 旱蓮木　397,439 | 佛指甲　1229 | 夜交藤　2069 | 枇杷葉　956,1076 |
| 豆油　1651 | 旱蓮草　398 | 佛桑花　361 | 夜合花　2083 | 長春花　036 |
| 豆根　1192,1655 | | | 夜明砂　2112 | 玫瑰花　869 |
| 豆黃　1653 | [丿] | **8畫** | 夜花藤　2093 | 附子　377 |
| 豆豉　1661 | | | 夜香牛　2089 | 附片　377 |
| 豆腐　1651 | 佗僧　876,1649 | [、] | 夜關門　2101 | 杷丹　954 |
| 豆蔻　1656 | 何首烏　040,419,2069 | | 油桐　2209 | 杷葉　956,1076 |
| 豆漿　1651 | 含羞草　396 | 於朮　1010,2234 | 油草　2208 | 杭白芷　967 |
| 豆角柴　1650 | 角莿片　114 | 羌活　109,269,1315 | 油魚　2210 | 杭菊花　259 |
| 豆豉草　1663 | 伸筋草　1219 | 祈蛇　085 | 油荣　2267 | 枝子　157 |
| 豆豉姜　1662 | 延胡　2159 | 泡沙參　917f | 油柑子　2203 | 枝核　153 |
| 豆腐渣　1652 | 延胡索　2159 | 炒附片　1046 | 油胡桃　2202 | 枝殼　154 |
| 豆蔻花　1657 | 牡荊　891 | 泥花草　1305 | 油桐子　2209 | 枝子頭　157 |
| 豆蔻殼　1657 | 牡蠣　730,892 | 波斯棗　1973 | 油桐根　2209 | 刺五加　1911A |
| 豆瓣綠　1659 | 牡丹皮　893,1474 | 河車　412,1840 | 油桐葉　2209 | 兩面針　738 |
| 豆腐渣果　1652 | 牡蠣殼　892 | 河蓮花　417 | 油荣子　2268 | 兩頭尖　739 |
| | 皂仁　1686 | 官連　553 | 油松節　2205 | 亞麻　521,1405 |
| [丨] | 皂尖　1684 | 官桂　674 | 油柑子根　2203 | 亞麻仁　2017 |
| | 皂角　1683 | 定經　1638 | 油柑子葉　2203 | 板朴　1037,1101 |
| 芍藥　1204 | 皂角子　1686 | 定心草　1808 | 油柑節虫　2203 | 板栗　729 |
| 芎藭　496 | 皂角莿　1684 | 定心散　1641 | 油桐木皮　2209 | 板藍根　1033 |
| 串珠酒餅　273 | 皂莿片　1684 | 定木香　1645 | 油荣子油　2206 | 阿片　004 |
| 芒硝　855 | 佛手　362 | 定經草　1638 | | 阿黃　002 |
| 芒果核　856 | 佛手片　362 | | | |

| | | | | |
|---|---|---|---|---|
| 阿膠 | 001,803,943,<br>1090 | 青果　216A,613 | 刺參　1899,1906 | 刺菱根　1895 | 芝麻　400 |

阿膠　001,803,943,
　　　1090
阿磺　002
阿魏　005
阿芙蓉　004
阿拉伯膠　003
東風菜　1801
東風橘　1800
東蒼朮　1680c
東綿麻　1805
東北土當歸　1791a
東北天南星　1622g
東化紅豆杉　1854
松子　1378a
松香　1378a
松根　1378a
松球　1378a
松節　1378
松蒿　1380
松蕈　1379
松藍　222d,1381
松蘿　1382
松花粉　1378a
松潘烏頭　1716c
青皮　221
青仙　215
青矾　781
青花　216

青果　216A,613
青荷　214
青蒟　209
青蒿　213
青箱　215
青黛　222
青藤　223
青礬　210
青蘭　217
青䕡　1549
青鹽　225
青木香　219,324a,1779
青皮子　221
青金石　207
青香薷　1242
青風葉　212
青風藤　212,404
青剛皮　732
青娘子　220
青蛇藤　1987
青筋藤　208
青葉膽　224
青箱子　215
青礦石　218,873
刺片　1902
刺李　1892
刺泡　1903

刺參　1899,1906
刺菱　1895
刺蜜　1898
刺糖　1898
刺藜　1891
刺人參　1885
刺三加　1904
刺五加　1939g
刺天茄　1909
刺石榴　1908
刺老鴉　1890
刺竹笋　1878
刺沙蓬　1905
刺玫花　1897
刺虎葉　1880
刺海松　1332
刺栗子　1894
刺桐花　1910
刺桐葉　1910
刺黃柏　1884
刺黃蓮　1883
刺梭羅　1887
刺蒬荼　1879
刺莓果　1897
刺梨果　1893
刺梨花　1893
刺梨根　1893
刺梨葉　1893

刺菱根　1895
刺草薢　1901
刺猬皮　1911
刺楸樹　1877
刺槐花　1881
刺蓋草　1886
刺蒺藜　72,1876
刺龍包　1896
刺五加皮　096
刺瓜米草　1887
刺果蘇木　1888
刺南蛇藤　1900
刺菓衞矛　1889
刺摩苓草　1899

[丨]

芸香　1450,2257,2258
芽戟　577
芮仁　1375
苂實　146
芥子　098,099
果皮　053
昆布　702
昇藥　1226
咖啡　095
岩白菜　2163A
岩筋草　1659
苡米　589
苡仁米　589

芝麻　400
芝麻殼　400
芭蕉根　113
芭蕉楊　1620
芙蓉　896
芙蓉花　368
芙蓉菊　080,451
芙蓉葉　369
味連　553
吳朮　1010
吳荑　2005
吳茱萸　1947
吳茱萸根　1947
吳茱萸葉　1947
芫青　220,1549
芫花　2245
芫胡　2159,2244
芫荽　524
芫荽子　2250
芫荽仁　2250
花粉　530
花椒　528
花木通　532
花乳石　531
花椒葉　529
花旗參　443
花蜘蛛　1689
花蕊石　531
明石　218,873

| | | | | |
|---|---|---|---|---|
| 明矾 971 | 竺黃 244 | 金沙牛 1529 | 金櫻頭 194 | 穿心蓮 278 |
| 明砂 2112 | 竺簧 244 | 金扭扣 1636 | 金鷄爪 163 | 穿破石 290 |
| 明黃 497 | 佩蘭 043,1059,1720 | 金花草 178 | 金龜子 1794 | 穿魚柳 1340 |
| 明雄 882 | 佩蘭葉 1059 | 金果蘭 180 | 金毛狗脊 182 | 穿山甲片 291 |
| 明礬 884 | 兒茶 313 | 金果攬 180 | 金釵石斛 1245a | 扁束 1086 |
| 明月砂 2255 | 兒茶鈎藤 314 | 金星草 355 | 金銀花葉 191 | 扁柏 1085 |
| 明礬參 884 | 狗脊 639 | 金桔乾 165 | 金銀花藤 191 | 扁郁 1084 |
| 虎杖 512 | 狗腎 647 | 金茯花 175,503 | 金錢松皮 166,1762 | 扁藤 1087 |
| 虎刺 527 | 狗寶 646 | 金剛藤 179 | 金鷄納皮 169 | 扁柏子 982 |
| 虎骨 517 | 狗鞭 647 | 金釵斛 161 | 金綫吊烏龜 176,1023 | 扁擔藤 1087 |
| 虎麻 827 | 狗肝菜 645 | 金鈕扣 184 | | 洋虫 2041 |
| 虎葛 1970 | 狗脊片 639 | 金絲草 174 | **9畫** | 洋芋 2060 |
| 虎膠 514 | 狗鈴草 2117 | 金精石 170 | | 洋油 1267 |
| 虎耳草 515 | 狗腳跡 644 | 金蓮花 181 | [、] | 洋葱 2058 |
| 虎舌紅 523 | 狗爪南星 1622c | 金銀花 190,878 | 洗皮 437,976 | 洋水仙 1311 |
| 虎骨膠 514 | 狗脊貫眾 639 | 金銀草 191 | 前胡 140 | 洋地黃 2054 |
| | 金山田七 0947A | 金銀藤 191 | 卷柏 295,542,1919 | 洋金花 335,2034 |
| [丿] | 金牛 183 | 金綫草 177 | 首烏 419,1285 | 洋雀花 2040 |
| | 金汁 168 | 金髮草 174 | 冠蟬 1174 | 洋耆草 2033 |
| 笋竹 1878 | 金砂 380 | 金橘乾 165,172 | 美人蕉 868 | 洋藿香 2046 |
| 知母 155 | 金釵 161 | 金錢草 167 | 活血丹 512,1664 | |
| 秈米 487 | 金斛 187 | 金礞石 873 | 津蒼朮 1680a | [一] |
| 爬山虎 1514,1900 | 金薄 185 | 金蟬花 162 | 兗州卷柏 2157 | |
| 忽地笑 1581 | 金不換 186 | 金鎖匙 188 | 神麯 1220 | 查(見13畫楂) |
| 肥皂子 331 | 金牛尾 137 | 金櫻子 192,195 | 神砂草 1637 | 查肉 016,017 |
| 使君子 1238 | 金牛草 183 | 金櫻肉 192 | 神黃豆 1221 | 查餅 017 |
| 委陵菜 1928 | 金石斛 187 | 金櫻根 194 | 神麯茶 1220 | 柯子 421,638 |
| 乳香 605,631 | 金古攬 180 | 金櫻膏 193 | 穿山甲 1157 | 眉豆 1014 |
| 乳糧石 2225 | 金耳環 173 | | | 柊葉 1807 |

272

海底椰　389A
海松子　1378b
海金沙　380
海金砂　380
海狗腎　383
海狗鞭　383
海南蒟　386
海風藤　352
海桐皮　392,926
海楓藤　382
海螵蛸　890
海螵蛸　387
海州常山　381
海南地黃連　1525b

[一]

起石　86,2032
蚤休　1685
核桃　420
桉葉　015
連翹　743
除蟲菊　255
枸刺木　1320
素馨花　1357
挺枝沙參　917g
栗殼　729
珠砂　1475
珠兒參　241
破石　290

破布葉　1104
破故紙　651,1103
真珠　048
真貝母　1051b
真珠母　049
夏天無　448
夏枯草　446
夏無踪　448
夏草冬蟲　311,449
秦皮　197
秦艽　196
秦椒　528
秦歸　1483
秦艽皮　196
桃仁　1501
桃葉　1501
桃樹　1501
桃樹皮　1501
桃葉珊瑚　1602
桃兒七　691A,1500A
桐木　1819
桐皮　392,1819
桐油　1824
桐根　1819
桐葉　1819
桐子油　1824
桐子花　1823
桔皮　122,263
桔白　121,262

桔紅　260
桔梗　119
桔絡　121,262
桔葉　123,265
桔紅紅　118
通草　1353,1822
通天草　1068,1821
通光散　1816
通花粉　1822b
通花根　1822b
通城虎　1808
通骨消　1815
通草花　1822b
通經草　1811
桂子　698
桂心　690
桂木　690,694
桂皮　696
桂枝　690
桂花　692
桂蒂　698
桂皮油　696
桂花耳　692
桂花油　692
桑白　1144
桑虫　1142
桑枝　1141
桑葉　1141

桑蛸　1143
桑螵　1143
桑白皮　1144
桑寄生　1140
桑椹子　1139
桑椹膏　1139
桑螵蛸　1143
桑蠹虫　1142
桑根白皮　1144
馬辛　432,1746
馬前　824
馬勃　835
馬胎　837
馬桑　836
馬渤　835
馬蝗　1297
馬蹄　838
馬寶　833
馬藍　222b
馬蘭　831
馬蘭　830
馬木通　675
馬甲子　823
馬先蒿　827
馬尾松　844
馬料豆　463
馬兜鈴　842
馬蜂窩　782

馬鈴薯　2060
馬齒莧　825
馬鞍藤　822
馬蹄金　839
馬蹄粉　838
馬蹄根　840
馬蹄草　822,841
馬蹄蕨　840
馬錢子　321,824
馬糞包　826
馬鞭草　834
馬蘭子　831
馬蘭花　831
馬蘭頭　830
馬纓丹　845,1988
馬尾黃蓮　843
馬蹄大黃　1406c

[丨]

茗　018,881
峨參　0947A
蚖青　1549
茴香　537,563
茹香　605
莕葉　721
茨實　146
茭白子　112
骨皮　655
骨碎補　657,1105,1376

烏鴉果 1760
烏鴉膽 1999a
烏橄欖 1969
烏龍根 1578
烏騷風 1987
烏薕連 1986
烏藥葉 2000
烏薇莓 1970
烏欖仁 712,1969
烏欖根 1969
烏欖葉 1969
烏奴龍膽 1981
烏柏根皮 1945
烏龍擺尾 1975
烏賊腹中墨 1994

**11畫**

[、]

商陸 1203
清膠 206
牽牛子 145
淫羊藿 2187
剪春羅 127
淩霄花 748
旋覆花 503
梁州大黃 1406b
寄奴 075,751

寄生 076
麻仁 829
麻黃 828
羚羊 750
羚羊角 750
粒花 569
粒紅花 569
望月砂 1925,2255
望江南 1921
涼粉果 735,1075
涼粉草 736
淮山 539,1199
淮通 909
淮山藥 539
密陀僧 876
密蒙花 872,874
密銀花 190,878
淡竹 1466
淡骨 387,1472
淡竹根 1466
淡竹筍 1466
淡竹殼 1466
淡竹葉 1467
淡豆豉 1477
淡味當藥 1480
鹿血 784
鹿尾 802

鹿角 777
鹿胎 793
鹿茸 786
鹿草 1741
鹿筋 776
鹿膠 775
鹿鞭 791
鹿目草 780
鹿耳苓 780
鹿耳韭 1599
鹿含草 783
鹿角膠 775
鹿角霜 777
鹿茸片 786
鹿茸末 786
鹿茸碎 608,786
鹿銜草 783

[一]

硃砂 252
硇砂 922
問荊 1929
梵天花 644
排錢草 1028
閉鞘薑 029
梔子 157,544
梔子根 157
雪山林 509

雪上一枝蒿 510
救必應 232
救兵粮 233
接骨木 120
接骨草 1498
陳皮 053
陳皮膏 054
陳棕炭 056
梅皮 867
梅花 867
梅莉 867
梅實 1977
軟棗 410
軟滑石 626
軟紫草 1862a
軟毛獨活 1748b
乾松 616
乾姜 611
乾薑 100,611
乾漆 610
乾木斛 898
麥冬 848
麥角 846
麥芽 849
麥斛 847
麥門冬 848
麥芽糖 592,850
麥冬蘇面 848

梧桐 1995
梧桐子 1995
梧桐花 1995
梧桐根 1995
梧桐淚 526
梧桐葉 1995
梧桐白皮 1995
陰香 2176
陰蠅 2180
陰行草 2178
陰地蕨 2186
陰香皮 2176
陰香根 2176
陰香葉 2176

[丨]

蛆 653,1960
國老 617
蚰虫 1142
莞花 2245
將軍 1406
蚯蚓 237
蔏麻 889
荷葉 214,422
崩大碗 769,1066
雀舌草 1624
蚺蛇皮 595

| | | | | |
|---|---|---|---|---|
| 野芋實 2153 | 野莧菜 2090 | 野席草根 2085 | 參丁 599 | 甜地丁 1551b |
| 野油麻 2152 | 野猪皮 2073 | 野核桃仁 2082 | 參碎 599 | 甜杏仁 1607,1607a |
| 野東菊 2140 | 野猪蹄 2073 | 野馬蹄草 2109 | 參葉 1222 | 甜菜葉 1630 |
| 野昇麻 2126 | 野黄皮 2095 | 野猪外腎 2073 | 參鬚 599 | 甜遠志 1637 |
| 野芝麻 2071 | 野黄瓜 2094 | 野猪頭骨 2073 | 參三七 1115 | |
| 野芫荽 2154 | 野黄豆 2105 | 野梨枝葉 2104 | 魚肚 2231 | **12畫** |
| 野花生 2092 | 野棉花 2111 | 野葡萄藤 2121 | 魚藤 2238 | [ 、 ] |
| 野花椒 2091 | 野菊花 2077 | 野鳳仙花 2079 | 魚鰾 2231 | |
| 野扁豆 2118 | 野辣子 2102 | 野鴉椿子 2145 | 魚首石 2233 | 渥丹 1190c |
| 野前胡 2070 | 野葡萄 1944,2120 | 野鴉椿花 2145 | 魚腥草 088,2218 | 遂仁 1375 |
| 野洋參 2146 | 野漆樹 2068 | 野鴉椿根 2145 | 假蒟 094 | 焙附 1046 |
| 野苧麻 2075 | 野慈菇 2143 | 野櫻桃根 2151 | 假貝母 1051a,1786 | 游草 2207 |
| 野首蓿 2113 | 野綠豆 2106 | 啤酒花 2072 | 假馬鞭 2226 | 寒水石 399 |
| 野兔屎 1703 | 野鴉椿 2145 | | 假硃砂 309 | 裙帶菜 702a |
| 野香茅 2088 | 野靛青 2133 | [ ﹁ ] | 假鷹爪 273 | 富貴草 509 |
| 野酒花 2072 | 野檳榔 2119 | | 甜瓜 1613 | 溫郁金 2213a |
| 野高粱 2098 | 野藿香 2096 | 兜鈴 842,1658 | 甜茶 1591 | 湖南地黄蓮 1525d |
| 野料豆 2105 | 野蘇麻 2128 | 犁頭尖 733,1736 | 甜草 1632 | 訶子 416,421,638 |
| 野烟葉 2149 | 野罌粟 2150 | 釣竿 1558 | 甜菜 1630 | 訶黎勒 416,421 |
| 野海椒 2080 | 野櫻桃 2151 | 釣魚竿 1558 | 甜橙 1592 | 補骨脂 658,1103 |
| 野海棠 2081 | 野鷄草 2067 | 梨皮 728 | 甜石榴 1627 | 補骨紙 1103 |
| 野馬肉 2108 | 野蘋茄 2132 | 梨乾 728 | 甜瓜子 1613 | 補骨碎 1105 |
| 野馬追 2107 | 野大豆藤 2129 | 透骨消 1664 | 甜瓜皮 1613 | [ 一 ] |
| 野素馨 2127 | 野山螞蟥 2123 | 透骨草 1665 | 甜瓜花 1613 | |
| 野茶子 2066 | 野西瓜苗 2084 | 側柏 1722 | 甜瓜根 1613 | 椶木 1896 |
| 野荔枝 2103 | 野百里香 1511 | 側柏葉 1722 | 甜瓜莖 1613 | 捲丹 1190a |
| 野麥子 2110 | 野洋烟根 2147 | 鳥不宿 926 | 甜瓜葉 1613 | 硝皮 473,1102 |
| 野梧桐 2144 | 野苦梨根 2100 | 鳥不踏 926 | 甜瓜蒂 1613 | 犀角 429 |
| | 野扇花果 2122 | 細辛 432 | | 琥珀 522 |
| | | 細葉石斛 1245c | | |

| | | | | |
|---|---|---|---|---|
| 草麻　1050 | **[丿]** | 猪鬃七　1563 | 無梗五加　1939i | 榅桲　1932A |
| 草蘚　1048 | | 絲瓜　1348 | 無患子皮　1956 | 椴樹根　2125 |
| 草麻子　1050 | 絡石　767 | 絲通　1353 | 無患子葉　1956 | 楂肉　016,017 |
| 草麻油　1050 | 筒朴　1101 | 絲綿　1349 | 無患樹皮　1956 | 楂餅　017 |
| 草麻葉　1050 | 飯豆　1014 | 絲白皮　533,1351 | 無患樹皰　1956 | 硼沙　1064 |
| 黑丑　315,401 | 筋骨草　991 | 絲瓜子　1348 | 無患子種仁　1956 | 硼砂　2256 |
| 黑竹　1839 | 鈎片　648 | 絲瓜皮　1348 | | 遠志　2242 |
| 黑參　505 | 鈎吻　649 | 絲瓜花　1348 | | 遠志肉　2242 |
| 黑棗　410 | 鈎藤　648 | 絲瓜根　1348 | **13畫** | 碎補　657,1105,1376 |
| 黑三稜　409,1127 | 象皮　461 | 絲瓜絡　1348 | **[、]** | 碎羚羊　750 |
| 黑心草　316 | 象貝　460,1051a | 絲瓜蒂　1348 | | 椿根　303 |
| 黑毛七　1572 | 象牙參　1763 | 絲瓜葉　1348 | 粳米　487,628 | 椿根皮　303 |
| 黑白丑　315,407 | 猴棗　427 | 絲瓜藤　1348 | 話梅　489 | 椿根白皮　303,1290 |
| 黑皮根　408 | 猴薑　885 | 絲通草　1822b | 溪黃草　082 | 雷丸　724,808 |
| 黑皮蛇　2185 | 猴子結　428 | 絲帶蕨　1352 | 新疆亞魏　005a | 雷蘑　722 |
| 黑老虎　405 | 番木瓜　320 | 絲棉木　1350 | 滇南星　1622f | 雷公木　2195 |
| 黑豆豉　1661 | 番木龞　321 | 無名子　1979 | 滇紫草　1862b | 雷公蛇　2164 |
| 黑附子　294,402 | 番石榴　323 | 無名異　883,1978 | 滑石　534 | 雷公藤　807 |
| 黑狗脊　403 | 番紅花　319,442 | 無花果　1955 | 滑石粉　535 | 椰子皮　2142 |
| 黑花蛇　1989 | 番瀉葉　318,483 | 無食子　904,1990 | 福花　367 | 椰子油　2142 |
| 黑面辰　406 | 猪母　155,251 | 無根藤　1958 | 福壽草　375 | 椰子殼　2142 |
| 黑面神　406 | 猪苓　247 | 無患子　1956 | **[一]** | 椰子漿　2142 |
| 黑面風　1233 | 猪牙皂　578,2022 | 無莿根　1996 | | 椰子瓤　2142 |
| 黑威靈　1715 | 猪古葱　2115 | 無葉藤　1958 | 槙桐　059 | 榆皮　464 |
| 黑骨頭　404 | 猪仔豆　618 | 無爺藤　2003 | 塘葛菜　1612 | 榆花　2235 |
| 黑脂麻　400 | 猪㙟蓮　1402 | 無漏子　1973 | 塊黃　497,1406c | 榆樹　2235 |
| 黑龍骨　404 | 猪屎豆　253 | 無槵子　900 | 榔榆　715 | 榆醬　2228 |
| | 猪龍草　248 | 無花果根　1955 | 隔山消　937,1009 | 榆仁醬　2235 |
| | | | 預知子　2212 | 榆白皮　2235 |
| | | | 搬倒甑　1829 | |

## 21畫

### [、]

鶯　2190
鶴蝨　418
麝香　1207
麝香草　1208

### [一]

霸王鞭　955B
攝石　1215
櫻根　194
櫻桃　2197
櫻額　2191
櫻桃水　2197
櫻桃枝　2197
櫻桃核　2197
櫻桃根　2197
櫻桃葉　2197
櫻草根　2198
櫻額梨　2191

### [丨]

蕻葖　2199
蠣殼　730
蠣殼粉　730
蠟梅花　710,1573

### [丿]

纈草　481

蠡實　831
繢豆皮　800
續隨子　139,500
續斷　501
續斷頭　501
雞連　073,553
雞蘇　1331
雞內金　074,924
雞爪參　163
雞血七　117
雞血藤　066
雞矢藤　077
雞卵黃　996
雞肫皮　074
雞冠花　071
雞屎藤　077
雞骨香　069
雞骨草　070
雞蛋殼　343
雞眼草　079
雞腸楓　060,068,950
雞爪三七　061
鐵（又見13畫鉄）
鐵　1562
鐵樹　1583
鐵包金　1578
鐵骨散　1946

鐵馬豆　1576
鐵馬鞭　1575
鐵海棠　1566
鐵草鞋　1587
鐵掃竹　1580
鐵莧菜　1569
鐵棒錘　1577
鐵絲七　1585
鐵筷子　1572
鐵腳雞　1564
鐵綫草　1570
鐵綫蓮　1568
鐵綫蕨　1567
鐵箍散　1571
鐵樹果　1584
鐵藤根　1586
鐵鞭草　1579
鐵皮石斛　1245e
鐵籬笆果　1574
鐵角鳳尾草　1563
鐵腳威靈仙　1565

## 22畫

### [、]

癬草　974
鷁鴣菜　042

### [一]

權花　361

## 23畫

### [、]

齏汁　063
欒華　806

### [丨]

鶯鶯蘭　1626
鱉甲　1080
鱉（又見25畫鼈）
蘿藦　764
蘿芙木　759
蘿蔔子　1113
蘿蔔仁　711,765
蘿蔔根　765
蘿藦莢　764

## 24畫

### [、]

鷹骨　2192
鷹頭　2192
鷹不伏　2193
鷹不泊　2193
鷹不撲　2195
鷹眼睛　2192

鷹嘴爪　2192
鷹不泊蔃　2194

### [一]

靈仙　737,1927
靈芝　745
靈砂　2174
靈香　747
靈脂　746
靈芝草　745
靈香草　747
靈陵香　747
靈霄花　748
鹽梅　993
鹽蛇　2164
鹽湯　2166
鹽膽水　2165
鹽麩子　2158
鹽麩木　2158
鹽麩葉　2158
鹽麩子根　2158
鹽麩木花　2158
鹽麩根白皮　2158
鹽麩樹白皮　2158
鼉　1670
鼉衣　1670
鼉豆　1672
鼉羌　109b
鼉砂　1670

蠶退　1670
蠶蛻　1670
蠶蛹　1670
蠶繭　1670
蠶豆花　1672
蠶豆莖　1672
蠶豆殼　1672
蠶豆葉　1672
蠶繭草　1671
蠶豆莢殼　1672

〔｜〕

鹼水　133
艷山薑　1430
鷇殼　423
鱧腸草　886

**25 畫**

〔一〕

欖仁　712

〔｜〕

觀音柳　58,677

籩甲　1080

籩虫　1082

籩裙　1081

籩（又見23畫鱉）

**26 畫**

〔一〕

驢鞭　804
驢皮膠　803
驢蹄草　841

**27 畫**

〔丿〕

鑽地風　405

**29 畫**

〔一〕

鬱金　2213
鬱金香　2214